全国高等中医药院校中药学类专业双语规划教材
Bilingual Planned Textbooks for Chinese Materia Medica Majors in TCM Colleges and Universities

中药炮制学实验

Processing of Chinese Materia Medica Experiment

（供中药学类、药学类及相关专业使用）
(For Chinese Materia Medica, Pharmacy and other related majors)

主　编　陆兔林　杨光明

主　审　禹志领　吴纯洁

副主编　金传山　杜　红　李慧芬

编　者（以姓氏笔画为序）

王　晖（天津中医药大学）
王法琴（南京中医药大学翰林学院）
叶喜德（江西中医药大学）
兰　卫（新疆医科大学）
杜　红（北京中医药大学）
李　芸（甘肃中医药大学）
李艳凤（黑龙江中医药大学）
李慧芬（山东中医药大学）
汪小莉（安徽中医药大学）
张朔生（山西中医药大学）
陈　红（福建中医药大学）
孟　江（广东药科大学）
禹志领（香港浸会大学）
彭　伟（成都中医药大学）
王金梅（河南大学）
石继连（湖南中医药大学）
田连起（河南中医药大学）
刘先琼（湖北中医药大学）
杨光明（南京中医药大学）
李兴华（中国药科大学）
李景丽（陕西中医药大学）
吴纯洁（成都中医药大学）
张　凡（辽宁中医药大学）
陆兔林（南京中医药大学）
金传山（安徽中医药大学）
修彦凤（上海中医药大学）
梁泽华（浙江中医药大学）
魏　晴（贵州中医药大学）

中国健康传媒集团
中国医药科技出版社

内容提要

本教材是"全国高等中医药院校中药学类专业双语规划教材"之一，内容分5章，分别是绪论、中药炮制验证性实验、中药炮制综合性实验、中药炮制设计性实验和中药饮片企业见习。本教材为书网融合教材，即纸质教材有机融合电子教材、教学配套资源（PPT、微课、视频、图片等）、题库系统、数字化教学服务（在线教学、在线作业、在线考试）。

本教材实用性强，主要供中医药院校中药学类、药学类及相关专业使用，也可作为研究生考试与医药行业培训的参考用书。

图书在版编目（CIP）数据

中药炮制学实验：汉英对照 / 陆兔林，杨光明主编 . —北京：中国医药科技出版社，2020.9
全国高等中医药院校中药学类专业双语规划教材
ISBN 978 – 7 – 5214 – 1870 – 5

Ⅰ. ①中… Ⅱ. ①陆… ②杨… Ⅲ. ①中药炮制学 – 实验 – 中医学院 – 教材 – 汉、英
Ⅳ. ① R283 – 33

中国版本图书馆 CIP 数据核字（2020）第 097097 号

美术编辑 陈君杞
版式设计 辰轩文化

出版 **中国健康传媒集团** | 中国医药科技出版社
地址 北京市海淀区文慧园北路甲 22 号
邮编 100082
电话 发行：010 – 62227427 邮购：010 – 62236938
网址 www. cmstp. com
规格 889 × 1194 mm 1/16
印张 17 1/4
字数 497 千字
版次 2020 年 9 月第 1 版
印次 2020 年 9 月第 1 次印刷
印刷 三河市万龙印装有限公司
经销 全国各地新华书店
书号 ISBN 978 – 7 – 5214 – 1870 – 5
定价 59.00 元

出版说明

近些年随着世界范围的中医药热潮的涌动，来中国学习中医药学的留学生逐年增多，走出国门的中医药学人才也在增加。为了适应中医药国际交流与合作的需要，加快中医药国际化进程，提高来中国留学生和国际班学生的教学质量，满足双语教学的需要和中医药对外交流需求，培养优秀的国际化中医药人才，进一步推动中医药国际化进程，根据教育部、国家中医药管理局、国家药品监督管理局等部门的有关精神，在本套教材建设指导委员会主任委员成都中医药大学彭成教授等专家的指导和顶层设计下，中国医药科技出版社组织全国50余所高等中医药院校及附属医疗机构约420名专家、教师精心编撰了全国高等中医药院校中药学类专业双语规划教材，该套教材即将付梓出版。

本套教材共计23门，主要供全国高等中医药院校中药学类专业教学使用。本套教材定位清晰、特色鲜明，主要体现在以下方面。

一、立足双语教学实际，培养复合应用型人才

本套教材以高校双语教学课程建设要求为依据，以满足国内医药院校开展留学生教学和双语教学的需求为目标，突出中医药文化特色鲜明、中医药专业术语规范的特点，注重培养中医药技能、反映中医药传承和现代研究成果，旨在优化教育质量，培养优秀的国际化中医药人才，推进中医药对外交流。

本套教材建设围绕目前中医药院校本科教育教学改革方向对教材体系进行科学规划、合理设计，坚持以培养创新型和复合型人才为宗旨，以社会需求为导向，以培养适应中药开发、利用、管理、服务等各个领域需求的高素质应用型人才为目标的教材建设思路与原则。

二、遵循教材编写规律，整体优化，紧跟学科发展步伐

本套教材的编写遵循“三基、五性、三特定”的教材编写规律；以“必需、够用”为度；坚持与时俱进，注意吸收新技术和新方法，适当拓展知识面，为学生后续发展奠定必要的基础。实验教材密切结合主干教材内容，体现理实一体，注重培养学生实践技能训练的同时，按照教育部相关精神，增加设计性实验部分，以现实问题作为驱动力来培养学生自主获取和应用新知识的能力，从而培养学生独立思考能力、实验设计能力、实践操作能力和可持续发展能力，满足培养应用型和复合型人才的要求。强调全套教材内容的整体优化，并注重不同教材内容的联系与衔接，避免遗漏和不必要的交叉重复。

三、对接职业资格考试，“教考”“理实”密切融合

本套教材的内容和结构设计紧密对接国家执业中药师职业资格考试大纲要求，实现教学与考试、理论与实践的密切融合，并且在教材编写过程中，吸收具有丰富实践经验的企业人员参与教材的编写，确保教材的内容密切结合应用，更加体现高等教育的实践性和开放性，为学生参加考试和实践工作打下坚实基础。

四、创新教材呈现形式，书网融合，使教与学更便捷更轻松

全套教材为书网融合教材，即纸质教材与数字教材、配套教学资源、题库系统、数字化教学服务有机融合。通过“一书一码”的强关联，为读者提供全免费增值服务。按教材封底的提示激活教材后，读者可通过PC、手机阅读电子教材和配套课程资源（PPT、微课、视频等），并可在线进行同步练习，实时收到答案反馈和解析。同时，读者也可以直接扫描书中二维码，阅读与教材内容关联的课程资源，从而丰富学习体验，使学习更便捷。教师可通过PC在线创建课程，与学生互动，开展在线课程内容定制、布置和批改作业、在线组织考试、讨论与答疑等教学活动，学生通过PC、手机均可实现在线作业、在线考试，提升学习效率，使教与学更轻松。此外，平台尚有数据分析、教学诊断等功能，可为教学研究与管理提供技术和数据支撑。需要特殊说明的是，有些专业基础课程，例如《药理学》等9种教材，起源于西方医学，因篇幅所限，在本次双语教材建设中纸质教材以英语为主，仅将专业词汇对照了中文翻译，同时在中国医药科技出版社数字平台“医药大学堂”上配套了中文电子教材供学生学习参考。

编写出版本套高质量教材，得到了全国知名专家的精心指导和各有关院校领导与编者的大力支持，在此一并表示衷心感谢。希望广大师生在教学中积极使用本套教材和提出宝贵意见，以便修订完善，共同打造精品教材，为促进我国高等中医药院校中药学类专业教育教学改革和人才培养做出积极贡献。

全国高等中医药院校中药学类专业双语规划教材
建设指导委员会

数字化教材编委会

主　编　陆兔林　杨光明

主　审　禹志领　吴纯洁

副主编　金传山　杜　红　李慧芬

编　者　（以姓氏笔画为序）

王　晖（天津中医药大学）
王法琴（南京中医药大学翰林学院）
叶喜德（江西中医药大学）
兰　卫（新疆医科大学）
杜　红（北京中医药大学）
李　芸（甘肃中医药大学）
李艳凤（黑龙江中医药大学）
李慧芬（山东中医药大学）
汪小莉（安徽中医药大学）
张朔生（山西中医药大学）
陈　红（福建中医药大学）
孟　江（广东药科大学）
禹志领（香港浸会大学）
彭　伟（成都中医药大学）
王金梅（河南大学）
石继连（湖南中医药大学）
田连起（河南中医药大学）
刘先琼（湖北中医药大学）
杨光明（南京中医药大学）
李兴华（中国药科大学）
李景丽（陕西中医药大学）
吴纯洁（成都中医药大学）
张　凡（辽宁中医药大学）
陆兔林（南京中医药大学）
金传山（安徽中医药大学）
修彦凤（上海中医药大学）
梁泽华（浙江中医药大学）
魏　晴（贵州中医药大学）

前　言

《中药炮制学实验》是“全国高等中医药院校中药学类专业双语规划教材”之一，是在全国高等中药学类专业双语规划教材建设指导委员会的指导下，为适应我国高等中医药教育发展的需要，全面推进素质教育，培养 21 世纪高素质创新人才，由南京中医药大学牵头组织全国 25 所中医药院校的同行专家、教授编写而成，可供全国高等中医药院校及综合院校、西医院校中医药学院的中药学类、药学类及相关专业使用。

本实验教材绪论部分主要包括中药炮制实验通则、中药炮制原辅料与仪器设备、中药炮制实验思路与方法等内容。为配合中药炮制学理论教学设立了中药炮制验证性实验、中药炮制综合性实验、中药炮制设计性实验等。本实验教材与其他实验教材相比，不仅实验数量有所增加，而且实验内容更加体现了传统炮制技术与现代实验研究的有机结合，所收录的与饮片生产企业相关的实验可以作为学生进行实习的参考资料。本教材编写遵循教学性、系统性和逻辑性三大原则，严格按照教学规律、突出重点、精简内容、严谨求实的要求。

本教材的绪论由杜红、李慧芬、杨光明、李艳凤编写，中药炮制验证性实验由陈红、田连起、刘先琼、叶喜德编写，中药炮制综合性实验由张朔生、李景丽、彭伟、魏晴、梁泽华、李兴华、石继连、孟江、李芸、修彦凤、兰卫编写，中药炮制设计性实验由王金梅、王晖编写，中药饮片企业见习由金传山、汪小莉编写，附录由张凡编写。全书由陆兔林、杨光明负责统稿，禹志领、吴纯洁负责最终审稿，王法琴协助。

本教材编写过程中，得到了参编院校各级领导的大力支持，在此深表谢意。

近年来中药炮制学学科发展迅速，科研成果日新月异，编写过程中疏漏之处在所难免，恳请各院校在使用本教材过程中，通过教学实践，不断总结经验，并不吝赐教，以便再版时修订提高。

编　者

2020 年 3 月

Foreword

One of "National bilingual teaching materials for Chinese medicine majors in higher institutions of Chinese medicine" ——*Traditional Chinese Medicine Processing Experiment* is edited under the guidance of National Committee of Experts on Teaching Materials for Higher Medical Education and according to the instructions of *Opinions of the Ministry of Education on the Construction of Undergraduate Textbooks for General Higher Education in the 13th Five-Year Plan*. This book is planning materials that China Medical Science and Technology Press entrusts Nanjing University of Traditional Chinese Medicine to lead the preparation of peer experts and professors from 25 Chinese medicine universities across the country. It can be used for national institute of advanced chinese medicine and department of pharmacy and related majors in colleges of traditional chinese medicine, western hospitals.

The introductory part of *Traditional Chinese Medicine Processing Experiment* mainly includes the general principles of Chinese medicine processing experiment, the raw materials and equipment of Chinese medicine processing, and the ideas and methods of Chinese medicine processing experiment. In order to cooperate with the theoretical teaching of traditional Chinese medicine processing, we have established confirmatory experiments of traditional Chinese medicine processing, comprehensive experiments of traditional Chinese medicine processing, and design experiments of traditional Chinese medicine processing. Compared with other experimental textbooks, this experimental textbook not only increases the number of experiments, but also the content of the experiments reflects the organic combination of traditional processing technology and modern experimental research. The collected experiments related to the manufacturer of the decoction pieces can be performed as students References for internships. This textbook complies with the three principles of teaching, systematic and logical, strictly in accordance with the teaching rules, highlighting the key points, streamlining the content and rigorous and realistic requirements.

The introduction of this textbook was written by Du Hong, Li Huifen, Yang Guangming, and Li Yanfeng. The verification experiment of traditional Chinese medicine preparation was written by Chen Hong, Tian Lianqi, Liu Xianqiong, and Ye Xide. The comprehensive experiment of traditional Chinese medicine preparation was made by Zhang Shuosheng, Li Jingli, Peng Wei, and Wei Qing. Written by Liang Zehua, Li Xinghua, Shi Jilian, Meng Jiang, Li Yun, Xiu Yanfeng, and Lan Wei. Designed experiments of traditional Chinese medicine prepared by Wang Jinmei and Wang Hui. Trainees of Chinese herbal medicine enterprises were prepared by Jin Chuanshan and Wang Xiaoli. The appendix was prepared by Zhang Fan. The entire book was written by Lu Tulin and Yang Guangming, and Wu Chunjie and Yu Zhiling were responsible for the final review with the assists of Wang Faqin.

Thanks for the strong support from the leaders of the participating institutions in the course of textbook compilation.

In recent years, the discipline of traditional Chinese medicine processing has developed rapidly, and the results of scientific research are constantly changing. Omissions in the compilation process are unavoidable. I urge all colleges and universities to continuously sum up your experience through teaching practices in the process of using this textbook, and not to enlighten us so that we can be revised during reprint improve.

Editor

March 2020

目录 | Contents

第一章　绪论 …… 1

第一节　中药炮制学实验通则 …… 1

Chapter 1　Introduction …… 5

Section 1　General Principles of CMMP Experimentation …… 5

第二节　中药炮制辅料与设备 …… 12

Section 2　Chinese Medicine Processing adjuvant and Equipment …… 24

第三节　中药炮制实验思路与方法 …… 42

Section 3　The ideas and methods for researches on Chinese medicine processing …… 47

第二章　中药炮制验证性实验 …… 56

实验一　净制、切制 …… 56

Chapter 2　Validation Experiment of Chinese Medicine Processing …… 59

Experiment 1　Cleaning and cutting …… 59

实验二　清炒法 …… 64

Experiment 2　Simple stir-baking …… 67

实验三　加固体辅料炒 …… 72

Experiment 3　Stir-baking with solid excipients …… 76

实验四　炙法 …… 82

Experiment 4　Stir-baking with liquid excipients …… 86

实验五　煅法 …… 93

Experiment 5　Calcining …… 96

实验六　蒸煮焯法 …… 100

Experiment 6　Steaming, boiling and blanching methods …… 102

实验七　复制法 …… 105

Experiment 7　Complex processing method …… 107

实验八　发酵法、发芽法 …… 110

Experiment 8　Fermenting and Sprouting methods …… 112

实验九　其他制法 …… 115

Experiment 9　Other methods …… 118

第三章　中药炮制综合性实验 …… 123
实验一　净制对牡丹皮有效成分含量的影响实验 …… 123
Chapter 3　Comprehensiveness Experiment of Chinese Medicine Processing …… 125
Experiment 1　Effects of Cleaning on the Content of Active Ingredients in Moutan Cortex …… 125
实验二　切制对甘草中成分含量的影响实验 …… 127
Experiment 2　Effect of cutting on the content of components in Glycyrrhizae Radix Et Rhizoma …… 129
实验三　炒黄对王不留行浸出物的影响实验 …… 132
Experiment 3　The influence of stir-frying to yellow on extractives of Vaccariae Semen …… 134
实验四　炒炭对槐米成分及止血作用的影响实验 …… 136
Experiment 4　The influence of carbonizing by stir-frying on chemical compositions and hemostatic effects of the Flos Sophorae Immaturus …… 139
实验五　砂炒对马钱子质量及毒性的影响实验 …… 143
Experiment 5　The effect of Sand-fried on quality and toxicity of Strychni Semen …… 146
实验六　酒炙对大黄成分及泻下作用的影响实验 …… 150
Experiment 6　Effects of stir fried Rhei Radix et Rhizoma with rice wine on composition and purgative activity …… 153
实验七　醋炙延胡索对延胡索乙素含量和镇痛作用的影响 …… 157
Experiment 7　The influence of stir-frying Corydalis Rhizoma with rice vinegar on the content of tetrahydropalmatine and its analgesic effect …… 160
实验八　煅制石膏质量评价实验 …… 164
Experiment 8　Experiment of calcined gypsum quality evaluation …… 166
实验九　煅淬对自然铜成分含量的影响实验 …… 169
Experiment 9　Experiment of effects of calcining and quenching on the composition of Pyritum …… 172
实验十　蒸制对黄芩成分含量的影响实验 …… 176
Experiment 10　The Influence of steaming on the Composition of Scutellariae Radix …… 178
实验十一　煮制川乌质量评价实验 …… 181
Experiment 11　The quality evaluation experiment of Processed Aconiti Radix …… 184
实验十二　制苦杏仁质量评价实验 …… 188
Experiment 12　The quality evaluation experiment of blanching Armeniacae Semen Amarum …… 191
实验十三　清半夏炮制降低毒性的实验评价 …… 195
Experiment 13　Experimental evaluation on attenuating toxicity of Pinelliae Rhizoma processed into Pinelliae Rhizoma Praeparatum Cum alumenine …… 199

实验十四 制霜对巴豆成分的影响实验 …… 205
Experiment 14 The effect of making frost-like powder on the composition of Crotonis Fructus …… 207

第四章 中药炮制设计性实验 …… 210
Chapter 4 Design Experiments of Chinese Medicine Processing …… 211
实验一 制何首乌饮片综合设计性实验 …… 213
Experiment 1 Comprehensive experiment design for decoction pieces of Polygoni Multiflori Radix …… 217
实验二 制草乌饮片综合设计性实验 …… 224
Experiment 2 Comprehensive experiment design for decoction pieces of Aconiti Kusnezoffii Radix Cocta …… 228

第五章 中药饮片企业见习 …… 234
Chapter 5 Noviciate in enterprises of decoction pieces …… 235

附录 …… 237
附录一 中药饮片生产质量管理规范 …… 237
Appendix …… 242
Appendix Ⅰ Good Manufacturing Practice for Chinese medicine decoction pieces …… 242
附录二 中药饮片 GMP 认证检查项目 …… 249
Appendix Ⅱ GMP certification inspection items for Chinese medicine decoction pieces …… 254

第一章　绪　论

中药炮制学是理论和实践并重的学科，其实验教学是中药炮制学教学过程中的重要环节，是学生或专业技术人员学习、实践并掌握中药炮制技术、工艺、质量标准以及现代中药炮制研究的必要手段，同时也是中药炮制学理论联系实际的重要途径。通过中药炮制学实验的具体实践，使学生掌握中药炮制的基本方法和基本技能，熟悉传统中药炮制的工艺技术和操作方法，加深对中药炮制理论的理解，培养学生求真务实的学习态度和独立分析问题、解决问题的能力。为传承、创新、发展中药炮制学理论与实践技能奠定坚实的基础。

PPT

第一节　中药炮制学实验通则

一、中药炮制学实验课程的性质与任务

中药炮制学实验是一门专业性强，具传统与现代特色的实验课程，是为了加深中药学及相关专业学生对中药炮制学这门课程理论知识的进一步理解，而采取的通过实际操作使学生得到系统实验技能训练的课程。中药炮制学实验具有涉及面广，综合性强，知识点多等特点。传统炮制技术的验证性实验中每一步均蕴含着炮制操作技能，综合性实验、设计性实验又充分融合了各种专业基础知识点和方法。只有将传统炮制技术与现代科学技术有机结合，才能揭示中药炮制的科学内涵，传承中药炮制的方法和技术。通过中药炮制学实验验证中药炮制理论内容，实现理论与实践相结合，对掌握中药炮制学知识和科学研究方法、培养实验技能及创新精神都具有重要作用。

二、中药炮制学实验目的

1. 通过中药炮制学的实验教学，使学生掌握中药炮制的基本操作方法和技能，结合化学、药理、毒理及现代科学技术进行中药炮制的实验研究，以阐述中药炮制的作用和原理，为中药炮制工艺规范化与饮片质量标准化研究奠定基础。

2. 将开放式实验教学与实训结合，使学生了解中药炮制常用的传统工具与现代生产设备，了解饮片质量分析仪器的基本原理、结构、性能，掌握规范的操作规程及仪器设备使用方法。

3. 通过中药炮制综合设计性实验，使学生进行完整的实验设计与操作，观察实验现象，做好实验记录，处理实验数据，撰写实验报告或论文等，培养学生分析问题和解决问题的能力、创新性思维和探索求知的精神。

4. 培养学生查阅和使用中药炮制相关文献资料的能力，了解国内外中药炮制研究科技动态及最新发展，剖析中药炮制学实验研究典型案例，理解炮制实验意图与设计原则，认识实验形成过程，分析实验中设置的条件的目的，掌握实验设计方法，培养学生的文献综述能力和实验方案设计能力。

三、中药炮制学实验规则

1. 实验前认真阅读实验教材，明确实验目的、要求、方法和操作步骤。结合实验内容复习相关理论知识，预测实验各步骤可能出现的情况。

2. 进入实验室必须穿好实验服，准备好实验仪器、试剂、药品、工具等，并保持实验室的整洁安静，注意维护实验台面和仪器的清洁，以利于实验进行。

3. 实验时认真听从实验指导教师对实验内容的讲解，明确实验原理、操作方法、注意事项等。严格遵守操作规程，特别是称取或量取药品，在拿取、称量、放回时应进行三次认真核对，以免发生差错。称量任何药品，在操作完毕后应立即盖好瓶塞，放回原处，凡已取出的药品不能再倒回原瓶；公共仪器（如抽滤装置、色谱仪等）和特殊试剂（显色试剂等）应按照实验要求在指定地点使用。

4. 实验中要以严肃认真的科学态度进行操作，认真观察，联系课堂讲授内容进行思考，对实验中出现的问题进行分析讨论，详细记录实验数据。实验记录要求简明扼要，完整、准确，字迹整洁。如实验失败时，先要找出失败的原因，考虑如何改正。

5. 严格遵守实验室的规章制度，包括报损制度、赔偿制度、清洁卫生制度、安全操作规则以及课堂纪律等。

6. 注意节约，爱护公物，尽力避免破损。实验室的药品、器材、用具以及实验成品，一律不准擅自携出室外。

7. 实验后须及时提交实验报告。实验报告的内容应包括实验名称、实验目的、仪器设备、试剂、使用的药材（饮片）及辅料、实验内容（包括实验原理、方法步骤、结果）、讨论（对实验结果的分析、实验操作中应注意的事项、对实验原理进行探讨等内容）。

8. 实验完成后应及时整理实验物品和仪器，检查水源、火源和电源，打扫实验室卫生，经指导教师同意后方能离开实验室。

四、中药炮制通则

中药炮制是按照中医药理论，根据药材自身性质，以及调剂、制剂和临床应用的需要，所采取的一项独特的制药技术。中药饮片系指中药材按法定的中药炮制规范生产的可直接用于中医临床调剂或制剂生产使用的处方药品。中药饮片的生产、流通、使用等应符合下列有关规定。

药材凡经净制、切制或炮炙等处理后，均称为“饮片”；药材必须净制后方可进行切制或炮炙等处理。饮片是供中医临床调剂及中成药生产的配方原料。用于中药饮片生产所需的中药材原料和辅料应符合相应的质量要求，炮制用水应为饮用水。中药饮片的生产应严格按照已颁布的中药饮片炮制规范进行，饮片的生产、包装和贮藏等管理应符合饮片企业 GMP 的要求。毒性中药（含按麻醉药品管理的中药）饮片应使用特殊包装，并应贴上相应的标记。饮片在运输、贮藏和使用过程中，应符合相关的规定。特别要注意防止污染、受潮、霉变、腐烂、变质及防虫等变异现象。

除另有规定外，中药炮制应符合下列有关要求。

（一）净制

净制即净选加工。可根据具体情况，分别使用挑选、筛选、风选、水选、磁选、摘、剪、切、刮、削、挖、剔除、酶法、剥离、挤压、焯、刷、擦、火燎、烫、撞、碾串等方法，以达到净度要求。

（二）切制

切制时，除鲜切、干切外，均须进行软化处理，其方法有喷淋、抢水洗、浸泡、润、漂、蒸、煮等。亦可使用回转式减压浸润罐，真空气相置换式润药箱等软化设备。软化处理应按药材的大小、粗细、质地等分别处理，分别规定温度（压力）、水量、时间等条件，应少泡多润，防止有效成分流失。切后应及时干燥，以保证质量。

切制品有片、段、块、丝等。其规格厚度通常如下。

1. 片　极薄片 0.5mm 以下，薄片 1~2mm，厚片 2~4mm。

2. 段　短段 5~10mm，长段 10~15mm。

3. 块　8~12mm^3 的方块。

4. 丝　细丝 2~3mm，宽丝 5~10mm。

其他不宜切制者，一般应捣碎或碾碎使用。

（三）炮炙

除另有规定外，常用的炮炙方法和要求如下。

1. 炒　分单炒（清炒）和加辅料炒。需炒制者应为干燥品，且大小分档；炒时火力应均匀，不断翻动。应掌握加热温度、炒制时间及程度要求。

（1）单炒（清炒）　取待炮炙品，置炒制容器内，用文火加热至规定程度时，取出，放凉。需炒焦者，一般用中火炒至表面焦褐色，断面焦黄色为度，取出，放凉；需炒炭者，一般用武火炒至表面焦黑色，可喷淋清水少许，再炒干。

（2）麸炒　先将炒制容器加热，至撒入麸皮即刻烟起，随即投入待炮炙品，迅速翻动，炒至表面呈黄色或深黄色时，取出，筛去麸皮，放凉。

除另有规定外，每 100kg 待炮炙品，用麸皮 10~15kg。

（3）砂炒　取洁净河砂置炒制容器内，用武火加热至滑利状态时，投入待炮炙品，不断翻动，炒至表面鼓起、酥脆或至规定的程度时，取出，筛去河砂，放凉。

除另有规定外，河砂以掩埋待炮炙品为度。

如需醋淬时，筛去辅料后，趁热投入醋液中淬酥。

（4）蛤粉炒　取碾细过筛后的净蛤粉，置锅内，用中火加热至翻动较滑利时，投入待炮炙品，翻炒至鼓起或成珠、内部疏松、外表呈黄色时，迅速取出，筛去蛤粉，放凉。

除另有规定外，每 100kg 待炮炙品，用蛤粉 30~50kg。

（5）滑石粉炒　取滑石粉置炒制容器内，用中火加热至灵活状态时，投入待炮炙品，翻炒至鼓起、酥脆、表面黄色或至规定程度时，迅速取出，筛去滑石粉，放凉。

除另有规定外，每 100kg 待炮炙品，用滑石粉 40~50kg。

2. 炙法　是待炮炙品与液体辅料共同拌润，并炒至一定程度的方法。

（1）酒炙　取待炮炙品，加黄酒拌匀，闷透，置炒制容器内，用文火炒至规定的程度时，取出，放凉。

酒炙时，除另有规定外，一般用黄酒。除另有规定外，每 100kg 待炮炙品，用黄酒 10~20kg。

（2）醋炙　取待炮炙品，加醋拌匀，闷透，置炒制容器内，炒至规定的程度时，取出，放凉。

醋炙时，用米醋。除另有规定外，每 100kg 待炮炙品，用米醋 20~30kg。

（3）盐炙　取待炮炙品，加盐水拌匀，闷透，置炒制容器内，以文火加热，炒至规定的程度时，取出，放凉。

盐炙时，用食盐，应先加适量水溶解后，滤过，备用。除另有规定外，每 100kg 待炮炙品，用食盐 2kg。

（4）姜炙　先将生姜洗净，捣烂，加水适量，压榨取汁，姜渣再加水适量重复压榨一次，合并汁液，即为“姜汁”，姜汁与生姜的比例为1∶1。或将生姜或干姜切制或捣碎附后加水煎煮两次，合并煎液滤过，取滤液适当浓缩后备用。

取待炮炙品，加姜汁拌匀，置锅内，用文火炒至姜汁被吸尽，或至规定的程度时，取出，晾干。

除另有规定外，每100kg待炮炙品，用生姜10kg或干姜3kg。

（5）蜜炙　先将炼蜜加适量沸水稀释后，加入待炮炙品中拌匀，闷透，置炒制容器内，用文火炒至规定程度时，取出，放凉。

蜜炙时，用炼蜜。除另有规定外，每100kg待炮炙品，用炼蜜25kg。

（6）油炙　羊脂油炙时，先将羊脂油置锅内加热溶化后去渣，加入待炮炙品拌匀，用文火炒至油被吸尽，表面光亮时，摊开，放凉。

3. 制炭　制炭时应“存性”，并防止灰化，更要避免复燃。

（1）炒炭　取待炮炙品，置热锅内，用武火炒至表面焦黑色、内部焦褐色或至规定程度时，喷淋清水少许，熄灭火星，取出，晾干。

（2）煅炭　取待炮炙品，置煅锅内，密封，加热至所需程度，放凉，取出。

4. 煅　煅制时应注意煅透，使酥脆易碎。

（1）明煅　取待炮炙品，砸成小块，置适宜的容器内，煅至酥脆或红透时，取出，放凉，碾碎。

含有结晶水的盐类药材，不要求煅红，但需使结晶水蒸发至尽，或全部形成蜂窝状的块状固体。

（2）煅淬　将待炮炙品煅至红透时，立即投入规定的液体辅料中，淬酥（若不酥，可反复煅淬至酥），取出，干燥，打碎或研粉。

5. 蒸　取待炮炙品，大小分档，按各品种炮制项下的规定，加清水或液体辅料拌匀、润透，置适宜的蒸制容器内，用蒸汽加热至规定程度，取出，稍晾，拌回蒸液，再晾至六成干，切片或段，干燥。

6. 煮　取待炮炙品，大小分档，按各品种炮制项下的规定，加清水或规定的辅料共煮透，至切开内无白心时，取出，晾至六成干，切片，干燥。

7. 炖　取待炮炙品，按各品种炮制项下的规定，加入液体辅料，置适宜的容器内，密闭，隔水或用蒸汽加热炖透，或炖至辅料完全被吸尽时，放凉，取出，晾至六成干，切片，干燥。

蒸、煮、炖时，除另有规定外，每100kg待炮炙品，用规定的辅料20~30kg。

8. 煨　取待炮炙品，用面皮或湿纸包裹，或用吸油纸均匀地隔层分放，进行加热处理；或将其与麸皮同置炒制容器内，用文火炒至规定程度取出，放凉。

除另有规定外，每100kg待炮炙品，用麸皮50kg。

（四）其他

1. 燀　取待炮制品，投入沸水中，翻动片刻，捞出，有的种子类药材，燀至种皮由皱缩至舒展、易搓去时，捞出，放入冷水中，除去种皮，晒干。

2. 制霜（去油成霜）　除另有规定外，取待炮制品，碾碎如泥，经微热，压榨除去大部分油脂，反复操作直到含油量符合要求后，取残渣研制成符合规定的松散粉末。

3. 水飞　取待炮制品，置容器内，加适量水共研成糊状，再加水，搅拌，倾出混悬液。残渣再照上法反复操作数次，合并混悬液，静置，分取沉淀，干燥，研散。

4. 发芽　取待炮制品，置容器内，加适量水浸泡后，取出，在适宜的湿度和温度下使其发芽至规定程度，晒干或低温干燥。注意避免带入油腻，以防烂芽。一般芽长不超过1cm。

5. 发酵　取待炮制品，加规定的辅料拌匀后，制成一定形状，置适宜的湿度和温度下，使微生物生长至其中酶含量达到规定程度，晒干或低温干燥。注意发酵过程中，发现有黄曲霉菌，应禁用。

Chapter 1 Introduction

Chinese Materia Medica processing (CMMP) is a discipline that places equal emphasis on theory and practice. Practical teaching plays an important role in CMMP teaching which is essential for students or professional technicians to learn, practice and master the technology, quality standards and state of the art research means about CMMP. It is also important to integrate the theory of CMMP with practice and refine theory through practice. The practical course of CMMP experimentation will allow students to master the basic CMMP methods and technologies, familiarize themselves with general CMMP skills and operation processes, strengthen their understanding of the CMMP theory, and finally cultivate their pragmatic learning attitude, independent analytic and problem solving ability. The course will lay a solid foundation for inheriting, innovating and developing the theory and practical technology of CMMP.

Section 1 General Principles of CMMP Experimentation

1. Nature and Mission of the Course

CMMP experimentation is a highly specialized practical course with both traditional and modern characteristics. CMMP experimentation deepens the understanding of theoretical knowledge and adopts course that allows students of Chinese pharmacy (pharmacology) and related majors to obtain systematic experiment skill training through practical operations. CMMP experimentation involves comprehensive knowledge of multi-disciplines. Each step of the confirmatory experiments in traditional processing consists of various processing skills. The new comprehensive and designing experiments fully integrate various specialized professional knowledge and methods. Only by combining the traditional processing technology with modern science and technologies, can the scientific connotation of CMMP be revealed and the methods and technologies be inherited and developed. Validation of CMMP theories through experimentation and combining CMMP theory with practice are of great significance for mastering the knowledge of CMMP, grasping scientific research methodologies, cultivating experiment skills and developing innovative CMMP.

2. The Purpose of CMMP Experimentation

2.1 By educating students about CMMP, students will be able to understand the basic operation methods and skills required to conduct research experiments. They will be able to combine chemistry, pharmacology, toxicology and modern scientific technologies to further elaborate the function and principle of CMMP, allaying the foundation for research on the standardization of processing technology and the quality control criteria of processed decoction pieces (Yinpian).

2.2 By combining the teaching of experiments with CMMP practical training, students will be enable to familiarize themselves with the traditional tools, commonly used modern production CMMP equipments, basic principles, structure and specifications of instruments for quality analysis of decoction pieces and the standardized operating procedures of instruments and equipment.

2.3 Through the application of comprehensive CMMP experiment design, students are expected to design complete experiments, carry out experiment operations, observe experiment phenomena, record experiment procedures and details, analyze experiment data and write experiment reports and research articles. The training will allow students to master the ability to independently analyze and solve problems and become motivated to be creative.

2.4 CMMP experimentation also trains students' ability to search and review literature and design experiment schemes. By comprehensively reviewing the CMMP literature, students can understand the domestic and international development status and trends of CMMP research. An in-depth analysis of typical CMMP experiments will help students understand their aims, principles, process, purpose and their settings and conditions. The students will master experiment methodologies, literature analysis and independent experiment design.

3. Rules of CMMP Experimentation

3.1 Students are required to read the experiment textbook carefully, clearly understand the experiment aims, requirements, methods and operating procedures prior to the practical class. Students should also review related theoretical knowledge and predict what may happen during each step of the experiment.

3.2 Upon entering the laboratory, students are required to wear laboratory coats, set up experiment equipment, prepare reagents, chemicals tools etc. The laboratory must be kept neat and quiet. The experiment table and instruments must also be well maintained and cleaned to facilitate the experiment.

3.3 Students are required to carefully listen to the instructor's explanation of the experiment, and fully understand the principles of the experiment, operation procedures and precautions. During the experiment, the operating procedures shall be strictly complied with. Special attention should be paid while weighing chemicals or drugs, and measuring liquid reagents. To avoid errors, during the picking up, weighing and returning of chemicals, reagents must be carefully checked three times. After weighing, bottles should be capped immediately and put back in their original place. Note that once the chemicals have been taken out, they cannot be returned to the original bottle. Public instruments (such as filtering equipment, chromatograph, etc.) and special reagents (chromogenic reagents, etc.) should be used at designated areas according to the requirements of the experiment.

3.4 Carry out the experiment operation with seriousness and scientific attitude and observe the experiment carefully. Think in relation to the contents of given lectures, discuss the problems that may arise during the experiment, and record experiment data in detail. The experiment records should be concise, complete, accurate and tidy. If the experiment fails, the cause of the failure must be identified and corrected in the subsequent experiments.

3.5 Strictly abide by the rules and regulations of the laboratory, including loss reporting rules, compensation rules, cleaning and sanitation rules, safety operating rules, and classroom discipline.

3.6 Be economical in the use of resources, care for public property, and avoid damage. Laboratory chemicals, equipment, tools and experiment products belong to the laboratory and they shall not be taken outside of the laboratory without authorization.

3.7 Submit experiment reports on time. The contents of experiment reports should include Title, Aims, Equipment, Reagents, Medicinal Materials (including Yinpian) and adjuvants, Experimental Contents (including the experiment principle, operation procedures, results), and Discussion (analysis of experiment results, matters needing attention in experiment operation, discussion in relation to experiment principles, etc.).

3.8 Return reagents and chemicals to their original place, tidy up laboratory supplies and equipment on time after the experiment. Carefully check the water, fire and power sources and make sure all are switched off. Clean up the laboratory and leave the laboratory with the consent of the instructor.

4. General Principle for Chinese Materia Medica Processing

CMMP is a unique pharmaceutical technology that processes crude Chinese medicine according to the TCM theory, the crude drug's individual nature, drug dispensing, pharmaceutical preparation, and clinical need of application. Processed decoction pieces (Yinpian) refer to the prescription drugs produced from crude drugs following the regulations of CMMP, which can be directly used in TCM clinical practice or pharmaceutical preparation. The production, distribution, and use of processed decoction pieces should comply with the following requirements.

Once crude drugs are processed by cleaning, cutting and other procedures, they are called 'decoction pieces'. Crude drugs shall firstly be cleaned properly before they are cut or further processed. Processed decoction pieces are the starting materials of drug dispensing and pharmaceutical preparation. The crude drugs and adjuvants used to prepare processed decoction pieces should be processed in compliance with the corresponding quality requirements. The processed decoction pieces of TCM must be produced strictly with the officially issued CMMP regulations. The production, packaging, storage and management of Yinpian should conform to the requirements of the GMP standard. Toxic drugs (including anesthesia drugs) should be specially packaged with appropriate labels. The delivery, storage and use of processed decoction pieces should abide by the corresponding regulations. They shall be kept dry and special attention should be paid to avoid contamination, dampness, rotting, deterioration and growth of mould or moth.

Unless specified otherwise, the processing should comply with the following requirements.

4.1 Cleaning

Refers to the cleansing of crude drugs as required. This is done through the selective use of methods like sorting, sifting, wind separation, water separation, magnetic separation, picking, shearing, cutting, scraping, paring, scooping, removing, enzyme hydrolysis, peeling, squeezing, blanching, brushing, rubbing, cauterizing, scalding, colliding, grinding etc., to achieve the drug purity requirement.

4.2 Cutting

Except drugs which must be prepared from fresh or dry form, crude drugs should be softened before cutting. Common softening methods include showering, washing quickly, soaking, moistening, rinsing, steaming and boiling, etc. Alternatively, this can be done with the use of softening devices such as rotary decompressed infiltration cans or gas phase replacement moistening chambers. Crude drugs shall be treated separately and appropriately according to their size, thickness, and hardness at a specified temperature, with specified quantity of water, and for a specified duration. Moistening is preferable to soaking because this will reduce the loss of active components. Drug pieces should be dried in time to guarantee their quality.

The format of drug pieces includes slices, sections, cubes, slivers, etc. Their sizes and thickness are generally as follows.

Slices

Cut less than 0.5mm of thickness for very thin slices, 1~2mm for thin slices, and 2~4mm for thick slices.

Sections

Sections are produced in 5~10mm of length for short sections and 10~15mm for long sections.

Cube

Chinese medicine cubes are in 8~12mm^3.

Slivers

2~3mm in width for narrow slivers, 5~10mm for broad slivers.

Crude drugs that are not suitable for cutting are generally pounded or crushed before use.

4.3 Processing

Unless otherwise specified, the general methods and requirements of processing are as follows.

4.3.1 Stir-frying

This is divided into simple stir-frying and stir-frying with adjuvants. Crude drugs should be dried and graded by size. During frying, drugs should be stirred frequently to ensure even and homogeneous heating, with controlled temperature, duration and required conditions.

Simple Stir-frying

Cleaned crude drugs are placed in a hot pot and stir-fried on a gentle fire for the specified extent. Processed material should be transferred to a clean, cold and dry container and left to cool. For drugs which need to be deeply fried, they shall be stir-fried on a medium fire until the cutting surfaces turn dark brown and fractures become brown. The stir-fried drugs are then removed from the heat and left to cool. For drugs which need to be carbonized, they shall be stir-fried on strong fire until the surface turns brownish-black. Spray some water onto the drugs to extinguish any spark and then fry to dryness.

Stir-frying with bran

Put wheat bran in a hot stir-frying pot and heat until the bran smokes. Put the crude drugs into the pot, stir quickly until the surface of the drugs turns yellow or dark yellow, take them out, remove the bran by sifting and leave to cool.

Unless otherwise specified, use 10~15kg of wheat bran per 100kg of crude drugs.

Stir-frying with sand

Put clean river sand in a stir-frying pot, heat on strong fire until the sand can move smoothly in the pot and then add the crude drugs, keep stirring frequently until the drugs' surface swells and turns crisp or to a specified extent. Stop heating and remove the sand by sifting and leave to cool.

Unless otherwise specified, use an appropriate quantity of sand just enough to cover the crude drugs.

If required quenching with vinegar, sift out the sand and dip the drugs into vinegar while hot until they become crisp.

Stir-frying with clam-shell powder

Place a required quantity of sift-selected, fine and clean clam-shell powder in a pot, and heat on a medium fire until the powder can move freely and smoothly in the pot. Add the crude drugs, keep stir-frying until the drugs expand into a ball shape, turn crispy with a yellow surface, take them out, remove clam-shell powder by sifting and leave to cool.

Unless otherwise specified, use 30~35kg of powdered clam-shell for every 100kg of crude drugs.

Stir-frying with talcum powder

Put a quantity of talcum powder into a stir-frying pot, and heat on a medium fire until the talcum powder can move smoothly in the pot. Add the crude drugs, keep stir-frying until the drugs expand, turn crispy with yellow surface or to another specified extent. Take them out immediately, remove the talcum powder by sifting, and leave to cool.

Unless otherwise specified, use 40~50kg of talcum powder per 100kg of crude drugs.

4.3.2 Stir-frying with liquid adjuvant

Refers to a method of mixing crude drugs with liquid adjuvant until the drugs are moistened, and then stir-fry them to a specified extent.

Stir-frying with wine

Mix the crude drugs with yellow rice wine, and leave to set for a while until the drugs are completely moistened. Put the drugs in a stir-frying pot, heat on a gentle fire to a specific extent, take the drugs out, and leave to cool.

Unless otherwise specified, use 10~20kg of yellow rice wine per 100kg of crude drugs.

Stir-frying with vinegar

Mix the crude drugs with vinegar, and leave to set until the drugs are completely moistened. Put the drugs into a stir-frying pot, heat to a pre-specified extent. Take the drugs out and leave to cool.

Unless otherwise specified, use 20~30kg of rice vinegar per 100kg of crude drugs.

Stir-frying with salt solution

Mix the crude drugs with salt solution, and leave to set until the drugs are completely moistened. Put the drugs onto a stir-frying pot, heat on a gentle fire to a pre-specified extent. Take the drugs out and leave to cool.

To prepare salt solution, dissolve salt in an appropriate quantity of drinking water and filter before use. Unless otherwise specified, use 2kg of salt per 100kg of crude drugs.

Stir-frying with ginger juice

Crush fresh clean ginger into paste, add an appropriate quantity of water, and squeeze to obtain ginger juice. Add another small quantity of water to the ginger residue and squeeze again. Combine the ginger juice from both preparations for use. The yield of ginger juice to fresh ginger shall be 1 : 1. Alternatively, add a quantity of water into sliced or crushed fresh or dried ginger, decoct twice, combine the decoction, filtrate, and concentrate to an appropriate volume as necessary.

Mix the crude drugs with ginger juice evenly. Then place the drugs into a stir-frying pot, heat on gentle fire until ginger juice is absorbed entirely or to a specified extent. Take the drugs out and leave to cool.

Unless otherwise specified, use 10kg of fresh ginger or 3kg of dried ginger per 100kg of crude drugs.

Stir-frying with honey

Dilute refined honey with an appropriate quantity of boiled water, add the crude drugs, mix well to evenly penetrate. Put the drugs in a stir-frying pot, heat on gentle fire to a specified extent, take the drugs out and leave to cool.

Use refined honey for processing. Unless otherwise specified, use 25kg of refined honey per 100kg of crude drugs.

Stir-frying with lamb fat

Heat lamb fat in a stir-frying pot until it melts, remove the residue, add the crude drugs and mix well, heat on gentle fire until the fat is completely absorbed and the drugs surface become shiny bright, take the drugs out, spread drugs and leave to cool.

4.3.3 Carbonizing

When crude drugs are carbonized, the nature of the drugs should be preserved. Carbonizing prevents ashing, and more importantly, re-ignition.

Carbonizing by sir-frying

Put crude drugs in a hot stir-frying pot, heat on strong fire until the surfaces become brownish-black, and the inner parts become dark brown or a specified extent. Spray a little water over the drugs to extinguish any spark, take out the drugs and dry in the air.

Carbonizing by calcining

Put crude drugs in a calcining pot, close tightly, heat them to a specified extent, leave to cool and take the drugs out.

4.3.4 Calcining

Calcine crude drugs thoroughly until they become crispy and easily crushable.

Calcining openly

Crack crude drugs into small pieces, put in a suitable container, and calcine thoroughly until the drugs become crispy, brittle, or red. Take the drugs out, leave to cool, and then grind to powder.

Mineral salts containing crystal water do not need to be calcined to red. Make sure to evaporate all the crystal water, or calcine until the drugs become honeycomb-like solid masses.

Calcining and quenching

Calcine crude drugs until they are red, dip them quickly into a specified liquid adjuvant (repeat as needed until the drugs are sufficiently crispy). Take the drugs out, dry and grind into powder.

4.3.5 Steaming

Classify crude drugs by size, add a quantity of water or liquid adjuvant as described for the individual drug, mix well and allow to stand until the drugs are completely moistened. Put the drugs in a suitable steaming container, steam to a specified extent. Take the drugs out, cool, mix with the steaming liquid, air dry to 60% dryness, cut into slices or sections as appropriate, and leave to dry.

4.3.6 Boiling

Classify crude drugs by size, add a quantity of water or liquid adjuvant as described for individual drug and boil the drug, cut the drug to check the extent of processing and stop boiling when the inner center of the drugs is non-white. Take the drugs out, air dry to 60% dryness, cut into slices and leave to dry.

4.3.7 Stewing

Mix crude drugs with specified liquid adjuvant as described for individual drug, put in a suitable container, seal tightly, stew thoroughly on a water bath or by steaming, or keep stewing until the adjuvant are completely absorbed. Leave to cool, take the drugs out, air dry to 60% dryness, cut into slices and leave to dry.

For steaming, boiling, and stewing, use 20~30kg of liquid adjuvant per 100kg of crude drugs, unless otherwise specified.

4.3.8 Roasting

Wrap the crude drugs with dough or wet paper, or separate the crude drugs into uniform layers with oil-absorbent paper, and heat the drugs. Alternatively, put crude drugs together with wheat bran in a stir-frying pan, heat on gentle fire to a specified extent, take the drugs out and leave to cool.

Unless otherwise specified, use 50kg of wheat bran per 100kg of crude drugs.

4.4 Other processing methods

4.4.1 Blanching

Put crude drugs in an ample amount of boiling water, stir for a short while, and take the drugs out. For certain seeds, blanch until the wrinkled testa become smooth and easily removable, take the drugs out, put into cold water, peel off the testa and dry in the sun.

4.4.2 Frosty (prepare frost-like powder by removing oil)

Unless specified otherwise, crush the crude drugs into a paste, heat slightly, and squeeze repeatedly until the majority of oil is removed and the content of the residual oil is meets the specified requirement. Pulverize the residue into a fairly dispersible powder as required for the individual drug.

4.4.3 Levigating

Put crude drugs in a container, add a quantity of water and grind to paste. Add a large amount of water, agitate, and decant the supernatant suspension. Repeat the operation several times with the residual drug. Combine the supernatant suspensions, leave to stand, separate the precipitate, dry, and pulverize into powder.

4.4.4 Sprouting

Put crude drugs in a container, soak in an appropriate quantity of water, and then take the drugs out. Let the seeds sprout to a specified extent at an appropriate temperature and humidity. Dry in the sun or at a low temperature. Avoid the contamination of grease and ensure the drugs do not become rotten. The sprouts are generally no longer than 1cm.

4.4.5 Fermenting

Thoroughly mix the crude drugs with the specified adjuvant, make a suitable shape, place them under an appropriate temperature and humidity, and let the microorganism grow until the enzyme content reaches a specified requirement. Dry in the sun or at a low temperature. The fermented products are forbidden to use when flavus is observed during fermentation.

PPT

第二节　中药炮制辅料与设备

一、中药炮制辅料

中药炮制辅料是指除主药以外具有辅助作用的附加物料。利用辅料炮制是中药炮制的特色，在炮制过程中，通过辅料与药物共同作用，达到减毒增效、缓和药性、改变药性或矫味等炮制作用；亦可利用辅料的中间传热作用，改变药物质地，促进成分转化，利于药效成分的溶出和吸收，最大限度地发挥中药饮片的治疗作用。辅料质量的优劣以及用法是否得当对炮制品的质量影响很大。

中药炮制常用的辅料一般分为液体辅料和固体辅料两大类。

（一）液体辅料

1. 炮制用水

（1）饮用水　为天然水经净化处理后所得的水，其质量应符合现行国家标准《生活饮用水卫生标准》。此为中药饮片生产用水最低要求，可以作为药材净制时漂洗用水，切制前软化处理时泡、润用水，煎煮药汁用水，炮制器具的清洁用水等。

（2）纯净水　为蒸馏水或离子交换、反渗透或其他方法制备的水。纯净水或冷开水可以作为液体辅料的稀释用水。饮片生产企业应定期监测生产用水的质量，饮用水每年至少一次送相关检测部门进行检测。

2. 酒　炮制用酒除另有规定外，一般用黄酒。酒应是具有生产资格企业的产品，并具生产企业提供的出厂质量检验报告单。黄酒质量应符合中华人民共和国国家标准《黄酒》（GB/T 13662-2018）要求；白酒质量应符合中华人民共和国国家标准《食品安全国家标准蒸馏酒及其配制酒》（GB 2757-2012）要求。

（1）色泽　黄酒应为琥珀色或淡黄色液体，光泽明亮，无悬浮物和沉淀物；白酒应无色、透明、无悬浮物和沉淀物。

（2）气味　黄酒具有黄酒特有的醇香，醇厚而稍甜，酒味柔和无刺激性，不得有辛辣、酸涩特异味。白酒口尝醇厚、无异味，无强烈刺激性，各味协调；取白酒滴几滴于掌心，稍搓几下，再嗅手掌，有溢香，不应有异味、不良气味存在。

（3）含醇量　黄酒含乙醇 15%~20%，白酒含乙醇为 50%~70%。

酒炙时，一般每 100kg 待炮炙品，用黄酒 10kg，必要时，可用适量冷开水或纯净水稀释。酒炖或酒蒸时，依据药用部位决定用酒量。

3. 醋　炮制用醋应为米醋或其他酿造醋，以陈醋为优，不得用化学勾兑醋。醋应该为具有生产资格企业的产品，并具有生产企业提供的出厂质量检验报告单。质量应符合中华人民共和国国家标准 -《食醋卫生标准》（GB 2719-2018）要求。

（1）色泽　取样品置于试管中，在白色背景下用肉眼观察，呈琥珀色或者棕红色。

（2）气味　将样品置于具塞容器中振摇，去塞后，立即嗅闻，应具有食醋应有的气味和醋酸气味，无其他异味。口尝酸味柔和，稍有甜味，无其他异味。

（3）性状　将样品置于试管中，在白色背景下对光观察其浑浊度，应澄清。然后将试管加塞颠倒检查应无悬浮物质。放置一定时间后，再观察应无沉淀。必要时取出静置 15 分钟后的上清液，借助放大镜观察，应无醋鳗、醋虱、醋蝇。

（4）理化检测　应达到规定要求。

醋制（包括醋炙、醋煮、醋蒸）时按规定用量取用，一般每 100kg 药材，用醋 20kg，需要时，用冷开水或纯净水稀释。

4. 蜂蜜　炮制用蜜应为炼蜜。炼蜜有嫩蜜、中蜜、老蜜之分，一般蜜炙的中药采用中蜜进行炮制，但对于炼蜜有特殊要求的药物应该按照要求进行蜂蜜的炼制。质量应符合《中华人民共和国药典》2020 年版一部“蜂蜜”项下要求。

（1）性状　为半透明、带光泽、浓稠的液体，白色至淡黄色或橘黄色至黄褐色，放久或遇冷渐有白色颗粒状结晶析出。气芳香，味极甜。

（2）相对密度　按韦氏比重法秤测定，相对密度 1.349 以上。

（3）酸度检查　需符合规定。

（4）淀粉和糊精检查　需符合规定。

（5）5- 羟甲基糠醛检查　需符合规定。

（6）还原糖　碱性酒石酸酮试液测定法测定，含还原糖不得少于 60%。

蜜制时，一般每 100kg 药物，用炼蜜 25kg。炮制药物时炼蜜需用适量冷开水稀释后，方可与药物拌润。

5. 盐水　传统炮制用盐为原盐（粗盐、大粒盐），其中所含成分比较复杂，如含氯化钠、氯化镁、氯化钾、氯化钙、硫酸钙、硫酸镁、硫酸钠等。现代炮制多用食盐精制盐，主要含有氯化钠，还含少量的氯化镁、硫酸镁、硫酸钙等。质量应符合中华人民共和国国家标准《食用盐卫生标准》（GB 2721-2015）要求。

盐制药物时，一般每 100kg 药材，用盐 2kg，盐制时应先将盐加适量纯化或冷开水溶解后，滤过备用（精制盐可直接溶解后使用）。

6. 姜汁　制备炮制辅料姜汁所用姜有生姜和干姜两种，一般首选生姜。姜应符合食用标准，无霉败、腐烂等变异现象。

姜汁的制备方法有两种：一是先将生姜洗净，捣烂，加水适量，压榨取汁，姜渣再加水适量重复压榨一次，合并汁液即为“姜汁”。二是将生姜或干姜切制或捣碎后加水煎煮两次，合并煎液滤过，取滤液适当浓缩后备用。姜汁可用纯净水或冷开水稀释。一般每 100kg 药材，用生姜 10kg 或干姜 3kg。

7. 胆汁　是动物的新鲜胆液，常用的有猪、牛、羊胆汁，以牛胆汁为最佳。胆汁为绿褐色、微透明的液体，略有黏性，有特异的腥臭气。

炮制用胆汁可直接用规定的鲜胆汁，也可以用胆膏粉，1g 胆膏粉相当于 10g 鲜胆汁，加纯净水或冷开水稀释后使用。

8. 羊脂油　为牛科动物山羊等的脂肪经低温熬炼而成。主要成分为油脂，皂化值 192~195，含饱和脂肪酸和不饱和脂肪酸等。

羊油脂使用前需要熬炼。取羊腹部脂肪，切块，加热熬炼，融化后，去渣滤取油脂即得。羊油脂冷却后为乳白色的固体，加热熔化为液体。羊油脂与药物同制后能增强补虚助阳作用。常用羊脂油炮制的药物有淫羊藿等。

9. 麻油　为芝麻科植物芝麻种子经压榨法得到的脂肪油；其质量标准依据《中华人民共和国药典》2020 年版一部“麻油”项下要求。

（1）性状　淡黄色或棕黄色的澄明液体；具芝麻油特有的香气，味淡。

（2）相对密度及折光率　相对密度 0.917~0.923；折光率 1.471~1.475。

（3）检查　酸值≤ 2.5；皂化值为 188~195；碘值 103~116；加热实验：取本品 50ml，依法检查，不得有沉淀析出；杂质≤ 0.2%；水分与挥发物≤ 0.2%。

炮制中主要用于油炸、酥制药物。如马钱子、三七、蛤蚧等。

10. 米泔水 为淘米时第二次滤过的灰白色混浊液体，为淀粉与水的混悬液，还含少量维生素等。若选用免淘米，因其已除去杂质，使用第一遍淘米水即可。由于米泔水易酸败发酵，应临用时收集。也可用大米粉 2kg 加水 100kg，充分搅拌代替米泔水使用。

由于米泔水对油脂的吸附作用，炮制时可选用米泔水浸苍术、白术等，以降低药物的辛燥之性。

11. 其他药汁 药汁类的液体辅料，按常规煎煮法制备，根据品种不同适当采用轻煎、重煎或一般煎煮法，煎煮两次，四层纱布过滤，合并煎液。

（1）吴茱萸汁 为吴茱萸的煎汁，主要用于炮制黄连等。

（2）黑豆汁 为黑大豆加水适量，煎煮去渣的黑色混浊液体，主要用于炮制何首乌。

（3）甘草汁 为甘草饮片煎煮去渣的黄棕色至深棕色的液体。常用于炮制远志、半夏、吴茱萸等。

（4）萝卜汁 为鲜萝卜切片加水煎煮所得的淡黄色煎液。常用于提净芒硝。

（二）固体辅料

1. 稻米 为禾本科植物稻的种仁。主要成分为淀粉、蛋白质、脂肪、矿物质，尚含少量 B 族维生素、多种无机盐及糖类。中药炮制多选用大米或糯米。应符合食用标准，无霉变，无泥沙。

2. 麦麸 为禾本科植物小麦的种皮，呈黄褐色。主要成分为淀粉、蛋白质、维生素等。炮制用麸无异味，无霉变，无泥沙。麦麸与药物共制能缓和药物的刺激性，降低其燥性或寒性，增强其健脾和中的作用，此外还有矫味、矫臭、赋色等作用。麦麸还能吸附油脂，用于麸炒和煨制药物。

3. 白矾 为硫酸盐类矿物矾石，经加工提炼制成，又称明矾。呈不规则的晶体，无色或淡黄白色，透明或半透明，有玻璃样光泽，质硬而脆，气微，味微甜而涩。易溶于水和甘油，不溶于乙醇。水溶液显铝盐、钾盐与硫酸盐的各种反应，主要成分为带有结晶水分子的硫酸铝钾。

白矾由矾石加工提炼而得，可直接用于炮制。

4. 豆腐 为豆科植物大豆种子经粉碎盐析而成的植物蛋白，为乳白色固体。主含蛋白质、维生素、淀粉等物质。一般选择新鲜的食用豆腐作为炮制辅料。豆腐与药物共制可降低药物的毒性，去除污物。常用豆腐制的药物有藤黄、珍珠、硫黄等。

5. 土 中药炮制常用的是灶心土、黄土、赤石脂等。灶心土又名伏龙肝，呈焦土状，黑褐色、焦黄色或砖红色，附有烟熏气。主含硅酸盐、钙盐及多种碱性氧化物。灶心土多在拆除锅灶、炉灶、砖窑时获得，使用前需除去表面浮尘，捣碎、研细，备用。黄土挖取后，置于锅中武火加热翻炒，除去水分、有机质，微生物等，备用。赤石脂为硅酸盐类矿物多水高岭石，主含四水硅酸铝，用前须打碎，研细粉。

6. 蛤粉 为帘蛤科动物文蛤、青蛤等的贝壳经粉碎后的灰白色粉末，主含氧化钙等物质。粉碎、过筛后备用。常用于炮制阿胶。

7. 滑石粉 为硅酸盐类矿物滑石族滑石，经精选、洗净，粉碎成细粉或水飞成细粉而得。为白色或类白色，有蜡样光泽，质软，细腻，手摸有滑润感，气微无味。主要成分为含水硅酸镁。中药炮制一般作中间传热体拌炒药物，使药物受热均匀，用于滑石粉烫和煨制药物。

8. 河砂 筛取中等粗细的河砂，淘尽泥土，除尽杂质，晒干。炮制前河砂还要经过武火翻炒，以除去有机杂质、微生物等。使用油砂的，再加入 1%~2% 的食用植物油拌炒至均匀，油烟散尽，砂色泽加深时，取出备用。常用于砂炒，如砂炒马钱子、砂炒鸡内金等。

9. 朱砂 为三方晶系硫化物类矿物辰砂族辰砂，经净选，再用水淘去杂石和泥沙而得，主要成分为硫化汞，常含单质汞。中药炮制用的朱砂需水飞成极细粉后使用，生产上常用球磨机研磨水飞成极细粉。

二、传统中药炮制工具及设备

中药炮制作为一门历史悠久的制药技术，我国的制药先辈们设计制造了大量适用于炮制的工具、设备。这些传统工具、设备在手工作坊时期，为保证饮片的质量起到了重要的作用，其中有些传统工具至今仍在使用，尤其是在小剂量、临方炮制时有着广泛的应用。

（一）碾捣、切制工具

1. 乳钵（研钵） 为研磨药物所用的工具，用于制取细粉，也可用于水飞、乳化等。大多为粗瓷制品，亦有石材、玉石、玛瑙等材质的，配有槌棒。乳钵大小不一，大号的直径有 50cm，深约 17cm，一般备有钵架；普通用直径 27cm，深 10cm，或直径 23cm，深 10cm 的乳钵；中号的直径 18cm，深 6.7cm；小号的直径 15cm，深 4.3cm，或直径 10cm，深 3.3cm（图 1–1）。

2. 冲钵（俗称铜冲筒、铜药冲、铜冲、铜杵） 冲钵包括冲筒及杵槌两部分。冲筒系铜制圆筒，高 23~26cm，直径 10~14cm，上有盖，盖顶有圆孔，铜杵槌由此穿过，可防止药物飞溅。适用于配方或少量捣杵药物，以熟铜制品为佳，生铜制品易破碎脱底（图 1–2）。

3. 铁研船（铁研槽、铁船、研槽） 多系用生铁铸成，分研槽、研盘两部分。研槽形状如船形，可大可小，一般以 1m 长、中部宽约 20cm 较适宜踏研。研盘在研船（槽）中以人力消研滚动时兼具截切、轧压和研磨等作用。铁研船占地少，单人即可操作，粉碎度较细，是一种传统的以人力为主粉碎药物的常用工具，对于小作坊生产，十分实用（图 1–3）。

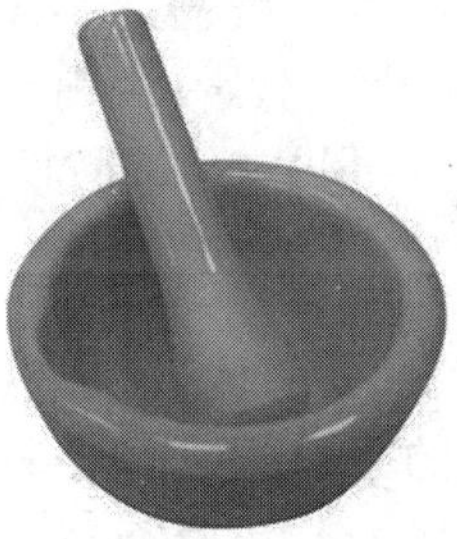
图 1–1 乳钵

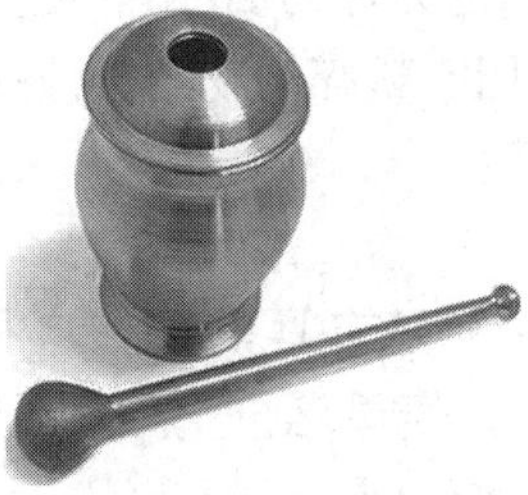
图 1–2 铜药冲

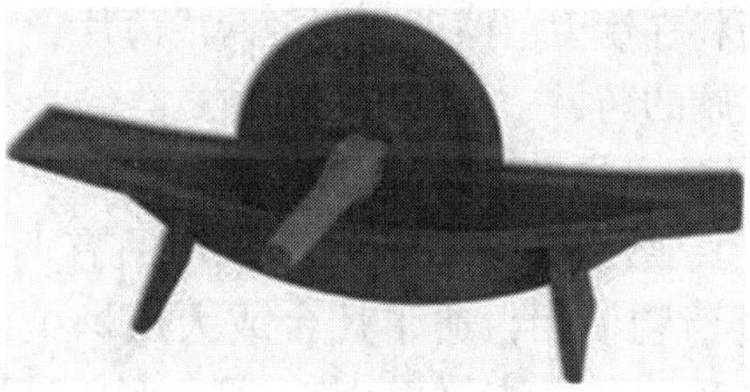
图 1–3 铁研船

4. 石磨、石碾 粉碎药物的工具，也可在除去果壳、木心等时使用。现在多用电动石磨碾药（图 1–4）。

5. 石臼 用粗糙的大石块凿成，方形或圆形，中有凹窝。大型的多用脚踏，系将石臼固定于一处，装置踏板一块，塔板前端正对石臼处，装一石杵，利用杠杆原理，撞击药物。小型的可用手舂，只需石臼和杵，不用木架等设备，适用于少量药物的粉碎（图 1–5）。

6. 磨池 由粗石凿成，形如砚台，长 27~34cm，宽 11~14cm，厚 6.7~10cm，四方平整，上面略凹，前端中部有突出小嘴，可流药汁。适用于水磨药物（图 1–6）。

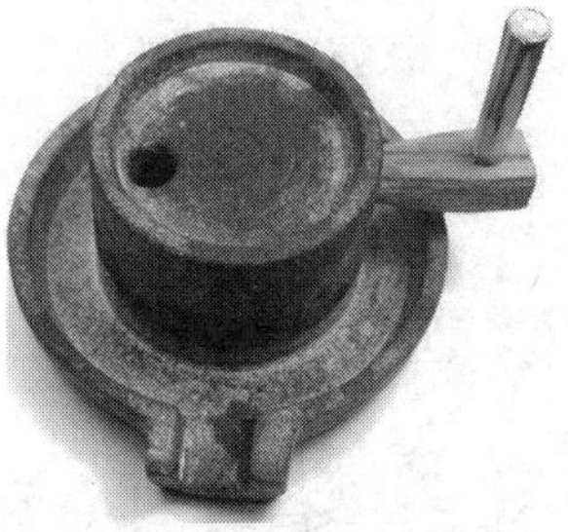
图 1–4 石磨

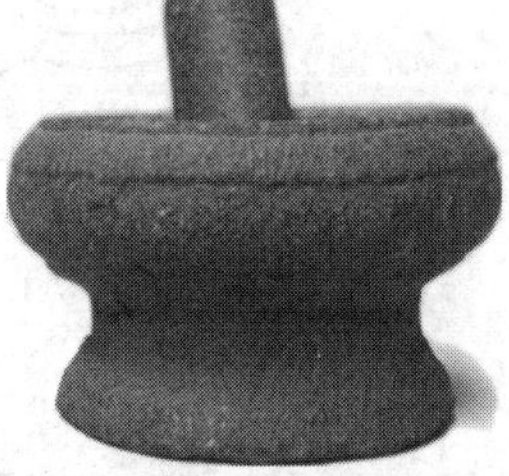
图 1–5 石臼

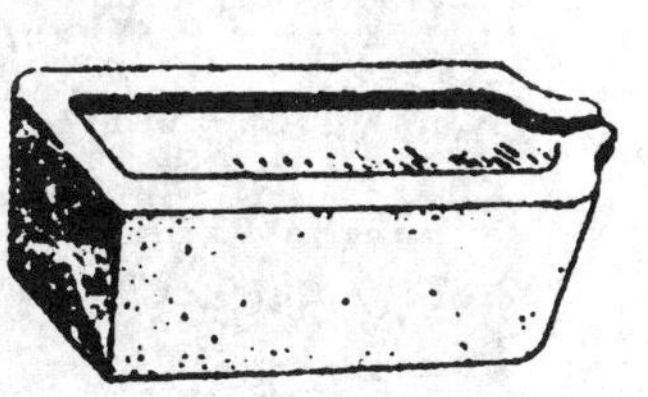
图 1–6 磨池

7. 切药刀 分刀身、刀床、刀脑三部分。刀身即刀片，又称刀叶子，略呈长方形，后上端竖立刀柄，稍向前弯，前下端微有小角突出（俗称刀鼻），上开一小孔，与刀床前端之刀脑相联合，组成铡刀状，为切制饮片的主要工具。简单的切药刀也有直接用片刀的。切药刀一般带有几种附件，即竹把子、刀撮子、竹簸箕、磨刀石等（图 1–7）。

此外还有竹刀、瓷片刀等，用于忌铁器药物去皮、核、瓤的加工处理。

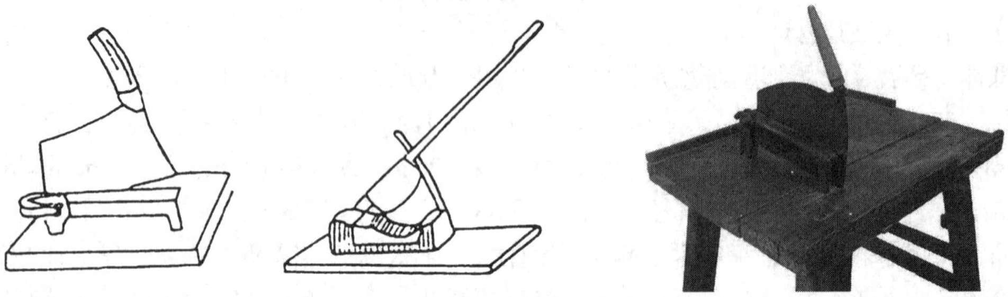

图 1–7 切药刀

8. 蟹爪钳（扁夹钳、槟榔钳） 由具有弹性的薄铁皮制成，上下对折，前端部有锯齿形咬口，宽 3~4cm，长约 16cm，为切药时钳夹药物所用，如制槟榔、青皮、山楂、泽泻等团块状的药物时（图 1–8）。

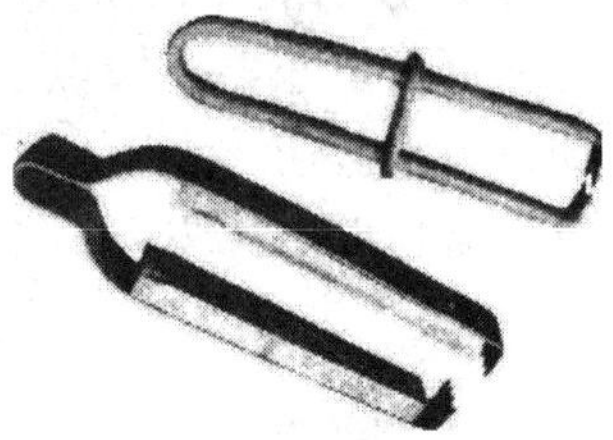

图 1–8 蟹爪钳

9. 镑刀 系在一块长 50cm、宽 6~7cm、厚 3~4cm 的木条上，每隔 1.5cm，装置高 3~4cm，宽度与木条宽度相同之刀片约 20 个。使用时药料在镑刀上擦动，即可镑成薄片。一般多用于粉碎动物角类或质地坚硬的药材，如犀角、沉香之类。

（二）炮炙设备及工具

1. 炒药锅、炒药灶 常用的有两种。一种是有耳的锅，口径较小，约 50cm，供炒、煅少量药物使用，适于灶台或大风炉上，比较方便灵活。另一种是无耳的平口锅，口径较大，66~100cm，供炒、煮、炮、煅、炙、蒸、煨、焙使用，多置于固定灶台上。

炒药锅有平放、斜放两种。南方一般习惯用平锅，药物接触锅面大，受热均匀；北方多用斜锅，药料常堆聚下方，受热不均，但翻炒、盛取药物比较便利。可用煤火或炭火作为热源炒药，如斜面灶；现代炒少量药多用电、煤气、液化气等加热源（图 1–9）。

炒药常配的工具有铁铲、扫帚、药匾、刷子等。

2. 煅药罐 阳城罐（以山西省阳城的陶罐著称而得名），俗称嘟噜，为陶制圆筒状罐子，中部膨大，口部与底部略小。阳城罐有大小数种，可根据需要选择（图 1–10）。

此外还有铁汤罐，上部呈圆筒状，下部较狭，直径 16~34cm，深度 26~50cm，适用于煅制容易爆碎的药物。煅药时常备铁钩，系铁制细圆杆，前端弯曲，成一双钩，为钩提煅药罐或翻动药物之用（图 1–11）。

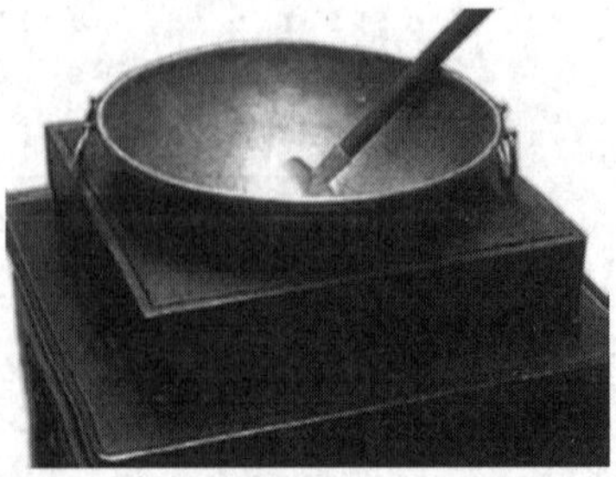

图 1–9 胡庆余堂“金铲银锅”

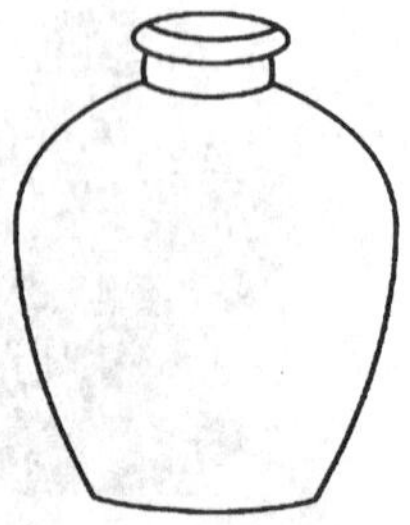

图 1–10 阳城罐

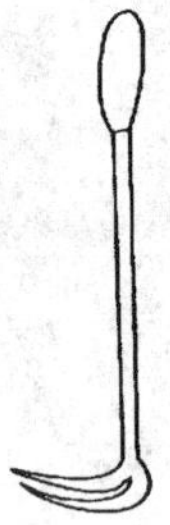

图 1–11 铁钩

3. **木蒸甑** 呈圆筒形，上面有盖，底部有屉，用以置锅上蒸制药物（图 1–12）。

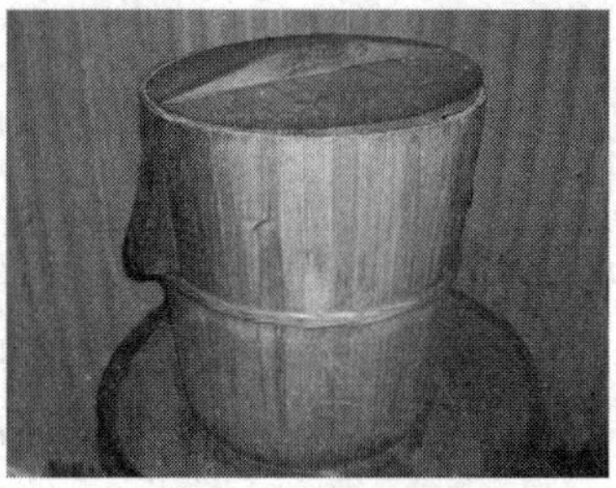

图 1–12 木蒸甑

（三）干燥设备

1. **木烘箱、木烘桶** 用于熏蒸药物，以防霉杀虫（图 1–13）。

2. **烘炕、烘房** 用于干燥药材和饮片。传统多用于木炭火加热，药物直接置于砖砌炕上进行干燥，尤其在阴雨、潮湿季节或者不能用晒法干燥的药材和饮片多用此法。也可在整个房间中加装回形散热铁管或火墙，药物置于药架上，使整个房间成为烘房来干燥药材和饮片。

3. **泛丸匾、竹匾** 用于盛装药物摊晾进行干燥，还可用作拌衣、泛制水丸等（图 1–14）。

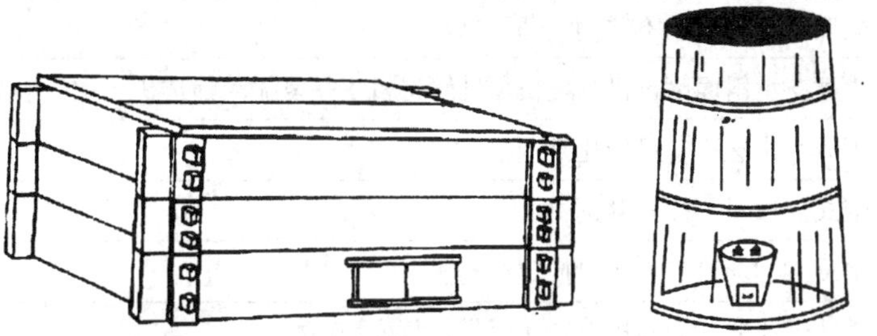

图 1–13 木烘箱、木烘桶

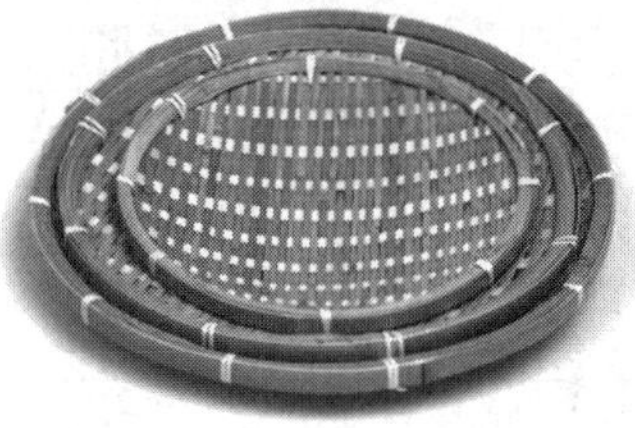

图 1–14 竹匾

（四）过筛及其他工具

1. **药筛** 用于筛选药物，进行大小分档，或除去药物中的碎屑、砂土，以及炒药后除去辅料等。药筛的孔眼大小有多种规格，可用竹编、马尾编、绢丝编、铜编、钢丝编等。

2. **剪刀、镊子、小刀等** 这些工具常用于挑选、净制药材。

3. **枳壳钳** 形如铡刀，上、下均为扁平阔厚之铁板，长约 33cm，宽约 7cm，两层对合面刻有斜形纵横交叉纹，下层前后端钉脚将钳固定在宽厚的木座上。钳的上层后端有木柄，前端有鼻，与下层的前端相连接，一般用于压扁枳壳一类的药物（图 1–15）。

4. **竹茹刀** 形狭长微弯，具有双柄，上方为刀背，下方为刀口，长约 40cm，宽约 10cm，专为刮取竹茹之用。

5. **龟刮板** 呈扁平条状，前端较阔，约 5cm，翘起呈钩形，有薄刀口，专为刮龟板或其他骨类药物皮肉筋膜所用。

6. **闸钳** 亦称铡剪，状如铡刀，刀厚而坚，形狭长，前端与下面垫条相连，供钳破坚硬药物之用（图 1–16）。

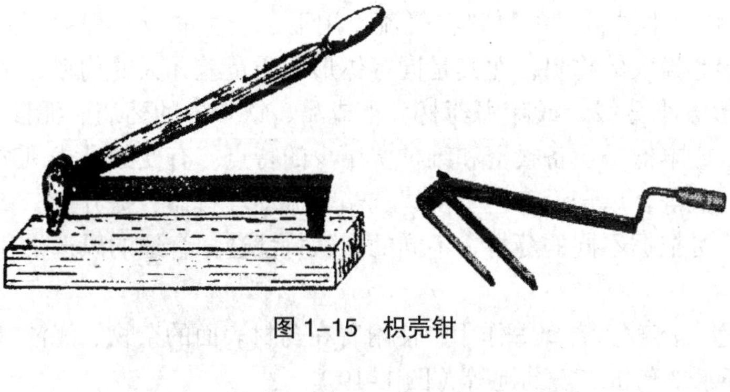

图 1–15 枳壳钳

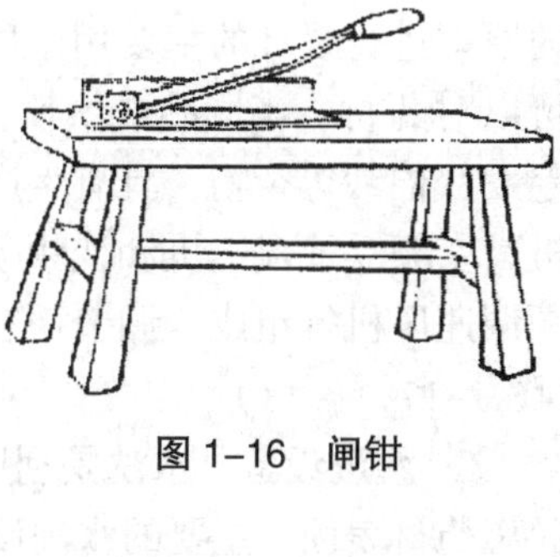

图 1–16 闸钳

三、现代中药炮制生产设备

随着时代的发展，中药炮制也逐步从传统的作坊式加工转向现代的机械化生产。因此，可以适应大生产的炮制设备应运而生。炮制设备是中药饮片企业的硬件基础。炮制设备发展到现在，已经研制出多种炮制设备供中药饮片生产企业使用，很大程度上解决了饮片规模化生产与传统炮制机具生产能力低的矛盾，为中药炮制的产业化和规模化做出了重要贡献。常用的炮制设备见表 1-1。

表 1–1　常用炮制设备一览表

制法	方式	常用设备
净制	风选	变频卧式风选机、变频立式风选机、变频吸风式风选机
	水洗	循环水洗药机、不锈钢洗药水槽
	筛选	柔性支承斜面筛选机、电机振动筛选机、往复振动筛选机
	挑选	不锈钢挑选机、机械化挑选机
	磁选	带式磁选机、棒式磁选机
切制	软化	水浸式润药机、气相置换式润药机
	往复切片	柔性带往复式切药机、金属履带往复式切药机
	旋转切片	转盘式切药机、旋料式切片机
碎制	破碎	颚式破碎机、挤压式破碎机（压扁机）
	粉碎	球磨机、锤式粉碎机
干燥	间歇干燥	封闭式烘干箱、敞开式烘干箱、滚筒式烘焙机
	连续干燥	网带式烘干机、转筒式烘干机
炒制	旋转式炒药	转筒式炒药机、转鼓式炒药机
炙制	炙药	转鼓式炙药机
	炙药	平转式炙药机
煅制	中低温	中低温煅药锅
	高温	反射式高温煅药炉
蒸煮	蒸	电加热蒸药箱、蒸汽蒸药箱、电汽两用蒸药箱
	煮	可倾式蒸煮锅

（一）净制设备

1. 风选设备　风选是利用不同形状、不同粒度的物料在气流作用下，产生的位移程度不同的原理进行设计的主要用于质量、体形差异大的物料，尤其是同等体形而质量差异大的物料，也可以对药材、半成品或饮片，按其体形大小分级，或除去药材、半成品、饮片中的药屑、泥沙、毛发、棉纱等杂物，具有生产能力大、成本低，设备投资和维护费用少的特点。有变频卧式风选机、变频立式风选机和变频吸风式风选机等。风选设备主要由风选箱、振动均料器、提升机、变频调速风机等组成。调节档有 2~5 档，可根据不同的药材、不同的形状特性选择合适的风选设备（图 1–17，1–18）。

2. 水洗设备　水洗是利用水的浸泡、溶解、卷离等作用，使附着在药材表面的杂物、泥沙等脱离药材表面。主要的水洗设备有循环水洗药机、洗药池等（图 1–19）。

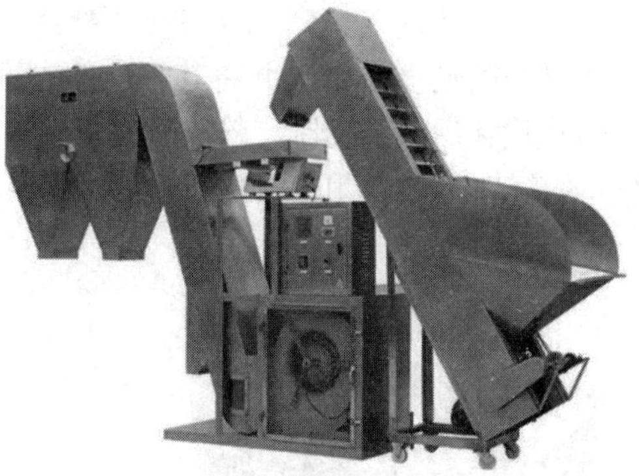

图 1-17　立式风选机

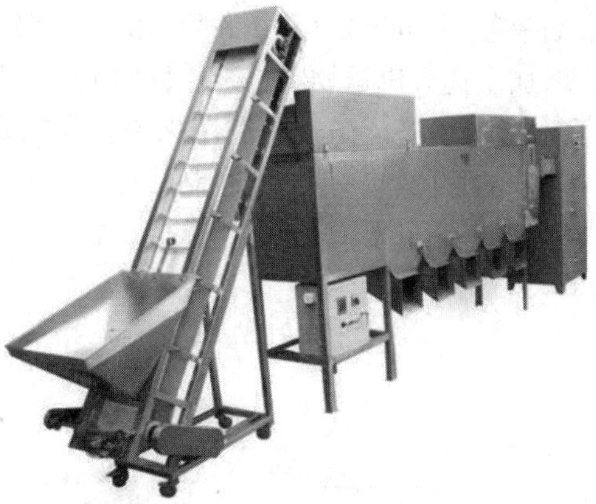

图 1-18　卧式风选机

循环水洗药机的主体部分是一壁面开有许多小孔的鼓式转筒，由电机通过皮带直接驱动转筒旋转。转筒下部是“V”型水箱，“V”型水箱的水经过泥沙过滤器由水泵将其增压，通过喷淋管、喷嘴喷向转筒内的药材。由于转筒一部分进入水箱，药材被充分浸泡，再通过喷淋水冲刷、转筒旋转使药材相互摩擦，使附着在药材表面的杂物脱落并被水流带走，达到清洗药材的目的。

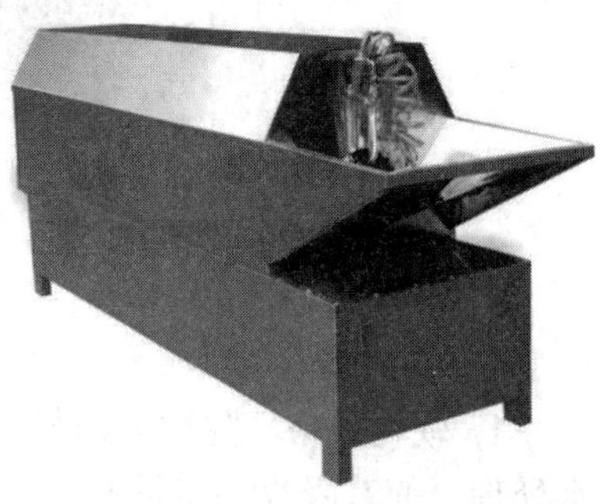

图 1-19　循环水洗药机

洗药池通常用混凝土制作，内衬不锈钢板。水池底部的排水管道与下水道相连，出口处装有放水阀，下水道上设置沉淀池，以避免泥沙堵塞下水道。进水管道上装有流量计和阀门，可以显示用水量和控制进水。水池的一个侧面通常设有小门，以方便用小车装载药材。在清洗过程中需要人工翻动、搅拌药材，以提高清洗效果。

3. 筛选设备　筛选是因物料（混合物）存在体形差异，物料与筛网之间的相对运动使小于筛网孔的物料与其他较大物料分离的一个过程。根据物料体形选择适当大小的网孔能达到较好的筛选目的。

根据筛网在驱动作用下产生的运动轨迹，筛选机分为柔性支承斜面筛选机、电机振动筛选机、往复振动筛选机。它们的运动轨迹分别是平面回转运动、上下往复运动、前后或左右往复运动。除了这些运动外，筛网必须与水平面成一定的倾斜角度才能使物料不断地前移。根据物料出口数目，有 2、3、4 出口之分。筛选设备一般由机架、传动装置、床身、筛网、出料斗等组成（图 1-20）。

4. 挑选设备　挑选是除去药材杂物的一种方法。被挑选的杂物包括缠绕、夹杂在药材中的杂物和非药用部位等。根据自动化程度高低，挑选设备分为不锈钢挑选台、机械化挑选机组。挑选

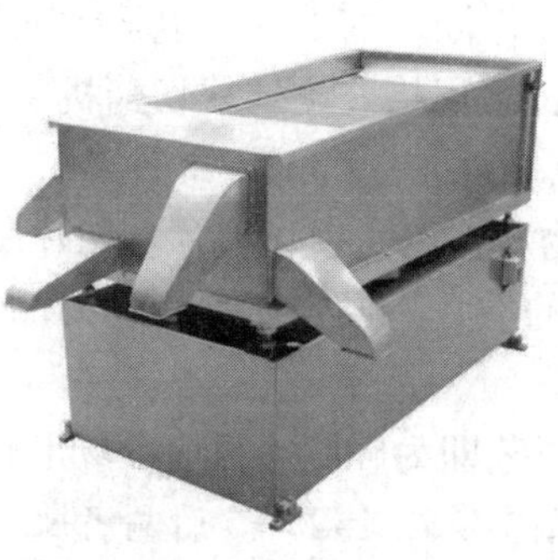

图 1-20　三层四出式平面回转式筛选机

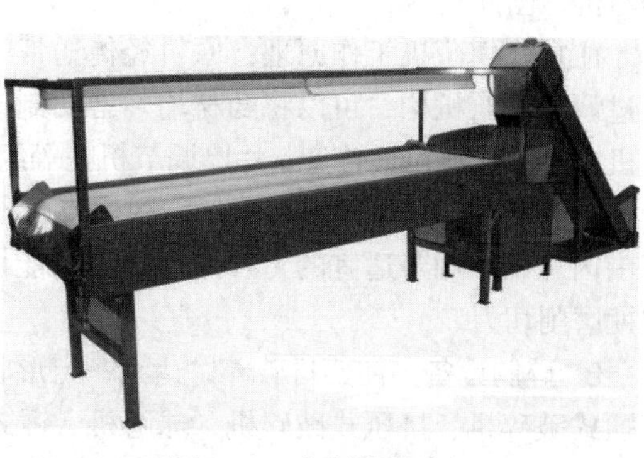

图 1-21　机械化挑选机

台台面一般为1m×2m，分平面、凹面、带落料孔三种形式，机械化挑选机组与不锈钢挑选台相比，增加了提升机送物料、杂质反向输送和磁选功能（图1–21）。

5. 磁选设备 磁选是利用强磁性材料吸附混合在药材中的铁质杂物，并将其分离的一种方法。磁选的目的，一是为了净制药材或饮片，二是为了避免损坏后续的切制、粉碎等加工机械。

磁选设备主要有带式磁选机、棒式磁选机。其主要部件是磁棒和振动均料器（图1–22，1–23）。

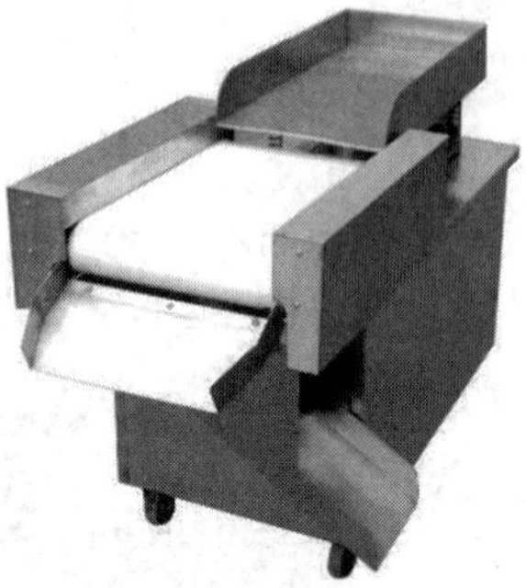

图1–22 带式磁选机

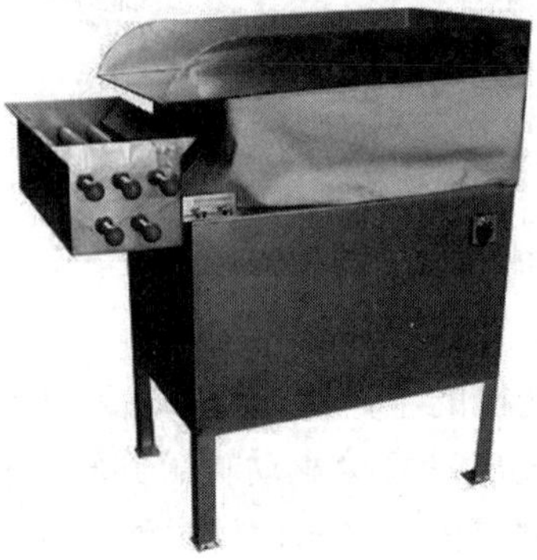

图1–23 棒式磁选机

（二）切制设备

1. 软化设备 除少数药材可趁鲜切制或干切外，大部分干燥的药材，切制前必须进行适当的水处理，使其吸收一定量的水分，达到质地柔软适中，以利于进一步切片。

现代常用的浸润软化机械设备有水浸式润药机、气相置换式润药机等，相比较而言，后者较为先进，其工作原理是利用抽真空减压的方法，抽取药材组织间隙中的气体，使其成为负压状态，然后，将水蒸气通入罐内，使其迅速、均匀地进入药材组织内部，提高软化效果。对难润药材可进行多次软化。气相置换式润药机是由方形箱体、气泵及充气式密封机构、真空泵及控制系统、各种电磁阀、报警装置等组成（图1–24）。

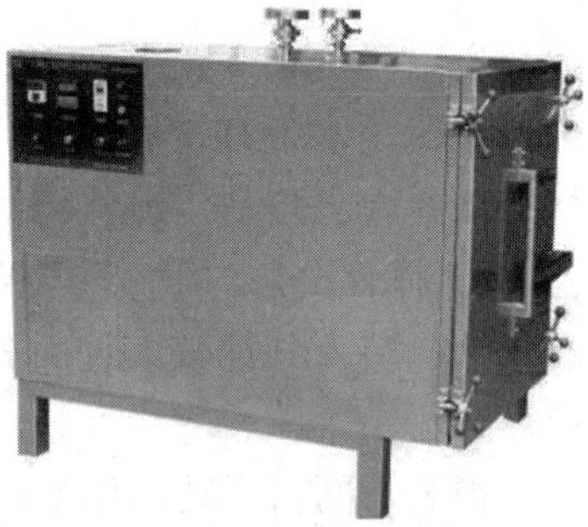

图1–24 水蓄冷真空气相置换式润药机

2. 切制设备 切制刀具的硬度远远高于药材，刀具接触药材并施加压力，刀刃陷入药材将其切开。刀刃与药材接触并产生相对运动是切制的基本条件。

现代切药机器种类较多，根据刀具和物料的相对运动方式，分为上下往复式和旋转式切制设备。属于上下往复式的切制设备有柔性带往复式切药机、金属履带往复式切药机等；属于旋转式切制设备的有转盘式切药机、旋料式切片机等。其他还有多功能切药机、刨片机等。

往复式切药机工作原理：原料经传送带间断送料，刀片作同步的上下往复运动而切断药材；通过调节进给机构，可以将药材均匀地切制成不同厚薄、长短规格。旋转式切药机主要由机架、电机、刀片、料斗、转盘、片厚调节机构等组成（图1–25）。

被切制的药材不能混有铁丝、铁块或石子之类的硬性物质，以免损坏刀片。切片厚度在一定范围内可调，调节适宜的刀片厚度和刀角能切出理想片形的饮片。要定期检测切刀的锋利程度，定期磨削切刀。

3. 碎制设备 使药材破碎，达到一定形状大小规格的工艺即为碎制。目前市场上破碎机主要有颚式破碎机、挤压式破碎机、球磨机、锤式粉碎机等（图1–26，1–27）。后两者属于细粉碎机械，能粉碎出更小更细的颗粒状药物。破碎的原理是通过撞击或挤压力，克服药物分子之间的作

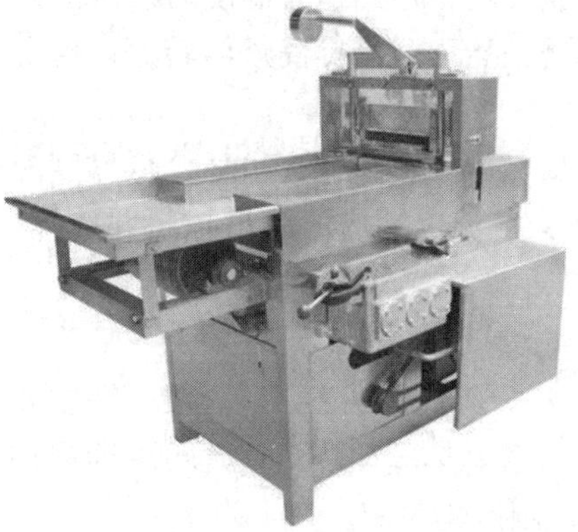

图 1-25　柔性带直线往复式切药机

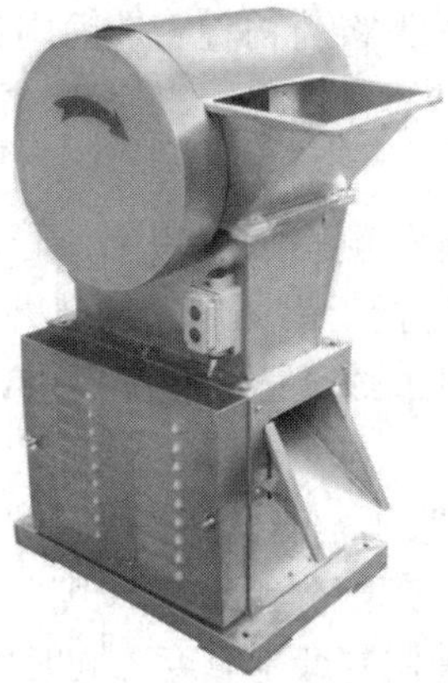

图 1-26　颚式破碎机

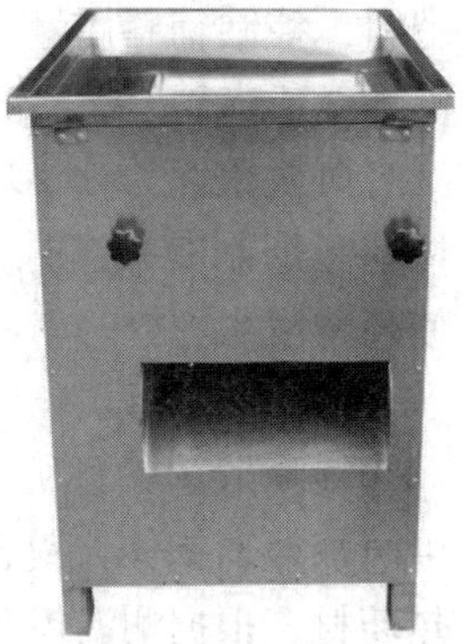

图 1-27　挤压式破碎机

用力，使其达到破碎或粉碎的效果。

（三）干燥设备

干燥原理是将热能作用于含水饮片，部分或全部水分从饮片中逸出而使饮片干燥的过程。根据饮片的烘干作业是连续的还是间歇的可分为连续烘干设备和间歇烘干设备。封闭式烘干箱、敞开式烘干箱和滚筒式烘干箱属于间歇烘干设备；网带式烘干机、转筒式烘干机和翻板式烘干机属于连续烘干设备（图 1-28）。

烘干设备主要由热源发生器、烘干箱体等组成。为药材提供热源的有蒸汽、电热、燃油及远红外线等。

在烘干过程中需要注意的是提供热源的温度不能过高，否则饮片会被烤焦或引起有效成分的损失或变化；另外，热源不能对饮片造成污染或起化学反应。

（四）炒制设备

常用的炒制设备有滚筒式炒药机、自控温鼓式炒药机、炒药锅等（图 1-29）。

炒药机由炒筒、炉膛、导流板、驱动装置、燃烧器、电控箱及机架等组成，物料由投料口进入，炒筒旋转使物料翻滚受热达到炒制的效果，当炒筒反向转动时，物料便自动排出炒筒外。

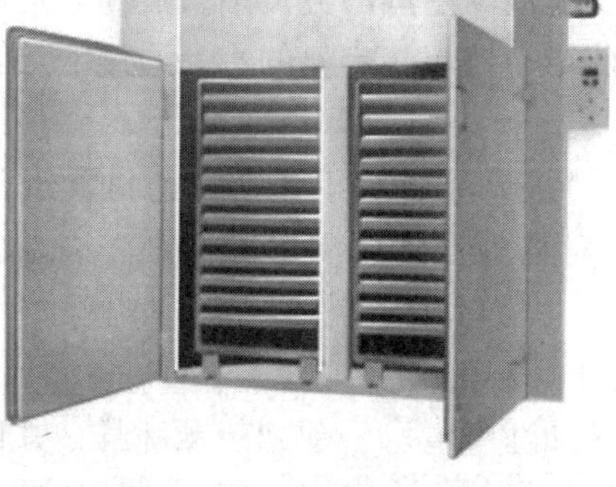

图 1-28　热风循环烘箱

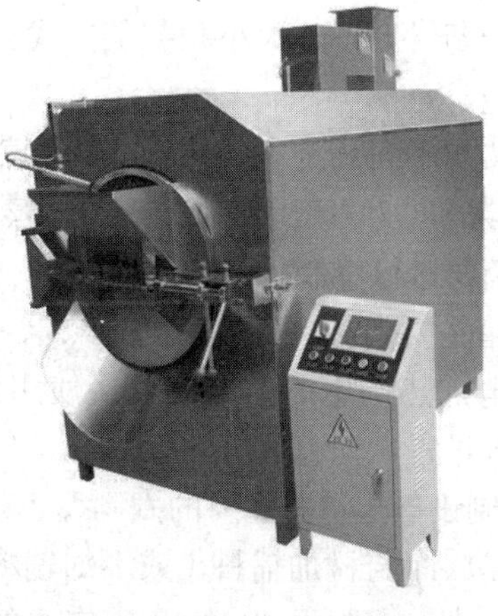

图 1-29　智能化红外控温炒药机

（五）炙制设备

炙制设备主要有炙药机与炙药锅两种（图 1-30）。

炙药机主体部分结构与炒药机相似，不同的是，热源的热能强度与炒筒转速低于炒药机，配套液体辅料喷淋装置，以便液体辅料喷淋、浸润、炒制等过程在同一设备完成，适合于醋、酒等低黏度液体辅料炙制。炙制过程先将药物置于炒筒内预热，慢速旋转，达到适宜温度时喷淋液体辅料，控制辅料用量，并保持炒筒慢速旋转，使药物浸润、闷透，然后适当提高炒筒转速，再升温炒至适当程度出料。

炙药锅锅体为半球形，锅体外侧是加热装置，适合蜂蜜等高黏度辅料炮制，也适合低黏度液体辅料炮制。操作时，先将药物置于锅体内，预热并搅拌药物，待温度适宜时喷淋辅料并搅拌，使药物浸润、拌匀、闷透，再升温炒至适当程度出料。

（六）煅制设备

根据煅药设备所能承受温度的高低分为中低温煅药锅、高温煅药炉（图 1–31）。煅药锅主要由电加热、锅体、锅盖及废气处理部分等组成。其工作原理是：由电热丝加热药锅，再由药锅加热药材，根据测温棒及温控器来控制煅制温度，同时由计时器控制煅制时间。

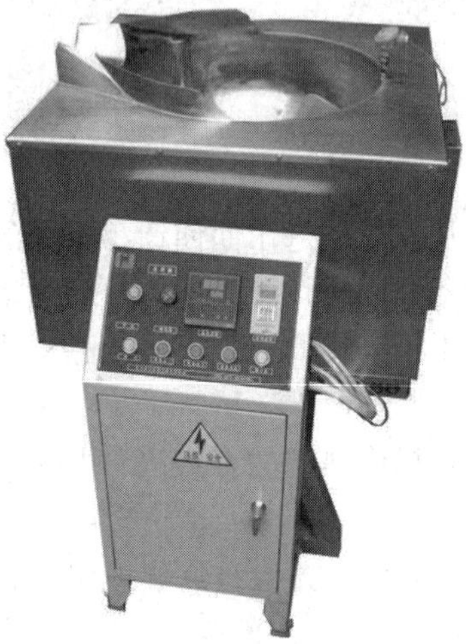

图 1–30 炙药锅

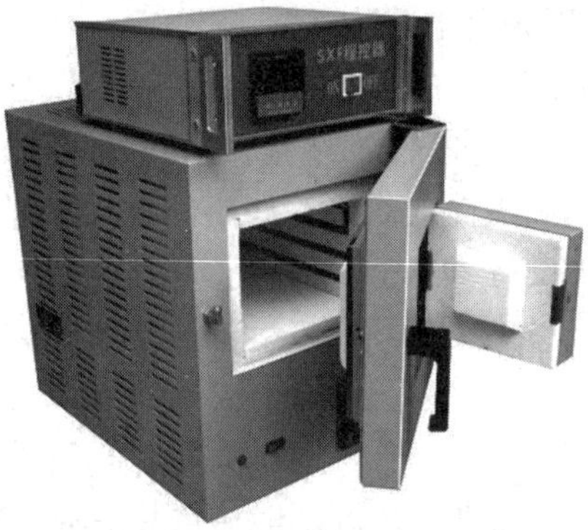

图 1–31 煅药炉

（七）蒸煮设备

1. 蒸制设备 蒸制原理为蒸汽作用于药材，由于蒸汽温度高与药材温度，蒸汽热量传递给药材，水蒸气因放热而液化成水，并被药材吸收。不断地通入蒸汽直至药材被蒸透。药材被蒸透的时间取决于药材形态、大小和装载方式，体型小、比表面积大、装载松散的药材易于蒸透，反之则不易蒸透。

根据热源不同分为电加热蒸药箱、蒸汽蒸药箱及电汽两用蒸药箱。蒸汽蒸药箱是由锅炉产生的蒸汽直接通入药箱蒸制的设备；电热蒸药箱是在药箱中放入一定量的水，通过电热管加热产生的蒸汽对药材进行蒸制的设备。

蒸药箱主要由控制系统、电加热器或蒸气管路、报警装置等组成。将药材置于密闭的箱体内，通过电加热产生的蒸气或直接使用外部的蒸汽对物料在常压下进行蒸制。进水、加热、报警、停机等过程自动完成（图 1–32）。

2. 煮制设备 目前主要的煮制设备是蒸煮锅（图 1–33）。

煮制是将净药材加辅料（或不加辅料）置锅内，加适量清水一起加热至沸腾，并保持沸腾的过程。其原理和蒸制类似，由于液态水的热容量和热传导能力大于水蒸气，故煮透的过程要快于蒸透。

（八）其他设备

除了上述用途较专一的设备外，还有很多通用的设备，如废气处理装置、干式除尘机、物料输送机、磨刀机等（图 1–34）。

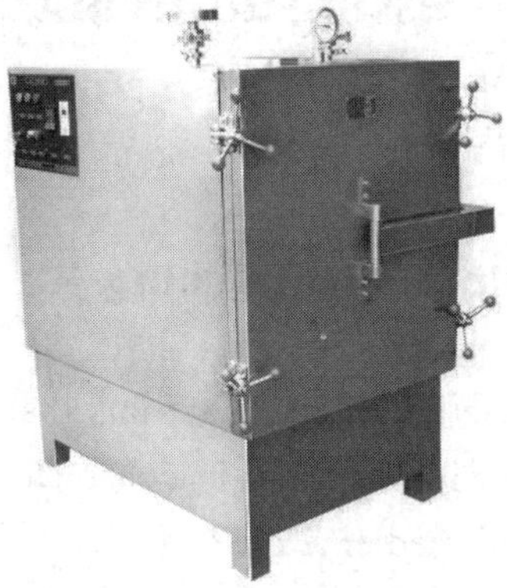

图 1-32　蒸药箱

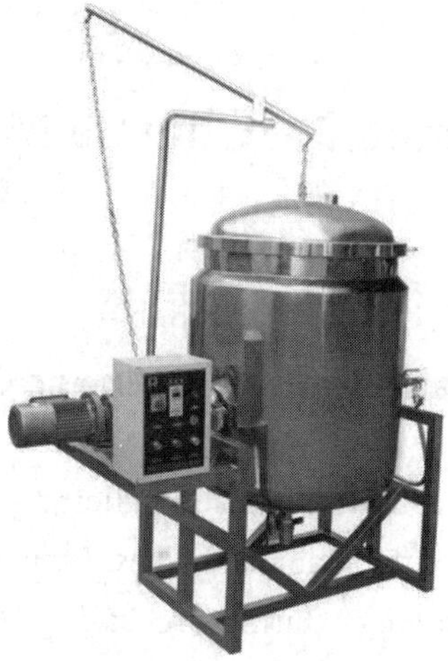

图 1-33　蒸煮锅

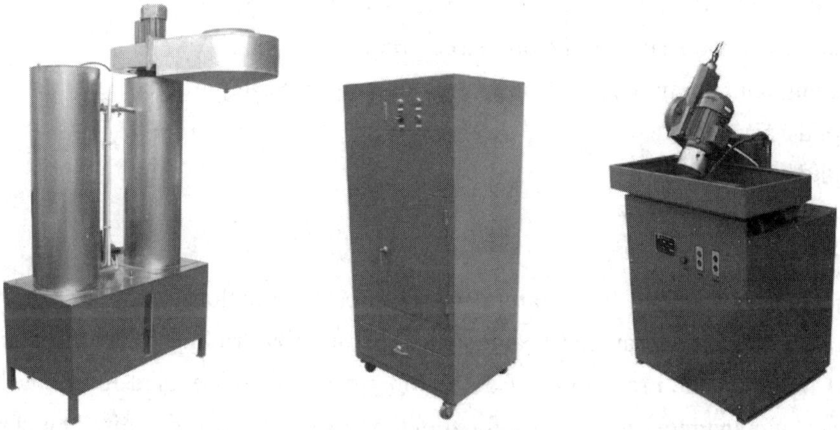

图 1-34　炮制其他设备

思考题

1. 简述炮制常用的液体辅料及其质量要求。
2. 简述传统炮制工具中磨池、木蒸甑、竹匾在药材的炮制中的用途。
3. 简述现代饮片生产中的干燥设备及其主要的工作原理。

Section 2 Chinese Medicine Processing adjuvant and Equipment

1. The adjuvant of Chinese herbal medicine processing

The adjuvants of Chinese medicine processing are the additional materials that have auxiliary functions besides the main medicines. Processing medicines with adjuvants is a characteristic of Chinese medicine processing. During processing, the adjuvant and medicine act together to reduce toxicity and synergize the effect, mitigating or changing the drug property, or modifying drug taste, etc. The intermediate heat transfer effect of the adjuvant can be used to change the texture of medicines, promote the transformation of ingredients, facilitate the dissolution and absorption of medicinal components, and maximize the therapeutic effects of decoction pieces. The quality of the adjuvants and their proper use have great influences on the quality of the processed products.

The adjuvants commonly used in Chinese medicine processing are generally divided into liquid adjuvant and solid adjuvant.

1.1 Liquid adjuvants

1.1.1 Water for processing

Drinking water

Drinking water is obtained from natural water after purification treatment. The quality of the water should reach the current national health standards for daily drinking water. This is the minimum requirement of water for the production of decoction pieces. It can be used for Chinese medicine as rinsing water, soaking and moistening water for softening treatment before cutting, the water for boiling medicine, and the cleaning water for the appliances and so on.

Purified water

It is distilled water or water prepared by ion exchange, reverse osmosis or other methods. Purified water or cold boiled water can be used as dilution water for liquid adjuvants.

The manufacturer of decoction pieces should regularly monitor the quality of production water, and the drinking water should be sent to the relevant inspection department for testing at least once a year.

1.1.2 Liquor

Unless otherwise specified, rice wine is generally used. The wine shall be produced by a qualified enterprise and have the factory quality inspection report provided by the manufacturer. The quality of rice wine should meet the requirements of rice wine (GB/T 13662-2018), which is the National Standard of the People's Republic of China. The quality of liquor should meet the requirements of Food Safety Standard of Distilled Liquors and Formulated Liquors(GB 2757-2012), which is the National Standard of the People's Republic of China.

Color

The color of rice wine should be amber light, yellow liquid or bright luster, without suspension and sediment. Liquor should be colorless, and transparent without suspension or sediment.

Odor

The smell of rice wine has a characteristic mellow slightly sweet aroma. The taste of the rice wine is mild and non-irritating, without any peculiar spicy, sour or astringent smell. The taste of liquor is mellow, without unpleasant odor or strong irritation. Upon taking several drops of liquor in the palm, rubbing several times, then sniffing the palm, there should be a pleasant fragrance not any unpleasant or bad odor.

Alcohol content

Rice wine contains 15%~20% ethanol. Liquor contains 50%~70% ethanol.

Unless otherwise specified, 10~20kg of rice wine will be used as adjuvant per 100kg of crude drugs. If necessary, it can be diluted with an appropriate amount of cold boiled water or purified water. When stewing or steaming with liquor, the amount of liquor depends on the medicinal part.

1.1.3 Vinegar

The vinegar for processing should be rice vinegar or other brewing vinegar. For this process, mature vinegar is the best. Chemical blending of vinegar is not allowed. Vinegar should be purchased from enterprises that have production qualifications and provide appropriate accompanying factory quality inspection reports. The quality should meet the requirements of the National Hygienic Standard for Vinegar of the People's Republic of China (GB 2719-2018).

Color

Take a sample, place it in a test tube and observe it with the naked eyes against a white background, the color shall be amber or brown-red.

Odor

Shake the sample in a container with a plug, smell immediately after removing the plug, the sample should have the odor of edible vinegar and acetic acid without other unpleasant odors. The taste should be sour, slightly sweet without other abnormal odor.

Character

The sample should be visualized in a tube against a white background under light. The sample should have no suspended material upon observation after the tube is plugged and shaken upside down. There should also be no suspended material in the sample after a certain period of time. If necessary, remove the supernatant after standing for 15 minutes. The sample should be free of vinegar eel, vinegar louse and vinegar fly when observed by a magnifying glass.

Physical and chemical testing

The sample should meet the requirements.

Unless otherwise specified, 20kg of vinegar will be used per 100kg of crude drugs. If necessary, it can be diluted with an appropriate amount of cold boiled water or purified water.

1.1.4 Honey

Honey for processing should be refined honey. Refined honey can be divided into under heated honey, appropriately heated honey and overheated honey. Generally, if medicines are required to be stir-baked with honey, the appropriate honey should be used. However, for medicines with special honey processing requirements, the honey should be refined in accordingly. The quality of honey should meet the requirements of honey in the 2020 edition of the Chinese Pharmacopoeia.

Character

Honey is a translucent, lustrous thick liquid. The color may vary from white to light yellow or orange to russet. When it is stored for a long time or cold, it will have white granular crystallization precipitation. It is also fragrant and very sweet.

Relative density

Measured by Wechsler's specific gravity method, the relative density is above 1.349.

Acidity inspection

Subject to regulations.

Starch and dextrin inspection

Subject to regulations.

5-hydroxymethyl inspection

Subject to regulations.

Reducing sugar

According to the alkaline tartrate ketone test method, the percentage of reducing sugar shall not be less than 60%.

Use refined honey for the stir-baking. Unless otherwise specified, 25kg of refined honey will be used per 100kg of crude drugs. Refined honey will be diluted with an appropriate quantity of cold boiled water before stir-baking.

1.1.5 Salt-water

The traditional processing salt is raw salt (crude salt, large grain salt), which contains complex components, such as sodium chloride, magnesium chloride, potassium chloride, calcium chloride, calcium sulfate, magnesium sulfate, sodium sulfate and so on. Refined salt is used in processing nowadays which mainly contains sodium chloride, but also contains a small amount of magnesium chloride, magnesium sulfate, calcium sulfate and so on. The quality should meet the requirements of the National Hygienic Standard for Edible Salt of the People's Republic of China (GB 2721-2015).

To prepare salt-water, salt is dissolved in an appropriate quantity of water and filtered (the refined salt can be directly dissolved before use). Unless otherwise specified, use 2kg of salt per 100kg of crude drugs.

1.1.6 Ginger juice

There are two types of gingers, i.e., fresh ginger and dried ginger, used in the preparation for ginger juice. Generally fresh ginger is preferred. Ginger should meet the food standards, and it should not be moldy, rotten or have other abnormal characteristics.

There are two ways to prepare ginger juice. First, crush fresh clean ginger in a container, add a quantity of water and squeeze to obtain the juice. Add a quantity of water to the ginger residue and squeeze again. Combine the juice for use. Second, cut or mash fresh ginger or dried ginger, add water and boil twice, combine the decoction and filter, take an appropriate concentration of filtrate for backup. Ginger juice can be diluted with purified water or cold boiled water. Unless otherwise specified, 10kg of fresh ginger or 3kg of dried ginger will be used per 100kg of crude drugs.

1.1.7 Bile

Bile refers to the fresh bile of animals. Bile comes from pigs, cows and sheep. Cows' bile is the best. Bile is a greenish-brown, slightly transparent liquid with a low viscosity. It has a characteristic fishy smell.

Both fresh bile and gallbladder paste powder can be used for Chinese medicine processing. 1g of gallbladder paste powder is equivalent to 10g of fresh bile. Dilute the gallbladder paste powder with purified water or cold boiled water before use.

1.1.8 Lamb sebum fat

Lamb sebum fat is refined from the fat of sheep and goats at low temperatures. The main components of sebum are fat with saponification values at 192~195, saturated and unsaturated fatty acids.

Sebum fat needs to be extracted before use, from the belly fat of sheep, which is cut into pieces and liquefied by heat. After melting, the fat residues are removed by filtering to obtain the fat. Sebum fat becomes a milky white solid upon cooling and melts into a liquid form upon overheating. Drugs stir-baked with sebum fat can enhance yang function and ameliorate tonic deficiency, and Folium Epimedii (Yinyanghuo) is a common TCM stir-baked with sebum fat.

1.1.9 Sesame oil

Sesame oil is extracted from sesame seeds by pressing. Its quality standards are specified in the Sesame oil section of 2020 edition of the Chinese Pharmacopoeia as the following.

Character

Character is a light yellow or brownish yellow clear liquid with the unique aroma of sesame oil and has a light taste.

Relative density and refractive index

Sesame oil has a relative density of 0.917~0.923, and a refractive index of 1.471~1.475.

Inspection and validation criteria

Sesame oil has a pH value of no more than 2.5 and a saponification value of 188~195. It also has an iodine value between 103~116. Heating experiment is taken out as following. Take 50ml of this product and heat up. Precipitation is not anticipated. The percentage of impurities must not exceed 0.2%. The percentage of water and volatile matter shall not exceed 0.2%.

Sesame oil is mainly used for frying and preparing crispy drugs, such as Semen Strychni (Maqianzi), Radix et rhizoma Noto ginseng (Sanqi) and Gecko (Gejie).

1.1.10 Rice-washed water

Rice-washed water is normally prepared and filtered after rice is washed for a second time and appears as a gray-white turbid liquid. It is a suspension of starch and water containing a small amount of vitamins. If clean rice is chosen with the impurities pre-eliminated, the first rice-wash water can be used. As the rice-washed water is prone to rancid fermentation, rice-washed water shall be freshly collected just before use. Alternatively, 2kg of rice flour may be added to 100kg of water as a replacement for rice-washed water.

Rice-washed water can help in the adsorption of oil and fat, and is used to process drugs such as Atractylodis rhizoma and Atractylodis macrocephalae rhizoma, so as to reduce their oil content.

1.1.11 Other medicine juice

The liquid adjuvant of medicine juice shall be prepared by conventional decocting method. According to different adjuvant, light decocting, heavy decocting or general decocting method may be used appropriately. The juice is decocted twice, combined and filtered with four layers of gauze.

Fructus evodiae (Wuzhuyu) juice

It is the decocting juice of Fructus evodiae (Wuzhuyu) mainly used for processing Rhizoma coptidis (Huanglian) and so on.

Black soybean juice

Black soybean juice is prepared by boiling black soybeans in an appropriate amount of water to produce a dark cloudy juice after the removal of dregs. It is mainly used for processing Radix polygoni multiflori (Heshouwu) .

Licorice juice

Licorice juice is prepared by boiling licorice in appropriate amount of water to produce a brown or dark-brown liquid after the removal of dregs. Combine the liquid from two preparations for use. It is mainly used for processing drugs such as Radix polygalae (Yuanzhi) , Rhizoma pinelliae (Banxia) and Fructus evodiae (Wuzhuyu) .

Radish juice

It is a light yellow decoction extracted from fresh radish, and which is commonly used to purify Natrii Sulfas（Mangxiao）.

1.2 Solid Adjuvant Materials

1.2.1 Rice

Rice is the kernel of paddy rice. It mainly contains starch, protein, fat and minerals, with a small amount of B vitamins, a variety of inorganic salt and sugar. Rice or glutinous rice is often used for TCM processing. It shall meet the edible standards, with no mildew or silt.

1.2.2 Bran

Bran is the yellow-brown wheat coat of the Gramineae plants. It contains starch, protein, vitamins and so on. The bran used for TCM processing shall have no odor, mildew, or sediment. Co-processing drug with bran can alleviate the irritation of the drug, reduce its dryness or coldness and enhance digestion. It also has the effects of neutralize bad odor, taste and coloring. Bran can also absorb oil and fats and be used for stir-baking and roasting.

1.2.3 Alum

Alum is made from the sulphate mineral alum after refinement. It is an irregular crystal, colorless or pale yellow-white, transparent or translucent, with glass-like luster, hard and brittle, slightly sweet and astringent with a light smell. It is soluble in water and glycerin but not in ethanol. Its aqueous solution shows various reactions of aluminum salt, potassium salt and sulfate salt. Its main ingredient is aluminum potassium sulfate with crystalline water molecules.

Alum is extracted from ettringite and can be directly used in TCM processing.

1.2.4 Bean curd

Bean curd is milky white solid vegetable protein from soybean seeds of leguminous plants and obtained by mechanical grinding and salt precipitation. It mainly contains protein, vitamin and starch. Generally, fresh edible bean curd is chosen as the processing adjuvant. Co-processing of drug and bean curd can reduce drug toxicity and remove dirt. Bean curd is often used to process drugs like Garcinia Morella Desv（Tenghuang）, Margarita（Zhenzhu）, Sulfur（Liuhuang）and so on.

1.2.5 Soil

The soil mostly used in TCM processing refers to the soil from the heart of a classical Chinese kitchen stove, loess, red halloysite etc. Kitchen stove soil, which is also known as Fulonggan, is smoky scorched earth and has a dark brown, brownish-yellow or brick-red color. Its main components are silicate, calcium salts and many alkaline oxides. Kitchen stove soil is primarily obtained during the renovation of an old-fashion kitchen, when the old-fashion cooker, stove and brick kiln are removed. Any dust on the old-fashion kitchen stove soil must be removed. The stove soil should be crushed, ground and set aside. The loess is heated on a strong fire and stir-fried in the pot to remove substances such as water, organic matters, microorganisms etc for use. Red halloysite is silicate mineral polyhydrate kaolinite, which mainly contains aluminum silicate tetrahydrate. It must be broken and ground into fine powder before use.

1.2.6 Clam powder

Clam powder is a grayish-white powder made from the shells of Meretrixmeretrix Linnaeus（Wenge）and Cyclina sinensis Gmelin（Qingge）etc. Its main component is calcium oxide. For example, shells are crushed and sifted to make a fine powder, and used for processing donkey-hide gelatin（E'jiao）.

1.2.7 Talcum powder

Talcum is a kind of silicate mineral talcium powder which is obtained after being carefully selected, washed, and pulverized into a fine powder. Talcum is white or white-like, has a waxy luster, is soft and delicate, feels smooth on the hand and is almost odorless. Its main component is hydrous magnesium silicate. It is generally used as an intermediate heat transfer agent to stir-bake the drug so that the drug is evenly heated. It is used for stir-baking and roasting.

1.2.8 River sand

The river sands of medium size are sifted, cleaned up to remove the soil and all impurities, and dried in the sun. The river sands must be stir-fried in strong fire to remove organic impurities and microorganisms, with 1%~2% of edible vegetable oil, until smoke has dispersed and the color has deepened. It is commonly used to stir-bake the drugs such as sand-fried Semen Strychni (Maqianzi) , sand-fried Corneum Endothelium Gigerii (Jineijin) , etc.

1.2.9 Cinnabar

Cinnabar is produced by scouring cinnabar ore and then washing away impurities and sediment. The main component is mercury sulfide, which often contains elemental mercury. The cinnabar must be levigated into fine powder, which is commonly grinded by ball mill.

2. The tools and equipment for the processing of Traditional Chinese Medicine

Traditional Chinese Medicine processing utilizes unique pharmaceutical technologies that have a long history. Chinese pharmaceutical practitioners have designed and manufactured a large number of tools and equipments suitable for processing. During the handicraft workshop period, these traditional tools and equipment played an important role in ensuring the quality of decoction pieces. Some of them are still in use today, especially in pharmacy for processing prescriptions in small quantity.

2.1 Milling tools and cutting tools

2.1.1 Mortar

The mortar is a tool for grinding medicine manually, which can be used for making fine powder and also for water grinding and emulsification processing together with mallets. Most of them are made of coarse porcelain, also some are made of stone, jade, agate, etc. The sizes of the mortars vary. The large ones may have a diameter of 50cm and a depth of about 17cm. They are usually equipped with a mortar stand. The common mortars have a diameter of 27cm with a depth of 10cm, or a diameter of 23cm with a depth of 10cm. The medium size is 18cm in diameter with a depth of 6.7cm. The small size ones are 15cm in diameter with 4.3cm in depth, or 10cm in diameter with 3.3cm in depth. The picture of a mortar is shown in figure 1-1.

2.1.2 Flush mortar (commonly known as copper flush mortar, copper medicine flush, copper flush, copper pestle)

The copper flush mortar consists of a bowl and a mallet. The flush is a copper cylinder with a height of 23~26cm and a diameter of 10~14cm. It has a cover with a round hole on the top. The copper pestle can pass through it to prevent the medicine from splashing out. It is suitable for formula or a small quantity of pestle medicine. Flush mortars made from wrought copper rather than raw copper which may break. The picture of a flush mortar is shown in figure 1-2.

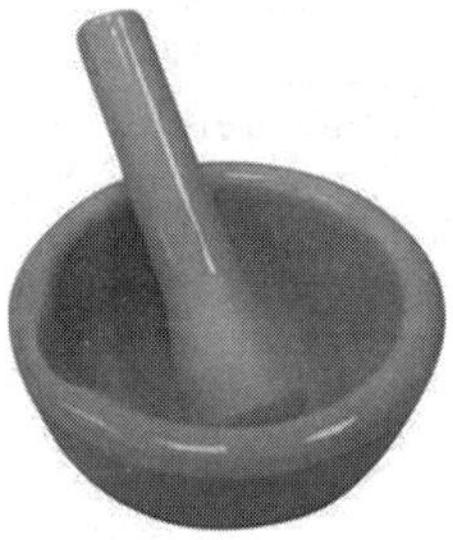

Figure 1-1 Mortar

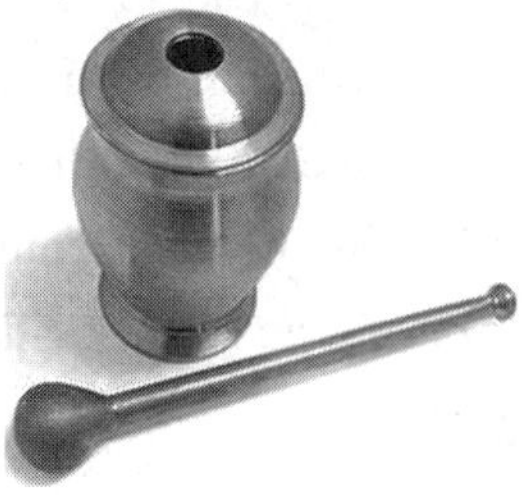

Figure 1-2 Flush mortar

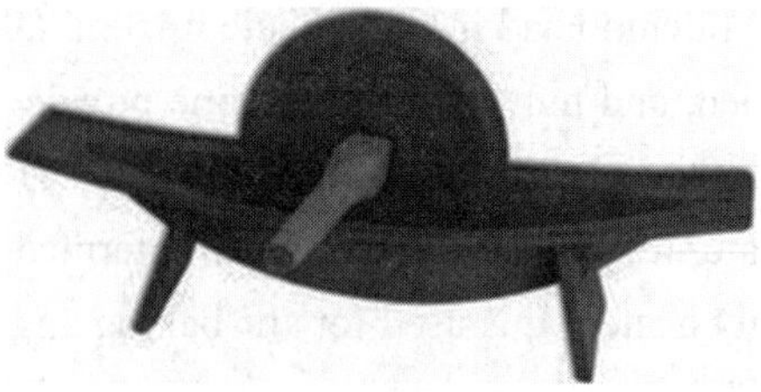

Figure 1-3 Iron ship mill

2.1.3 Iron boat mill (iron grooves, iron ship, grinding tank)

Most of the iron ship mills are cast with raw iron. They are divided into the grinding groove and the grinding disc. The boat-shaped grinding groove can be large or small. It is generally easier to operate with a length of 1m and a width of about 20cm in the middle. Grinding discs have the functions of cutting, rolling compacting and grinding. The iron boat mill occupies a small area, can be operated by one person, and has a fine crushing degree. It is a traditional tool for pulverizing drugs based on manpower. It is very practical for small workshop production. The picture of an iron boat mill is shown in figures 1-3.

2.1.4 Stone mill, stone roller

A stone mill is a tool for pulverizing medicine, which can also be used to remove nut shells or wood hearts. Electric stone mills are often used nowadays to grind the medicine. The picture of a stone mill is shown in figure 1-4.

2.1.5 Stone mortar

Stone mortars are chiseled with large rough stones. Its shape can be square or round with a round pit in the middle. The large stone mortars are often pedal-operated. A stone mallet (pestle) is attached to a pedal and pointed to the center of the fixed stone mortar. The device hits the drug according to the principle of leverage. Small stone mortars are often operated manually with a stone pestle suitable for crushing a small amount of medicine. The picture of a stone mortar is shown in figure 1-5.

2.1.6 Grinding well

Grinding well are chiseled from rough stone, shaped like an inkstone, with 27~34cm in length, 11~14cm in width, 6.7~10cm in depth. The bottom square is flat and the top is slightly concaved. The middle of one side has a small protruding mouth to allow the flow of processed medicinal juice. It is suitable for water-milled drugs. The picture of a grinding pool is shown in figure 1-6.

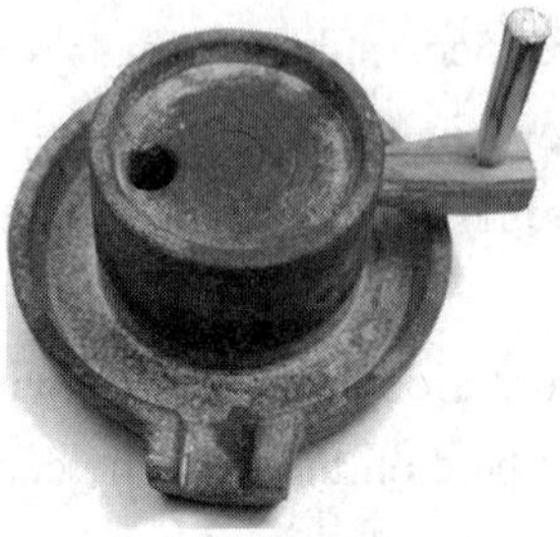

Figure 1-4 Stone mill

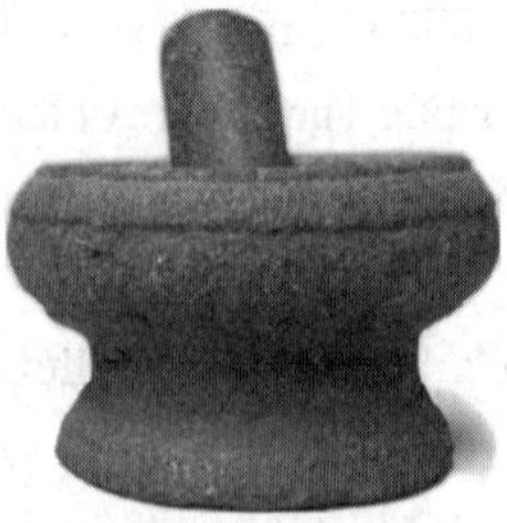

Figure 1-5 Stone mortar

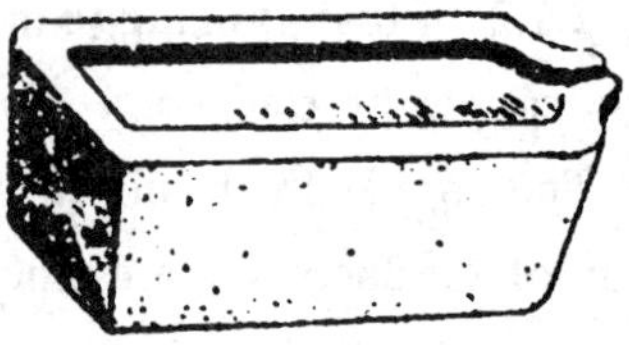

Figure 1-6 Grinding pool

2.1.7 Medicine-cutting knife

The medicine-cutting knife is divided into three parts, they are the knife body, the knife bed and the knife head. The knife body is a blade which is slightly rectangle shaped. The upper end of the blade stands upright and bends slightly forward. There is a small angle protruding at the lower end of the front (commonly known as the nose).The blade is connected with the knife head to form a guillotine. This is a main knife device for producing Yinpian. There is also a simple knife for cutting medicine. The medicine knife usually comes with multiple attachments, namely bamboo handles, knife handles, bamboo shavings, sharpening stones, etc. The picture of medicine knifes are shown in figure 1–7.

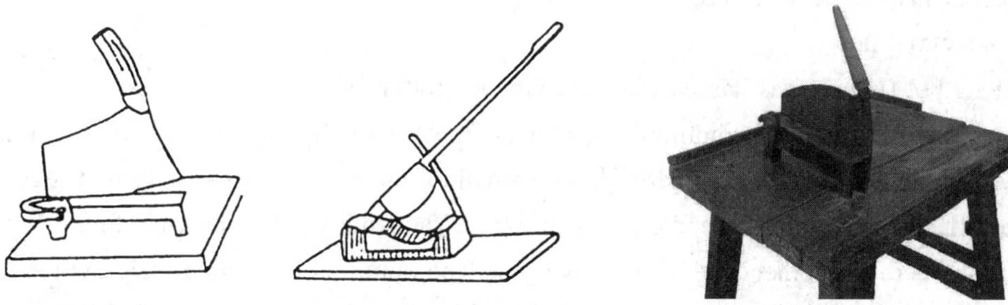

Figure 1–7 Medicine–cutting knifes

In addition, there are bamboo knives, porcelain knives and so on, which are used for the processing of peeling, removing nucleus and flesh, which are used for medicine preparations that preferably require that an iron knife not be used.

2.1.8 Crab claw foreceps (flat clamp, betel nut clamp)

Crab claw foreceps, 3~4cm in width and 16cm in length, are made of flexible thin iron, folded up and down, with a serrated bite at the front end. They are used to clamp drugs when cutting medicines, such as Arecaesemen (Binglang) , Viride Pericarpium Reticulatae Citri (Qingpi), Fructus Crataegi (Shanzha), and Rhizoma Alismatis (Zexie) and other large materials which are not easily handled by hand. A picture of Crab claw foreceps is shown in figure 1–8.

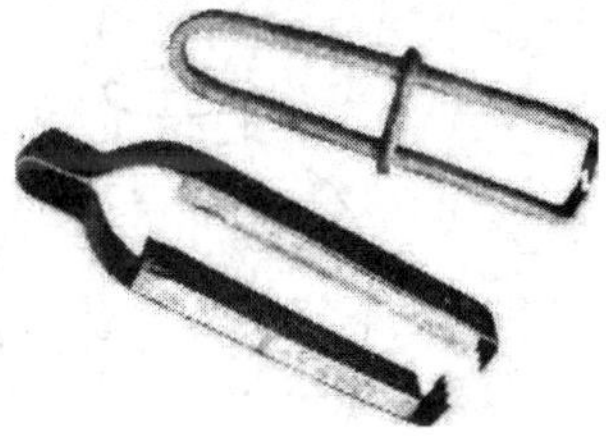

Figure 1–8 Crab claw foreceps

2.1.9 Pound knife

A Pound knife is attached to a wooden strip with a length of 50cm, a width of 6~7cm and a thickness of 3~4cm. On the strip, there are an array of approximately 20 blades (with strip width and 3~4cm height) in every 1.5cm of the strip. When the medicine is rubbed on the pound knife during use, the medicine can be sliced. It is generally used to crush animal horns or hard texture medicinal materials, such as Rhinoceros cornu (Xijiao) , Resinatum Lignum Aquilariae (Chenxiang) , etc.

2.2 Processing equipment and tools

2.2.1 Stir-frying pot, stir-frying stove

There are two kinds of common stir-fry pots. One is a pot with ears, which has a small caliber of about 50cm. It is convenient and flexible to use on a kitchen stove or blast furnace for frying or calcining a small amount of drugs and can be used on a cooking. Another is an earless flat pan with a larger caliber of 66~100cm, mostly placed on a fixed stove bench. They can be used for stir-frying, boiling, calcining, frying, steaming, braising, and baking of Chinese medicine.

There are two types of stir-frying pots, horizontally and obliquely placed. In the south of China, most of them are flat pans. Horizontally placed pots have the advantage of a large contact surface and even heating. In the north of China, inclined pots are often used, where the medicines are often piled up at the lower part of the pot. The heating may not be even, but they are more convenient for stirring/frying and the medicine is easy to collect. The energy sources for heating can be coal fire or for such as bevel stove. Nowadays, for frying small amounts of medicine, electricity, gas, liquefied gas and other heating sources are used as appropriate. The picture of a Golden Shovel and Silver Pot is shown in figure 1-9.

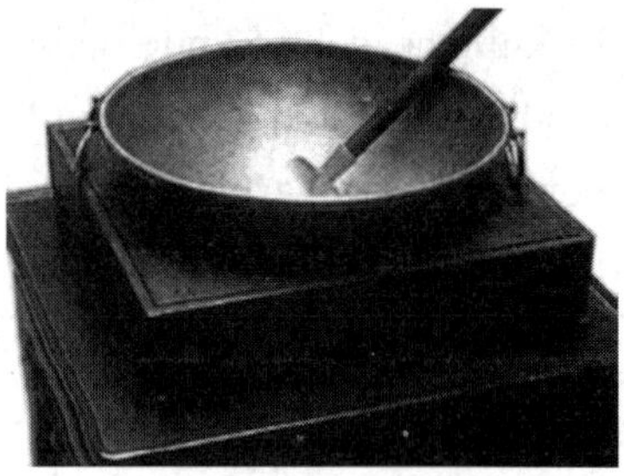

Figure 1-9 Hu Qingyutang's "Golden Shovel and Silver Pot"

The common tools for stir-frying medicine with pots are shovel, broom, medicine plaque, brush, and so on.

2.2.2 Calcined pot

Yangcheng pot (which was named after the famous pottery pot in Yangcheng, Shanxi Province), commonly known as Dulu, is a cylindrical pottery pot with the middle part expanded and the top and bottom parts slightly smaller. There are different sizes of Yangcheng pots, which can be selected according to needs. The picture of a Yangcheng pot is shown in figure 1-10.

In addition, there is another type of iron soup pot. The upper part is cylindrical, and the lower part is narrow, with the diameter of 16~34cm and the depth of 26~50cm. They are suitable for processing medicines which are easily broken when calcining. An iron hook is often prepared for calcining medicine, made of a thin round iron rod. Its front end is curved to form a double hook which is used to lift the calcining medicine from the pot or to mix the medicine. The picture of iron hook is shown in figure 1-11.

2.2.3 Wood steamer

A wood steamer has a cylindrical shape with a cover on the top and a drawer at the bottom, which is used for steaming medicine in the pot. The picture of a wood steamer is shown in figure 1-12.

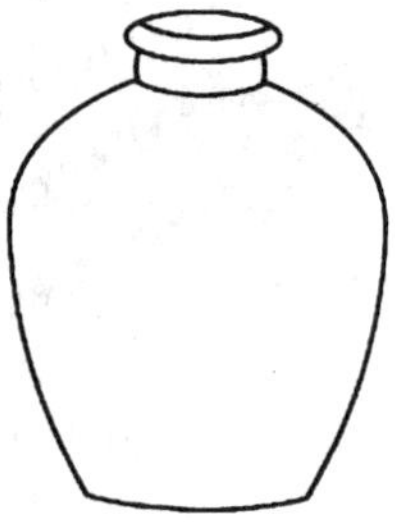

Figure 1-10 Yangcheng pot

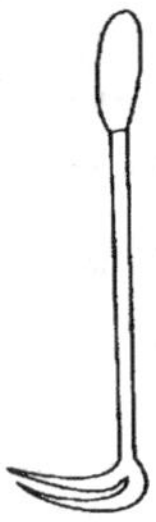

Figure 1-11 Iron hook

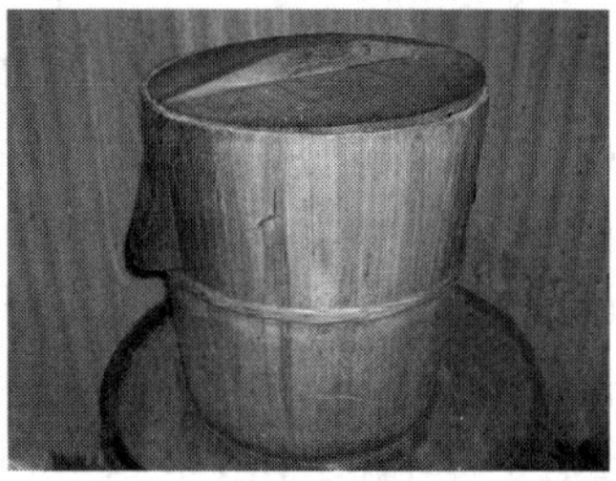

Figure 1-12 Wood steamer

2.3 Drying equipment

2.3.1 Wooden oven and wooden drying barrel

They are used for fumigating drugs to prevent mildew and insects. The picture of a wooden oven and a wooden drying barrel are shown in figure 1-13.

2.3.2 Drying bench and drying room

Both are used for drying medicinal materials and decoction pieces. Traditionally, medicines are directly placed on a brick bench, which can be heated up with charcoal for drying, especially in the rainy, wet seasons, or for medicinal materials and decoction pieces that cannot be dried in the sun. A drying room is installed with retro-shaped heat-dissipating iron pipes on the floor or wall in the entire room, and medicine can be placed on racks, so that the entire room becomes an oven to dry the medicinal materials and decoction pieces.

2.3.3 Pill rolling plaque and bamboo plaque

Both are often containers made of bamboo that can be used to hold medicines for air drying. It can also be used for coating adjuvants on drug surface and rolling medicine into pills. The picture of bamboo plaque is shown in figure 1-14.

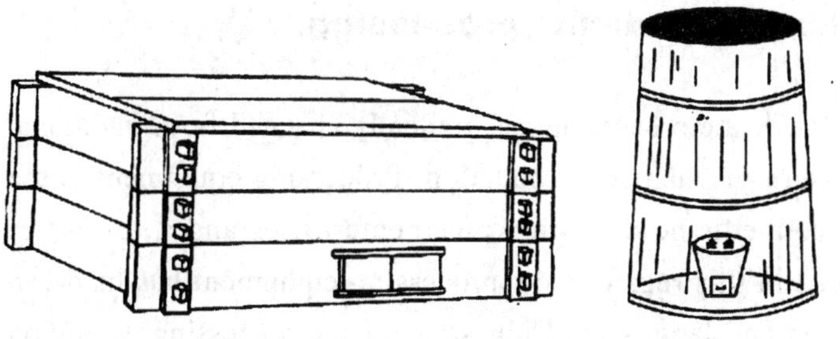

Figure 1–13 Wooden oven, wooden drying barrel

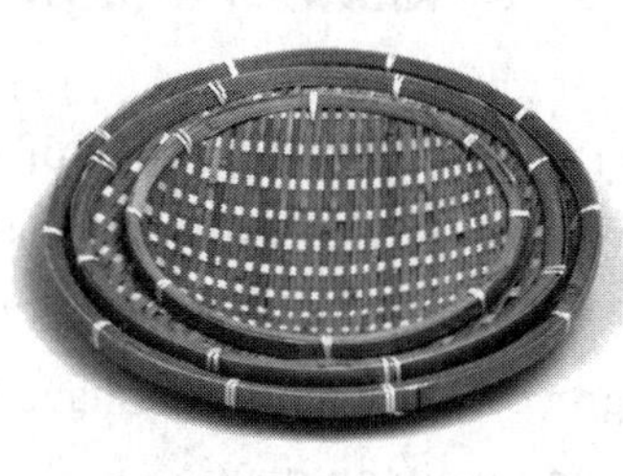

Figure 1–14 Bamboo plaque

2.4 Sifting and other tools

2.4.1 Medicine sieve

Medicine sieve is used for sorting medicines by size, or removing debris, soil/sand from medicines, and removing supplementary materials after the frying processing. There are various specifications of the medicine sieve with different hole sizes, which can be made of bamboo, horsetail hair, silk, copper and steel wire.

2.4.2 Scissors, tweezers, knife, etc.

These tools are often used to select, clean medicinal materials and remove unwanted parts.

2.4.3 Fructus anurantii pliers

The shape of the Fructus anurantii pliers is like a guillotine knife. The upper and lower parts are flat and thick iron plates. They are approximately more than 33cm long and about 7cm wide. The opposite surfaces of the two layers are obliquely engraved with vertical and horizontal cross lines. Both ends of the lower part are fixed on a wide and thick wooden base by nails. The front ends of both parts are connected through a hole. The back end of the upper plier has a wooden handle. They are generally used for crushing drugs with hard shells. A picture of a shell plier is shown in figure1–15.

2.4.4 Caulis bambusae knife

The shape of a Caulis bambusae knife is narrow and slightly curved, with two handles. The upper part is the back of the knife, and the lower part has a sharp edge. They are about 40cm long and 10cm wide and specially used for scraping Caulis bambusae.

2.4.5 Turtle scraper

The shape of the turtle scraper is a flat strip of about 5cm long with a wide front end. It bends like a hook with a thin blade. It is specially used for scraping the tortoise shell or other medicine to separate bone, skin and fascia.

2.4.6 Brake pliers

Brake pliers, also known as the guillotine shears, are shaped like a pliers.It is thick and strong, narrow and long in shape. The front end is connected to the underlying pad strip. Brake pliers are used for breaking hard drugs. The picture of brake pliers is shown in figure 1–16.

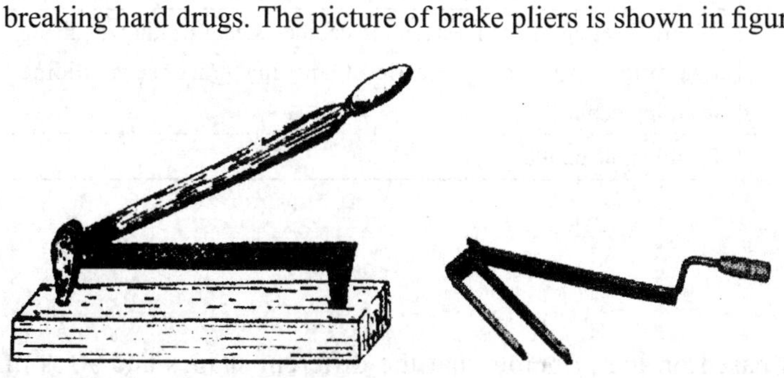

Figure 1–15 Shell pliers

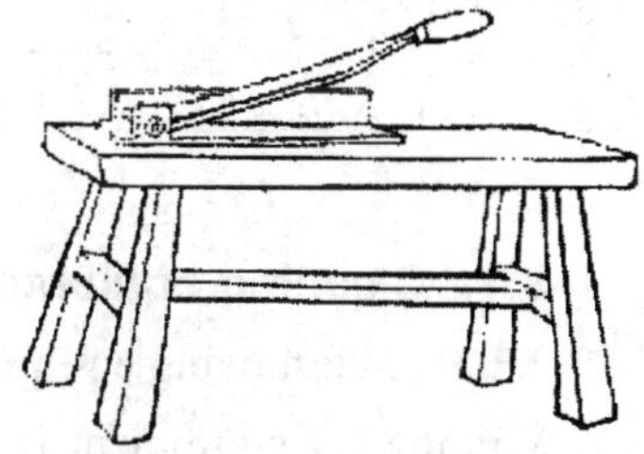

Figure 1–16 Brake pliers

3. Modern equipment for Chinese Medicine processing.

With the progression of time, Chinese medicine processing has gradually changed from traditional workshop processing to massive scale modern mechanized production. Processing equipment is the hardware foundation of traditional Chinese medicine decoction piece enterprises and a variety of processing equipments have been developed in this regard. New processing equipment has made an important contribution to the industrialization and large scale Chinese medicine processing. Common equipment for Chinese medicine processing is shown in Table 1-1.

Table 1-1 List of common equipment for Chinese medicine processing.

Processing method	the way	Common equipment
Cleaning	Winnowing	Variable frequency horizontal winnowing machine, variable frequency vertical winnowing machine, variable frequency suction winnowing machine
	Washing	Circulating water medicine washing machine, stainless steel medicine washing sink
	Sifting	Flexible support inclined plane sifting machine, motor vibration sifting machine, reciprocating vibration sifting machine
	Selection	Stainless steel picking tables and mechanized sorting units
	Magnetic separation	Belt magnetic separator and bar type magnetic separator
Cutting	Softening	Water immersion medicine moistening machine, gas phase replacement moistening machine
	Reciprocating cutting	Flexible belt reciprocating medicine cutter, metal crawler reciprocating medicine cutter
	Rotary cutting	Rotary disk type medicine cutter, rotary material slicer
Crushing	Crushing	Jaw crusher, extrusion crusher,
	Breaking	Ball mill, hammer crusher
Drying	Continuous drying	Hermetically sealed drying cabinet, open type drying cabinet and roller type drying cabinet
	Intermittent drying	Mesh belt dryer, rotary dryer
Stir-baking	Roller type	Roller type stir-baking machine, automatic temperature drum type stir-baking machine
Frying	Stir-frying	Drum type stir-frying medicine
	Stir-frying	Horizontal rotation stir-frying machine
Calcining	Medium and low temperature	Medium and low temperature calcining pot
	High temperature	Reflection type high temperature calcining furnace
Steaming and boiling	Steaming	Electric heating medicine steaming cabinet, steam heating medicine steaming cabinet and electric steam dual-purpose medicine steaming cabinet
	Boiling	Tiltable type cooking pot

3.1 Cleaning equipment

3.1.1 Winnowing equipment

Winnowing equipment is designed based on the principle that the different shapes and sizes of materials produce different degrees of displacement under the action of air flow. It is mainly used for materials with large differences in quality and body shape, especially materials with the same body shape but quite different quality. It can also classify medicinal materials, semi-finished products or pieces according to their size, or remove the debris, sediment, hair, cotton yarn and other sundries in medicinal materials, semi-finished products and pieces. It has the characteristics of large production capacity, low cost and low equipment investment and maintenance expenses. There are variable frequency horizontal winnowing machine, variable frequency vertical winnowing machine and variable frequency suction winnowing machine, etc. The winnowing equipment is mainly composed of air separation box, vibration equalizer, hoister and variable frequency speed regulating fan, etc. The adjustment range is from two to five, which can be selected according to different medicinal materials and different shape characteristics. The picture of vertical winnowing machine is shown in figure 1−17. The picture of a horizontal winnowing machine is shown in figure 1−18.

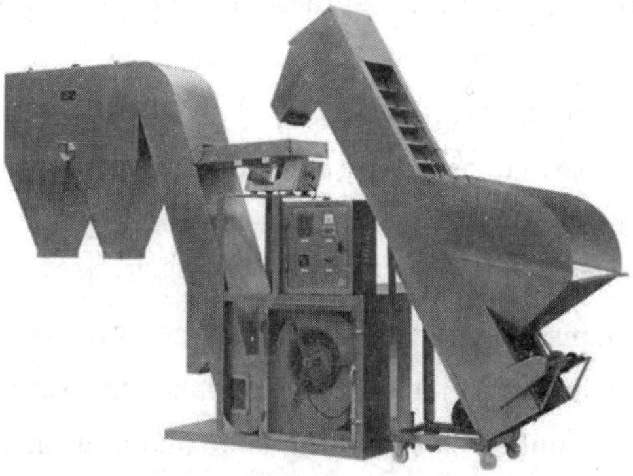

Figure 1−17 Vertical winnowing machine

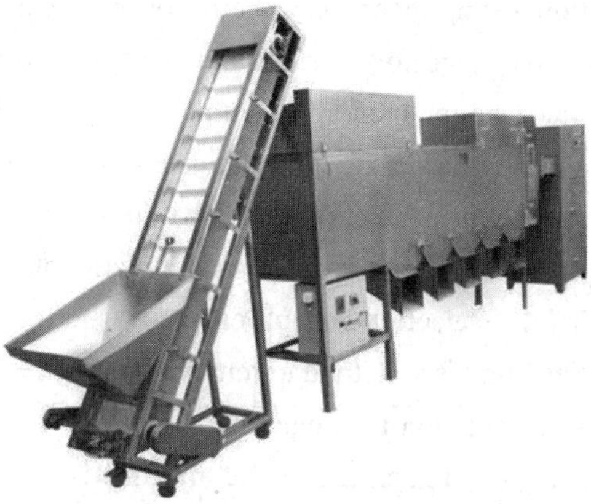

Figure 1−18 Horizontal winnowing machine

3.1.2 Washing equipment

Water washing is a process that allows for the soaking, dissolution, rolling away etc of medicinal material owing to the action of water, so that the impurities and sediment attached to the surface of the medicinal material can be separated from the surface of the medicinal materials. The main water washing equipment includes circulating water washing machines, medicine washing pools, etc. The picture of a circulating water medicine washing machine is shown in figure 1−19.

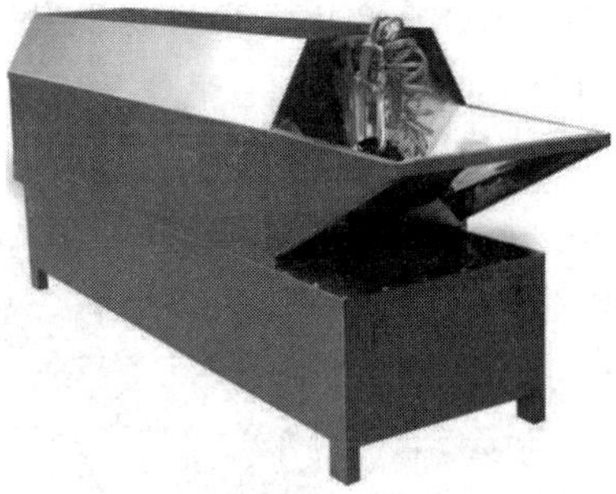

Figure 1−19 Circulating water medicine washing machine

The main part of the circulating water washing machine is a drum with many small holes on the wall surface, which is directly driven by a motor and belt. The lower part of the drum is a "V" type water tank; the water in the V-shaped water tank is pressurized by the water pump through the sediment filter and sprayed to the medicinal materials in the rotary drum through the spray pipe and nozzle. As part of the drum enters the water tank, the medicine is fully soaked, then the medicinal materials are rubbed against each other by spraying with water and rotating the drum so that the sundries attached to the surface of the medicinal materials fall off and are taken away by the water flow, so as to achieve the purpose of cleaning the medicinal materials.

The pool for washing medicine is usually made of concrete and lined with stainless steel plates. The drainage pipe at the bottom of the pool is connected with the sewer, the outlet is equipped with a drain valve, and the sewer is equipped with a sedimentation pool to avoid sediment blocking the sewer. The water inlet pipe is equipped with a flow meter and valve, which can display water consumption and control water inflowing. One side of the pool usually has a small door to facilitate the loading of medicine by a trolley. In order to improve the cleaning effect, it is necessary to manually turn and stir the herbs in the cleaning process.

3.1.3 Sifting equipment

Sifting is a process in which materials smaller than the sieve mesh are separated from other larger materials by relative movement between the materials and the sieve mesh due to the physical shape difference of the mixture of materials. Selecting the appropriate mesh size according to the shape of the material can achieve better sifting results.

According to the motion track of the sieve cloth under the driving action, machines can be divided into flexible support inclined plane sifting machines, motor vibration sifting machines and reciprocating vibration sifting machines. Their motion tracks are a plane turning motion, up and down reciprocating motion, back and forth or left and right reciprocating motion. In addition to these movements, the sieve cloth must be inclined at a certain angle to the horizontal plane to allow the material to move forward continuously. According to the number of exists for the material, there are types of 2, 3 and 4-exit machines. Sifting equipment generally consists of a frame, transmission device, bed, sieve cloth, discharge hopper, etc. The picture of a three-layer four- exit plane rotary sifting machine is shown in figure 1-20.

3.1.4 Selection equipment

Selection is a method to remove impurities from medicinal materials. The selected impurities include impurities and non medicinal parts that are intertwined or mixed in medicinal materials, etc. According to the degree of automation, the machine is divided into a stainless steel picking table and a mechanized sorting unit. The selection table surfaces are generally 1m × 2m, which are divided into three types, i.e., flat surface, concave surface and surface with hole. Compared to the stainless steel picking table, the mechanized sorting unit adds a material conveying function owing to the elevator, impurities reverse conveying function and magnetic separation function. The picture of a mechanized sorting machine is shown in figure 1-21.

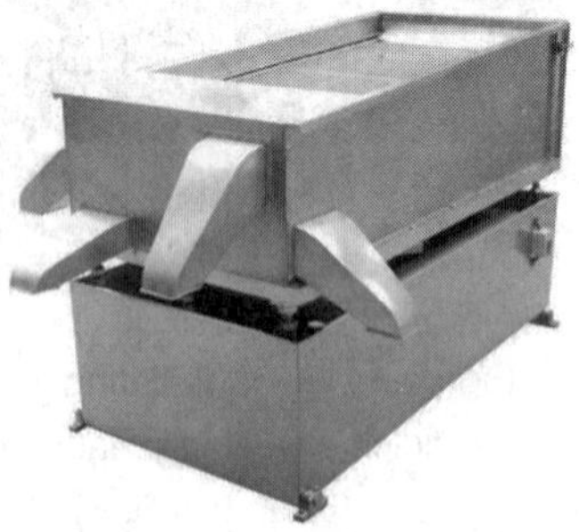

Figure 1-20 Three-layer four-exit plane rotary sifting machine

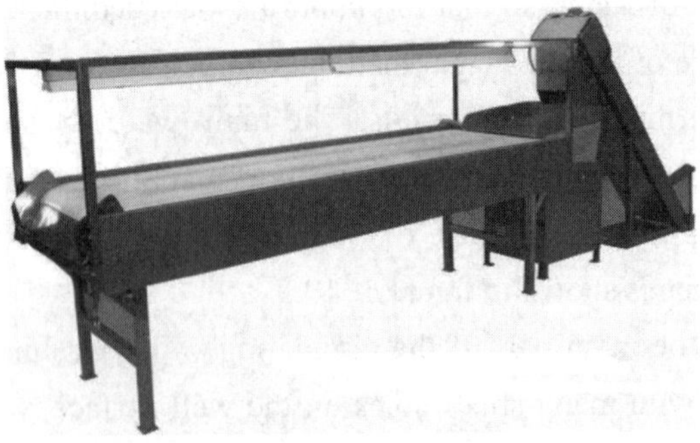

Figure 1-21 Mechanized sorting machine

3.1.5 Magnetic separation equipment

Magnetic separation is a method that uses strong magnetic materials to adsorb and separate iron impurities mixed in the medicinal materials. The purpose of magnetic separation is to clean materials and decoction pieces, and to avoid damaging subsequent cutting, crushing and other processing machines.

The magnetic separation equipment mainly includes belt magnetic separator and bar type magnetic separator. Its main components are a magnetic rod and a vibration equalizer. The pictures of the two types of separators are shown in figure 1–22 and 1–23.

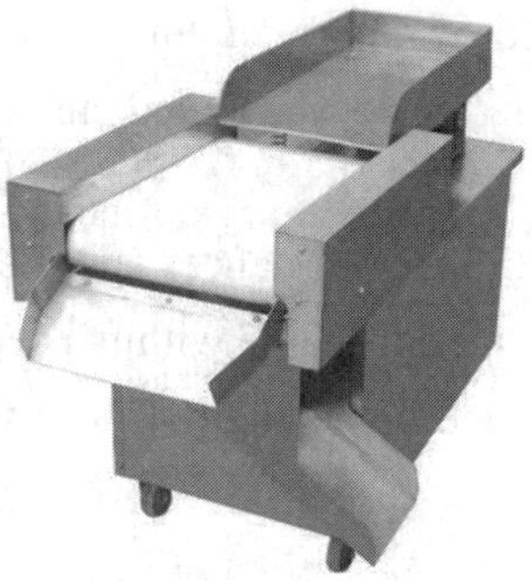

Figure 1–22 Belt magnetic separator

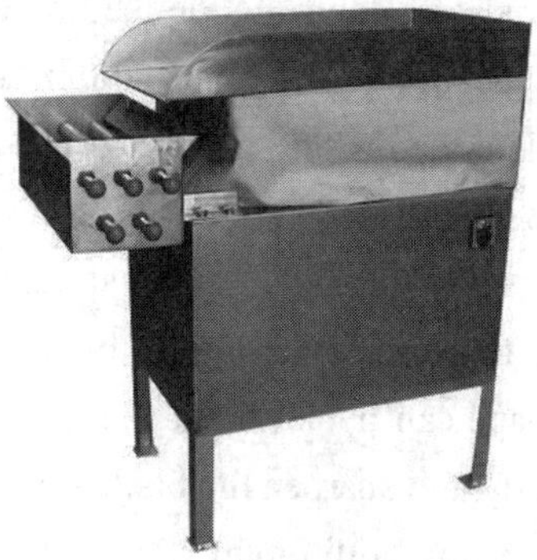

Figure 1–23 Bar type magnetic separator

3.2 Cutting equipment

3.2.1 Softening equipment

Except for a few drugs, which can be prepared from fresh or dry forms, most of the dried crude drugs must be softened before cutting to make them absorb a certain amount of water and achieve a soft and moderate texture to facilitate further slicing.

Modern commonly used infiltration and softening machines include water immersion medicine moistening machines, gas phase replacement medicines moistening machines, etc. Comparatively speaking, the latter is more advanced. Its working principle is to extract the gas in the tissue gap of medicinal material by vacuum decompression, creating a negative pressure state. Then, the water vapor is introduced into the tank so that it quickly and evenly enters the tissue of the medicinal material, to improve the softening effect. Medicinal materials which are difficult to soften can be softened many times. The gas phase replacement medicine moistening machine is composed of a square cabinet, air pump and inflatable sealing gear, vacuum pump and control system, various solenoid valves, alarm devices, etc. The picture of a chilled water storage vacuum gas phase replacement type medicine moisturizing machine is shown in figure 1–24.

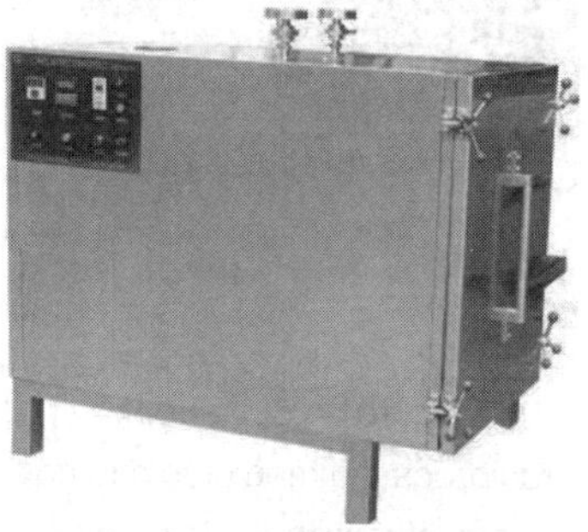

Figure1–24 Chilled water storage vacuum gas phase replacement type medicine moisturizing machine

3.2.2 Cutting equipment

The hardness of the cutting tool is much higher than that of the medicinal material. The tool contacts the medicinal material and exerts pressure, and the blade enters the medicinal material and cuts it. The basic condition of cutting is such that the blade contacts with the medicinal materials and generates relative movement.

There are many kinds of modern medicine cutting machines. According to the relative movement mode of the cutting tools and the materials, cutting machines are divided into vertical reciprocating and rotary cutting equipment. The up and down reciprocating cutting equipment includes a flexible belt reciprocating medicine cutter, a metal crawler reciprocating medicine cutter, etc. The rotary cutting equipment includes a rotary disk type medicine cutter, a rotary material slicer, etc. There are other multifunctional cutting machines, chippers, etc.

Working principle of reciprocating cutter: The raw materials are intermittently fed through a conveyor belt, and the blades make synchronous up and down reciprocating movements to cut off the medicinal materials, by adjusting the feeding gear, the medicine can be evenly cut into different thickness and length specifications. The rotary cutter is mainly composed of a rack, motor, blade, hopper, rotary table, slice thickness adjusting gear, etc. The picture of a linear reciprocating medicine cutting machine with a flexible belt is shown in figure 1-25.

The medicinal materials to be cut should not be mixed with hard substances such as iron wire, iron blocks or stones to avoid damaging the blade. The slice thickness is adjustable within a certain range. The optimal slice shape can be cut by adjusting the blade thickness and blade angle. Check the sharpness of the blade regularly and sharpen the blade regularly.

3.2.3 Crushing equipment

Crushing is the process of breaking medicinal materials to a certain shape, size and specification. At present, the main crushers in the market include jaw crusher, extrusion crusher, ball mill, hammer crusher, etc. The picture of a jaw crusher is shown in figure 1-26. The extrusion crusher is shown in figure 1-27. The latter two belong to fine crushing machines, which can crush smaller and finer granular drugs. The principle of crushing is to overcome the force between drug molecules through impact or extrusion, so as to achieve the effect of broken and crushing.

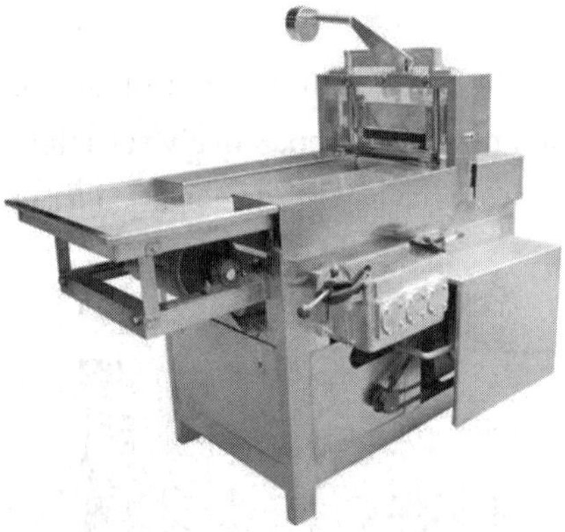

Figure1-25 Linear reciprocating medicine cutting machine with flexible belt

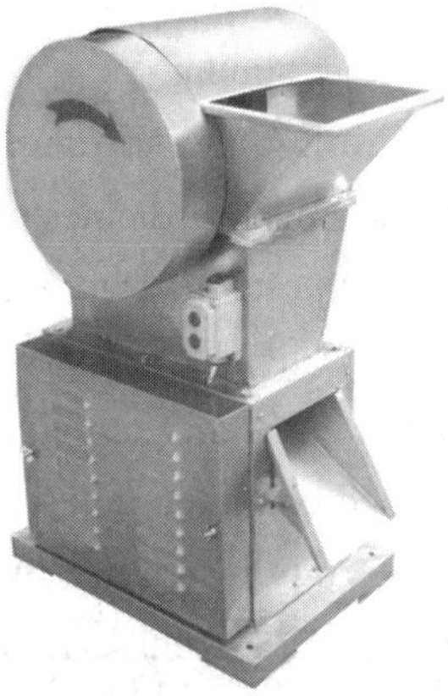

Figure 1-26 Jaw crusher

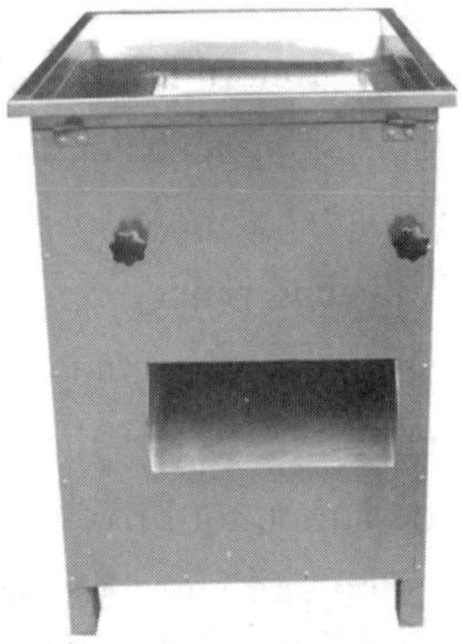

Figure 1-27 Extrusion crusher

3.3 Drying equipment

The drying principle is a process in which heat energy is applied to the water-containing decoction slices so that the water partially or complete escapes from the slices to dry them. Drying equipment can be divided into continuous drying equipment and intermittent drying equipment. Hermetically sealed drying cabinets, open type drying cabinets and roller type drying cabinets belong to intermittent drying equipment. Mesh belt dryers, rotary dryers and turning type dryers belong to continuous drying equipment. The picture of a hot air circulation oven is shown in figure 1-28.

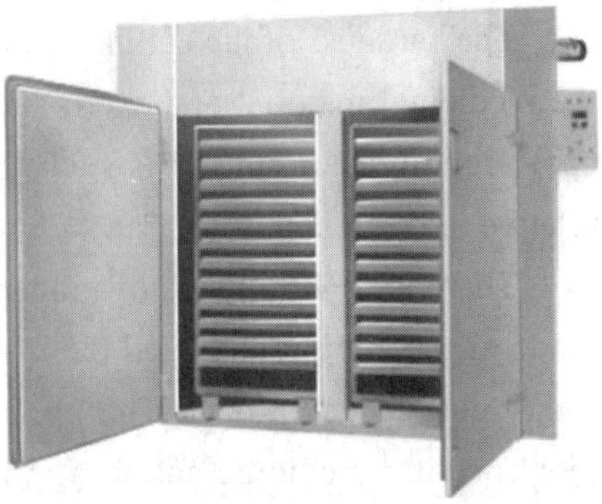

Figure 1-28 Hot air circulation oven

The drying equipment is mainly composed of a heat generator, drying cabinet, etc. There are several heat sources, such as steam, electric heat, oil and far infrared ray to provide heat for medicinal materials.

During the drying process, it is important to note that the temperature of the heat source should not be too high, otherwise the slices will be burnt or there may be a loss material or changes to the active ingredients. In addition, heat sources should not contaminate or react to the slices.

3.4 Stir-baking equipment

Commonly used stir-baking equipment includes roller type stir-baking machines, automatic temperature control drum type stir-baking machines, stir-baking pots, etc. The picture of an intelligent infrared temperature control stir-baking machine is shown in figure 1-29.

The stir-baking machine is composed of a stir-baking cylinder, a furnace, a flow guide plate, a driving device, a burner, an electric control cabinet, a rack, etc. The medicines are fed into the machine via the feeding inlet, and the stir-frying cylinder rotates so that the medicine rolls and get heated to achieve the effect of stir-baking. When the stir-frying cylinder rotates in reverse, the medicine is discharged automatically from the stir-frying cylinder.

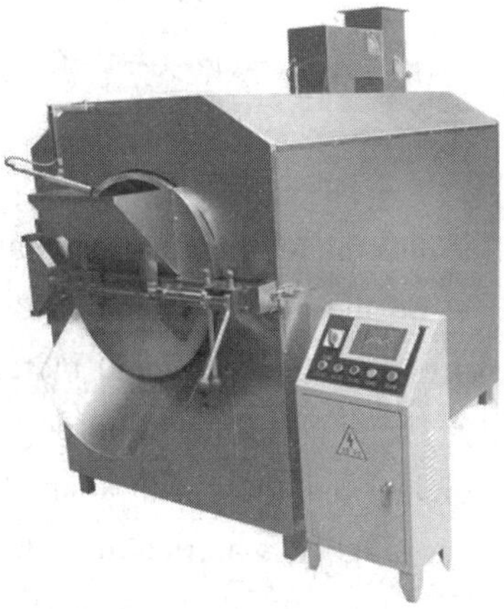

Figure 1-29 Intelligent infrared temperature control stir-baking medicine

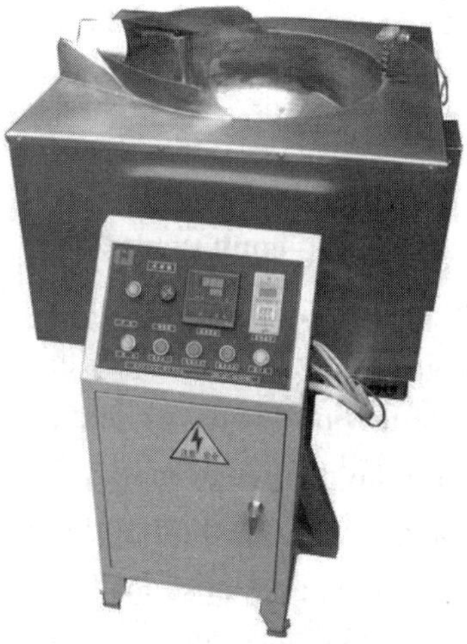

Figure 1-30 Frying pot

3.5 Frying equipment

There are mainly two kinds of frying equipment, medicine frying machines and medicine frying pots. The picture of a frying pot is shown in figure 1-30.

The structure of the main part of the medicine frying machine is similar to that of the stir-baking machine, except that the intensity of the heat source and the speed of the frying cylinder are lower than those of the stir-baking machine. It is equipped with a spray device for liquid adjuvants, so that the process of liquid adjuvant spraying, moistening and frying can be completed in the same equipment. It is suitable for processing with vinegar, rice wine and other low-viscosity liquid adjuvants. In the liquid adjuvant-frying process, the medicine is preheated by rotating slowly in the frying pot. When appropriate temperatures are reached, certain amounts of liquid adjuvant will be sprayed on to the medicine. The frying pot is kept rotating slowly to get the medicine infiltrated and moistened thoroughly. The speed of the frying pot is increased accordingly, and then the temperature is raised to fry the medicine to an appropriate degree.

The main body of a medicine frying pot is hemispherical, the outside of the pot body is the heating device, which is suitable for processing with honey and other high-viscosity adjuvants, and also suitable for processing with low-viscosity liquid adjuvants. When operating, medicine is preheated and stirred in the pot. When appropriate temperatures are reached, the adjuvant will be sprayed on to the medicine and stirred to make the medicine infiltrated, well mixed and moistened thoroughly. The temperature is then raised to fry the medicine to an appropriate degree.

3.6 Calcining equipment

According to the temperature, calcining equipment can be divided into medium and low temperature calcining pots and high temperature calcining furnaces. The picture of calciner is shown in figure 1-31. A calcining pot is mainly composed of an electric heater, pot body, pot cover and an exhaust gas treatment section. The working principle is that the pot is heated by an electric heating wire, and then the medicine is heated in the hot pot. The calcination temperature is controlled by a temperature measuring rod and temperature controller, while the calcination time is controlled by the timer.

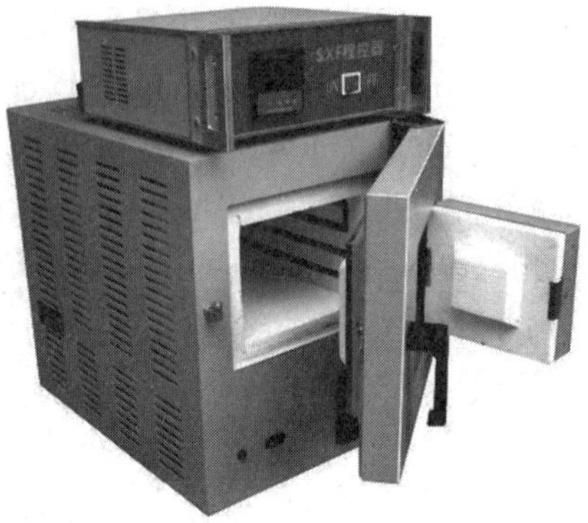

Figure 1-31 Calciner

3.7 Boiling and steaming equipment

3.7.1 Steaming equipment

During steaming, steam acts on the medicinal materials. Because the temperature of steam is higher than that of the medicinal material, the steam heat is transferred to the medicinal material. The water vapor is liquefied into water by releasing the heat, and is absorbed by the medicinal materials. Keep steaming until the medicinal materials are steamed thoroughly. The time of steaming depends on the shape, size and loading method of the medicinal materials. Medicinal materials with a small size, large specific surface area and loose loading are steamed easily and thoroughly, materials that do not fit this description are often more difficult to steam.

Depending on the different heat sources, steaming cabinets are divided into electric heating, steam heating and electric steam dual-purpose medicine steaming cabinets. A steam heating medicine steaming cabinet is a device in which steam generated by the boiler goes directly through the cabinet. The electric heating medicine steaming cabinet is a device that can generate steam through the vaporization of water in the cabinet via electric heat pipes.

Medicine steaming cabinets mainly consists of a control system, a electric heater or a steam pipeline, an alarm device, etc. Medicinal materials are placed in a sealed cabinet, and then steamed under atmospheric pressure directly with external steam or steam generated by the electric heating. The processes of water inflowing, heating, alarm and termination are completed automatically. The picture of a medicine steaming cabinet is shown in figure 1-32.

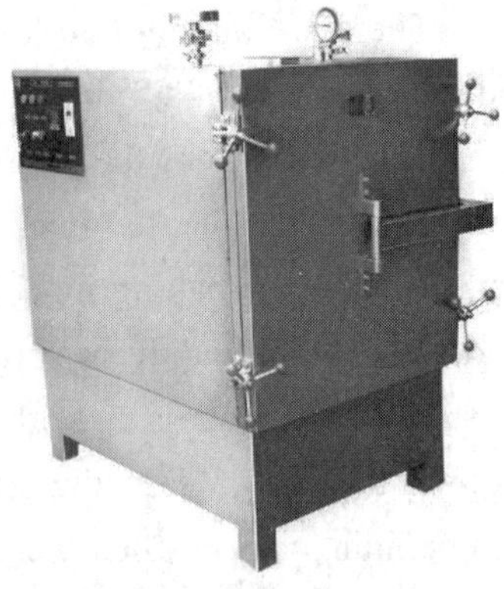

Figure 1-32 Medicinal material steaming cabinet

3.7.2 Boiling equipment

At present, the main boiling equipment is a boiling pot. The picture of boiling pot is shown in figure 1-33.

Boiling is the process of adding raw medicinal materials with or without adjuvants in a pot, adding an appropriate amount of water and heating to boil, and maintaining the boiling process. The principle is similar to that of steaming. Because the heat capacity and heat conduction capacity of liquid water are greater than those of water vapor, boiling is faster than steaming thoroughly.

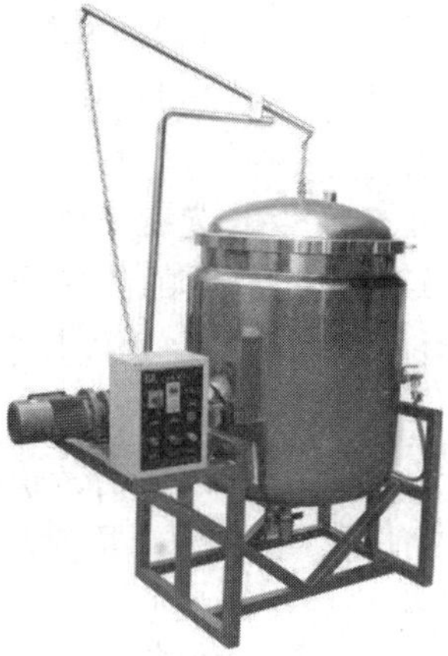

Figure 1-33 Boiling pot

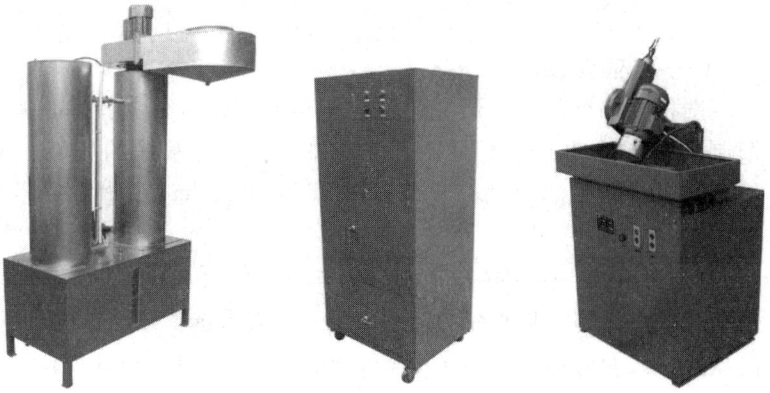

Figure 1-34 Other processing equipments

3.8 Other equipment

In addition to the above equipment for specific purposes, there are a lot of general purpose equipments, such as exhaust gas treatment devices, dry type dusting machines, material conveyors, knife sharpeners, etc. A picture of several other processing equipments is shown in figure 1-34.

Questions

4.1 Briefly describe the common liquid adjuvants for processing and their quality requirements.

4.2 Briefly describe the use of traditional processing tools such as grinding pond, wood steamer and bamboo plaque in the processing of medicinal materials.

4.3 Briefly describe the drying equipment in the production of modern decoction pieces and its main working principle.

第三节 中药炮制实验思路与方法

一、实验研究选题

（一）选题原则

选择中药炮制实验研究课题，即确定实验研究的具体目标和研究内容。恰当的选题是中药炮制实验课成功的重要因素之一，并代表研究水平的高低。中药炮制实验研究选题的程序及原则与其他领域的研究选题基本相同，必须坚持实用性、可行性、科学性、创新性、效益性的原则。

1. 实用性 科学技术是第一生产力，科研选题不能离开行业的需求，否则，难以权衡其价值。对中药炮制实验研究的选题来说，应着重选择毒性饮片、贵重饮片、炮制前后作用差异较大的饮片，以及生熟异制的饮片等。只有了解了这些中药炮制前后理化性质和药理作用的变化以及这些变化的临床意义，才能正确地指导和促进炮制方法的改进、制订饮片质量标准、提高药品质量、确保临床用药安全有效。

2. 可行性 坚持选题的可行性或可能性原则，即考虑完成课题的条件。选题时分析课题的难易程度，预期达到课题目标所必须具备的客观条件，要从研究方案、研究人员组成、仪器设备、研究经费、主客观条件的相互结合与联系等方面进行综合考虑。对中药炮制实验研究来说，实验科研人员必须有较坚实的中医药知识，同时具有较丰富的现代科学知识和技能。只有将中医中药传统理论、经验与现代科学知识、技能结合起来，其研究成果才能为中医药人员所接受。

3. 科学性 科学研究本身就具有科学性。科学性的核心是实事求是，违背事实和客观规律就没有科学研究的意义。目前中药炮制研究选题多数是验证传统炮制理论和方法，但其中也有的是误传误用。例如，《中国药典》1985年版规定龟以腹甲入药，名为龟板，经对部分历史文献资料调查，元、明以前，龟上甲与下甲皆可入药，后因种种原因龟上甲被废弃。因此从龟上、下甲能否等重量替代入药，以何种方法炮制的饮片最佳的角度，立项进行系统研究。其成果为恢复龟上甲药用提供了文献依据和实验依据。《中国药典》从1990年版起规定，龟以背甲（上甲）及腹甲（下甲）入药，名为龟甲。由此看来，选题必须进行广泛深入地调查和课题检索，在反复分析研究的基础上，很慎重地确定科研课题，避免将一些没有足够的、可靠的科学依据的课题轻易地确定下来，造成人财物的浪费。

4. 创新性 是否符合中医药理论，是否充分利用现代科学知识和手段，有无自己的设计特色，决定了中药炮制研究是否具有创新性，也关系到研究成果能否被中西医药人员接受和推广应用。因为方剂是调整体内系统平衡的最优化治疗系统，也是中医临床用药的一大特点，所以将中药炮制纳入方剂中进行研究的选题思路具有较强的创新性，值得借鉴。

5. 效益性 效益包括科学效益、社会效益和经济效益。对中药炮制研究来说，科学效益应是第一位的。所谓科学效益就是选题对学科在学术上、科学价值上的推动作用，是社会效益和经济效益的基础和保证。因为中药炮制受历史条件和科学文化水平的限制，其炮制方法比较原始，工艺比较简单，理论阐述亦较简略。如果不探讨中药炮制的科学内涵和临床意义，就不能指导和促进炮制方法的改进。例如，药材“去芦”问题，历代医药学家认为“芦”为非药用部位，“去芦者免吐”，故应去除。通常认为要去芦的药材包括人参等有数十种，因为人参贵重，参芦占全人参药材的12%~15%，弃之可惜。所以历年来投入了很大的精力研究人参是否去芦的问题，对人参芦与人参主根进行系统的研究比较，具有明显的科学效益，而且对参芦的综合开发利用会带来很大的社会效益和经济效益。经化学成分、药理和毒理研究，以及临床观察，结果皆表明，人参芦与人参主根中人参皂苷的种类基本相同，但含量却比主根高 2~3 倍，挥发油亦比主根高 3 倍多。参芦具有与主根和全参相同的药理作用，对实验动物有相似的抗疲劳、耐缺氧、耐高温、耐低温、抗利尿、镇痛等作用。参芦与人参根或参芦总皂苷与人参根总皂苷具有相似的降低心率和血管阻力，增加血流量，提高实验动物各种组织中 Na^{+}–K^{+}–ATP 酶活性，抑制 Mg^{2+}–ATP 酶活性的作用；对 cAMP 和 cGMP 的含量具有双向调节作用。研究尚未发现参芦的化学成分中含有催吐成分。药理实验表明，人参芦对催吐药物敏感的动物家鸽、猫、狗、猴并无催吐作用。参芦与主根的急性和亚急性毒性实验结果也相似。故《中国药典》1995 年版已改为人参不去芦应用。

（二）选题途径

1. 从当前炮制研究存在的问题选题　中药炮制研究选题，首先应对当前选题的动态趋势以及存在的问题等进行认真的调查研究，才能广开思路，找准目标。公开报道的资料中，可以发现炮制研究存在的问题有如下方面。

（1）对同一种中药的炮制研究结论截然不同。例如，关于乳香的活血镇痛的活性成分，有认为是其所含的树脂，建议应炮制去油药用。亦有认为其镇痛作用的有效部位是挥发油，应生用或提取挥发油药用。因此，乳香的有效成分和炮制方法还有待于研究和验证。

（2）对同一种中药选用何种辅料炮制，看法不一。例如，《中国药典》2020 年版延胡索项下收载醋炙或醋煮延胡索，因为醋炙延胡索的水煎液中总生物碱量较酒炙高出一倍多。但又有报道，醋炙、酒炙延胡索均能提高其水煎液中总生物碱和延胡索乙素的煎出量，酒炙品的止痛作用仅次于醋炙、酒蒸。酒蒸能否代替醋炙，值得进一步研究。

（3）对同一种中药选用何种炮制工艺，看法不一。例如，白芍的加工，《中国药典》2020 年版规定芍药采后洗净，除去头尾及细根，置沸水中煮后除去外皮或去皮后再煮、晒干。但据报道，未经加工的原芍药含 3.02% 芍药苷，而刮皮后降至 1.49%，认为白芍不必刮皮。亦有报道认为，芍药外皮中不仅含有与白芍相同的化学成分，也含有其他独特的化学成分。因此，把去皮只视为是除去栓皮或非药用部位是不合适的，不可省去除外皮这一道工序。据此，白芍是否要去外皮尚需深入研究。

（4）对炮制程度缺乏客观指标。目前多数中药炮制程度仍靠传统经验判断，缺乏客观指标。如对熟地黄的炮制方法有单蒸、加酒蒸。酒蒸又有笼蒸、罐炖、九蒸九晒，炮制程度至黑润。实际生产中很难掌握一致。有报道地黄中梓醇的存在是其晒干或蒸干变黑的原因，且梓醇具降血糖、利尿、缓泻作用。因此，目前至少可根据经验鉴别，结合梓醇的含量，作为熟地炮制质量控制指标之一。

（5）实验研究结果不符合传统炮制理论。传统炮制理论有精华，也有糟粕，需用现代实验方法验证和发展。如传统认为"泽泻滋阴利水盐水炒"（《得配本草》），但有实验表明，泽泻的生品、酒炙品、麸炒品均有利尿作用，唯独盐制品利尿作用并不明显。可是《中国药典》历年版本皆收载泽泻盐制品，因此，对泽泻盐炙的问题尚需进一步研究。

（6）只注意宏量成分，不注意微量成分。如有实验认为，紫硇砂经醋制后是较纯的氯化钠，含量达 98% 以上，因此想利用食盐代替紫硇砂药用。古人认为硇砂能"消五金八石，腐坏人肠胃"，炮制是"杀其毒及去其尘秽"。现代研究认为，紫硇砂有治疗癌症的作用，其生品对小鼠 S_{180} 肉瘤有抑制效果，而普通食盐是没有此种作用的。因此认为，紫硇砂中抗癌活性成分可能是除 NaCl 以外的微量离子，这一问题有待研究探讨。

（7）不加分析的依法炮制未必完全合理。目前所说的依法炮制基本上是"遵古炮制"，没有通过现代科学的验证。例如，乌头与附子虽同出于一种植物，可是加工方法大不相同。《中国药典》历次版本皆规定附子采后加工成盐附子、黑顺片、白附片。盐附子入药用尚需制成淡附片。据报道，附子采后经水洗、胆巴泡、煮、剥皮、切片、漂片、蒸片、烘片等加工炮制处理过程，总生物碱量损失 81.30%。乌头、附子的炮制目的是减毒，而其毒性与乌头所含总生物碱的含量不成平行关系，主要决定于双酯型乌头碱的水解或分解程度，故为减少附子中乌头总碱因浸泡过度流失，是否可改用加压蒸法炮制，使双酯型乌头碱类分解成毒性低的苯甲酰单酯型乌头碱类和几乎无毒性的乌头原碱类等而减毒，值得研究。

2. 从中药已知的特种成分入手选题 凡是中药中特种成分性质比较清楚者，就可以寻找到其定性定量方法，进一步对该中药炮制前后此种成分进行分析比较。例如，栀子中除含栀子苷类成分外，近来研究发现尚含熊果酸。熊果酸具有明显的安定与降温作用，为栀子的解热、降温有效成分，可用高效液相色谱法色谱法测定栀子不同炮制品中栀子苷、熊果苷的含量。

3. 从中药效用或毒副作用入手选题 中药炮制的目的主要是增强药效或消减其毒副作用。用什么指标来衡量中药效用或毒副作用才符合中医药理论，这是值得探讨的问题。例如，黄芪自《神农本草经》以来，就认为对痈疽有效，用于内托排脓。在千金内托散和托里消毒散等方剂中皆配有黄芪。日本学者久保、堀田等研究证明，黄芪的抑菌作用强，并认为此抑菌成分可能是 L-3- 羟基 -9- 甲氧基紫檀素。因此可用抑菌作用为指标验证生黄芪托毒排脓、生肌的科学性。有相当一部分中药是通过增强机体抗御疾病的能力而起作用的。

毒性中药一般可分为两种类型，一类是其毒性成分与治疗成分不一样，须通过炮制将毒性成分去除，如巴豆中巴豆毒素、蓖麻子中蓖麻毒蛋白等。另一类既是有毒成分又是治疗成分，要通过炮制使其达到一定的含量，或转变成毒性较低的物质。如马钱子中马钱子碱和士的宁，乌头、附子中乌头碱，斑蝥中斑蝥素等。对毒性成分和有效成分尚不清楚的中药，可选择主要药效学和毒理学指标，同时做各种炮制品的对比研究。

4. 从中药配伍理论和技术展开联想 中药配伍应用是中医用药的特点之一，通过配伍可起到增效或解毒等作用。运用中药配伍理论和经验，可以创造出新的炮制品。例如《全国中药炮制规范》1988 年版收载三黄汤制炉甘石，既是传统炮制品，也为创制新的炮制品提供了思路。有人在研究由黄连、黄柏、大黄、甘草组成的复方对金黄色葡萄球菌代谢的影响过程中发现，黄柏对细菌 RNA 的合成有强烈抑制作用，大黄对细菌的乳酸脱氢酶抑制最强，黄连强烈抑制细菌呼吸和核酸的合成。推想以三黄汤制炉甘石，是从多种途径影响细菌的代谢环节，可增强炉甘石生肌消炎作用。再如，吴茱萸水制黄连，是“左金丸”配伍理论在炮制中的应用。

5. 从历代医药典籍中寻找选题 阅读历代医药典籍不仅是搜集炮制历史沿革资料所必需，而且也是炮制研究选题的一种重要途径。在阅读中往往受到启发，触类旁通，提出自己的课题。例如，自古以来认为半夏生品有毒，能“戟人咽”“令人吐”，需以水长期浸泡去毒。清代赵学敏在《本草纲目拾遗》中曾指出，“今药肆所售仙半夏。惟将半夏浸泡。尽去其汁味……全失本性……是无异食半夏渣滓，何益之有。”从实验亦可看出，半夏有毒物质不溶或难溶于水，短期浸泡不能达到去毒的目的，长期浸泡则水溶成分损失达 88.1%。醇溶成分损失为 87.5%，氯仿、甲醇溶出成分损失为 76.6%，生物碱损失为 50%。有报道，半夏经高温（115℃，150 分钟；121℃，100 分钟）或高压（132~152kPa/cm^2，2 小时）处理均能破坏其毒性，且工艺简便。在半夏有效成分和有毒成分尚不明确的情况下，半夏的水浸泡工艺能否用高压高温替代，值得深入研究。

6. 将其他学科理论和技术引进中药炮制学 应用化学、药理学、微生物学、免疫学、生物化学、物理学等近代科学技术，对中药炮制的原理、方法、工艺等方面进行研究。例如，采用薄层层析和紫外分光光度法以及高效液相色谱仪等测定白芍 5 种炮制品中芍药苷、丹皮酚、苯甲酸的含量，用化学动力学方法建立首乌清蒸过程中蒽醌成分随时间变化的动力学方程，用免疫学方法探讨大黄对人血清抗原抗体反应及抗体形成作用的影响，用酶学理论和技术对大黄 4 种不同炮制品中胰蛋白酶、胃蛋白酶、胰脂肪酶、胰淀粉酶的活性进行测定等，皆取得可喜的成果。

二、实验设计

（一）设计方法

1. 以中医临床疗效为设计的出发点 中药作用是中医在长期的临床实践中积累总结出来的。对中药作用的认识和研究，绝不能拘泥束缚于单纯某种化学成分或适合纯化学成分的某种药理模型进行研究，而忽视中药的特性。例如，中药四季青内服有清热解毒作用，在体外实验却无抑菌作用。因此，用什么指标来衡量中药效用或毒副作用才能符合中医药理论，这是值得探讨的问题。又如，清热解毒类中药的抗感染作用，往往不是因为它们有直接的抗微生物作用，而是与其免疫调节有关。再如，麦芽、神曲、山楂、鸡内金等消导药，习惯上皆炒至焦香后入药，如果单用所含酵素类成分来解释它们的消食作用，就具有很大的局限性。因为淀粉酶、蛋白酶等经加热炒制后或入煎剂会受到破坏，即使不被完全破坏，经口服后在胃酸的作用下，淀粉酶（最适 pH 为 6.8）也会失活。有的药物炒至焦香后，亦具有一定的苦味，轻微的苦味能对舌尖味觉神经及胃肠黏膜产生一种缓和的刺激作用，通过反射机能可纠正胃肠衰弱现象，以改善消化功能。单用化学成分或药理指标来研究和评价中药炮制的作用是不够完善的，必须以中医临床疗效为依据，设计适宜的成分指标和药理实验模型。

2. 以“证”的模型研究中药炮制原理 辨证论治是中医的特点，而证是根据患者整体宏观表现归纳总结出来的。同病可以异证，因而须异治；异病也可以同证，因而须同治。目前，在中药炮制药理研究中，多数以“证”为基础。因此，有些研究结果不能为中医药人员所接受。如镇痛实验常用“小鼠热板法”或“小鼠醋酸扭体法”。对延胡索等活血止痛、木香等理气止痛、肉桂等散寒止痛、独活等祛风止痛、蚤休等消肿止痛是否皆适合，答案可能是否定的。再如，大多数炭药是用于止血。因此，多用出血、凝血时间为指标来研究炭药，也是不全面的。因为炭药尚有其他多方面的作用，即便是出血，其出血原因各异，有因血热妄行而出血，有因瘀血而出血，有因脾不统血而出血，有因阴虚阳亢而出血，又有外伤性出血，消化道出血，呼吸道出血等。

从临床上发现热证患者的交感神经－肾上腺系统机能活动增强，而寒证患者则相反。经研究，用寒凉药（黄连、黄芩、黄柏等）长期喂养大鼠也可出现交感神经－肾上腺系统机能活动降低现象，造成“寒证”模型。而用温热药（附子、干姜、肉桂等）喂养大鼠则该系统的机能活动增强，造成“热证”模型。日人久保等研制出太阳病的动物模型，以观察桂枝汤的疗效；为观察小青龙汤的抗变态反应作用，又建立了另一种变态反应发作的太阳病模型。这样的动物模型，为我们研究中药炮制开阔了思路，提供了借鉴。

3. 将中药炮制纳入方剂中进行研究 方剂是调整体内系统平衡的最优化治疗系统，也是中医临床用药的一大特点。药物通过配伍组方可起到增效、减毒、缓和药性或产生新药效等作用。单味中药的研究结果往往与该药在方剂中的研究结果不完全一致，有的甚至截然相反。这也是中药炮制研究成果不易推广应用的原因之一。因此，将白芍的炮制纳入芍药甘草汤中进行研究，初步阐明了一些问题。5 种白芍组成的芍甘汤中均不含丹皮酚。芍药苷含量除酒炒白芍的芍甘汤外，皆明显高于生白芍煎液，说明甘草可提高方中芍药苷的煎出量。方中用白芍生品或清炒品、麸炒品芍药苷含量高，二者间无显著差异，但麸炒白芍的芍甘汤中苯甲酸含量最低，故对脾胃虚弱患者似更适宜。白芍各种炮制品不会降低芍甘汤中甘草次酸的煎出量。方中用生白芍鞣质含量最低，甘草与白芍混合煎煮液中鞣质含量明显低于分煎液的合并值。又因芍甘汤中鞣质含量的高低与其抗炎作用强弱不成平行关系。故芍甘汤制剂时可合煎。

（二）设计注意

1. 坚持均衡对照，随机化和重复的原则 要提高研究效率，保证科研结果的正确性和可靠性，试验设计时就应坚持均衡对照、随机化和重复的原则。对照的设计要按照“齐同对比”的原则，即除了探索的因素之外，研究组与对照组的各种条件要尽可能的相同，才能对比。文献有用生药10g与该药的炭药10g进行出血、凝血时间的比较，以说明该药制炭后止血效果是增强还是减弱，这就不是齐同对比。因生药10g，制炭后不能得到炭药10g。目前普遍存在的是对用不同方法或不同辅料炮制的各种炮制品，不按各种炮制品得率和平衡水分折算取样，而是各种炮制品的取样量与原生药等量，这也不是齐同对比。

随机化就是把研究对象分为几组，使分入研究组与对照组的机会均等，以便使系统误差减少到最低限度。违反随机化原则的做法在炮制研究中存在，如样品粉碎后只过一种筛目的筛，不规定上下限，取样时不随机化；动物分组先抓到的（不活泼者）为一组，后抓到的（活泼者）为另一组；实验观察顺序不随机化等。

做到随机化不易，需要研究者尽最大努力。这是研究者的责任，也反映研究者的科研道德。为什么有的研究结果别人不能重复出来，虽原因很多，但与随机化原则坚持不够有很大关系。

重复是保证科研结果可靠的重要措施之一。重复有两层含义：一是指实验过程是多次重复进行的；二是指设计中提出的方法、结果，别人也能重复出来。因为科学真理任何时候都不怕重复。1963年曾报道槐花炒炭后芦丁大量损失，但鞣质增加4倍，并认为槐花炒炭后止血作用增强，可能是鞣质增加的缘故。此后，虽然曾有槐花炒炭后鞣质不仅未增加，反而下降的报道，但进一步研究证明前面的报道是正确的，并观察到纯芦丁受热后也确可转化生成鞣质，此种转化与受热温度和时间密切相关。炮制研究中要得到重现性结果，是很不容易的。这与炮制的火候、时间、饮片大小厚薄、样品液的提取条件、实验操作技术等有密切关系。不能根据一两篇实验报道，就轻易否定前人几千年来的炮制理论和技术。

2. 正确看待和选用数理统计方法 科研中所收集到的各种数据要不要使用统计处理，以往存在着两种不同的看法：一种看法认为数理统计万能，把它说得玄而又玄；另一种看法认为数理统计是数学游戏，持怀疑态度。这些都有其片面性，适当地、正确地应用数理统计方法，可以使数据更接近于事实，这对于认识事物的本质是很必要的。例如，有人应用某药治疗手足癣病20例，治愈10例，就得出结论说治愈率为50%。这显然是不可信的。经数理统计处理可知，10/20的实际可能范围是27%~73%（P=0.05），而不一定是50%。

由此可见，炮制研究中适当地应用数理统计方法是很有必要的。但必须指出，数理统计的运用，只能对已得数据进行科学处理，它无法证明数据来源是否正确。数理统计不能代替科学思维，更不能代替辩证唯物主义的分析。

炮制研究中得来的测量资料或计数资料常需进行统计学处理。选用的假设检验方法应符合其应用条件。计量资料的比较常用t检验，计数资料的比较常用X^2检验。同为计量资料，配对设计与完全随机设计（成组比较）t检验方法也不相同。如某药材炮制前后实验指标的比较，应为配对资料比较，若用成组比较的t检验方法处理，则不但浪费信息，还可能得出错误的结论。不能用大样本的u检验代替小样本的t检验，也不能用一般的t检验代替方差不齐的检验。

Section 3 The ideas and methods for researches on Chinese medicine processing

1. Selecting research topics

1.1 Principles for selecting topics

The selection of a viable scientific research topic concerning Chinese medicine processing requires that the specific objectives and research content be clear. Proper topic selection is one of the most important factors in determining the success of the practical course on Chinese medicine processing and represents the level of research. The procedures and principles for Chinese medicine processing research are essentially the same as those in other fields, which involve practicality, feasibility, scientificity, innovation and efficiency.

1.1.1 Practicality

Before selecting a scientific research topic the needs of the industry must be taken into consideration, otherwise, the research topic will be of low value. The focus of the research topic should be placed upon Chinese medicines that have high toxicity, high value, and different functions before and after processing as well as those medicines that need to be prepared specifically owing to their crude or processed nature, etc. Only after understanding the changes in the physical and chemical properties and pharmacological effects of Chinese medicine, before and after processing, and mastering the clinical significance of these changes, can we properly guide and promote the improvement of processing methods. Furthermore, by enhancing our understanding, the formulation of quality standards for prepared slices and the quality of Chinese medicines can be improved. The safety and effectiveness of Chinese medicines for clinical application can be consequently assured.

1.1.2 Feasibility

Persist in the principle of feasibility or possibility for topic selection, that is, to consider the conditions for completing the project. When selecting the topic, one should analyze the difficulty of the project, and the objective conditions needed to achieve the expected goal of the subject. Comprehensive consideration should be given to the design of the project, the qualification of researchers, instruments and equipment, research funds, and the combination of subjective and objective conditions, etc. For projects concerning the processing of Chinese medicine, researchers must have a profound knowledge of Chinese medicine and a wealth of modern scientific knowledge and skills. Only by combining the traditional theory and experience of Chinese medicine with modern scientific knowledge and skills can the research results be accepted by Chinese medicine personnel.

1.1.3 Scientificity

The core aim of science is to seek truth from facts. Scientific research is meaningless if facts and objective laws are violated. At present, most research topics focus upon verifying traditional processing theory and methods, but some results are misreported or misused. For example, the 1985 edition of the Chinese pharmacopoeia stipulated that only the abdominal shell of tortoise should be used as medicine, Guiban in Chinese. While according to some ancient literature, before the Yuan and Ming dynasties, both the abdominal shell and the back shell of the tortoise could be used as medicine. Owing to the information in the 1985 edition, the back shell of the tortoise gradually became less commonly used. Therefore, a systematic study was carried out to clarify whether the abdominal shell and the back shell of the tortoise could be used in clinics at equivalent weights, and by what kind of processing could the best medicine be obtained. The results provided a literature and experimental basis for the medicinal use of both the abdominal shell and the back shell of the tortoise. Subsequently, in the 1990 edition of the Chinese pharmacopoeia, the term, tortoise shell, now refers to both the back (upper) and belly (lower) armor of the tortoise. From this point of view, the research topic must be determined carefully based on extensive and thorough investigation and literature review and on the basis of repeated analyses and research, to avoid wasting human resources and funds due to inadequate and unreliable subject planning.

1.1.4 Innovation

Do the research indicators and methods conform to the theory of Chinese medicine? Does the project make full use of modern scientific knowledge and means? Is the research design distinctive? All the aforementioned determine if the topic is innovative or not, and whether the research achievements can be accepted and popularized by Chinese and western medical personnel. As TCM prescriptions focus upon the optimization of treatment strategy to adjust balance in the body, and is also a major feature of the clinical use of Chinese medicine, applying the knowledge from Chinese medicine processing research to TCM prescriptions is a highly innovative approach that is worth learning.

1.1.5 Profitability

Benefits include scientific benefits, social benefits and economic benefits. For the study of Chinese medicine processing, the scientific benefit should be the first consideration. The so-called scientific benefit is that the selected research subject may promote the disciplines academic and scientific value. This is the basis and guarantee of social and economic benefits. Because the development of Chinese medicine processing is limited by poor historical conditions and scientific levels, the processing methods are relatively primitive, the processing techniques are rather simple, and the state of processing theory is also too brief. If the scientific connotation and clinical significance of Chinese medicine processing are not discussed, the processing method cannot be guided and promoted. For example, the problem of "get rid of rhizoma (Lu in Chinese)" of Chinese medicines. Ancient medical experts considered "Lu" as a non-medicinal part, "People won't vomit without Lu", so "Lu" should be removed. It is generally believed that the rhizoma of dozens of medicinal herbs should be removed, including ginseng. But since ginseng is very precious, it is a big waste to discard the rhizoma of ginseng which accounts for 12%~15% of the total ginseng, therefore, great efforts have been devoted over the years to the research on whether the rhizoma of ginseng should be eliminated or not, and a systematic comparison between the rhizoma and taproot of ginseng will result in obvious scientific benefits, and the comprehensive development and utilization of the rhizoma of ginseng will bring great social and economic benefits. Research on chemical compositions, pharmacology and toxicology, and clinical observation, show that the types of ginsenosides in the rhizoma and taproot of panax are basically the same, while the content in the rhizoma is 2~3 times higher than that in the taproot, and the volatile oil in rhizoma is more than 3 times higher than that in the taproot. The rhizoma of ginseng has the same pharmacological actions as the taproot and the whole ginseng, and has similar anti-fatigue, anti-hypoxia, anti-high temperature, anti-low temperature, anti-diuretic and analgesic effects in animal experiments. The total saponins of panax ginseng rhizoma and panax ginseng root have similar effects in lowering heart rate and vascular resistance, increasing blood flow, improving the enzymatic activity of Na^+–K^+–ATP in various tissues of the animal model in experiments, and inhibiting the enzymatic activity of Mg^{2+}–ATP. They also have a bidirectional regulating effect on the content of cAMP and cGMP. No emetic components are found in the chemical components of ginseng rhizoma. Results of pharmacological experiments showed that the ginseng rhizoma had no emetic effect on domestic pigeons, cats, dogs and monkeys which were sensitive to emetic drugs. The results of acute and subacute toxicity tests of the rhizoma and the taproot of ginseng were also similar. Owing to these finding, the 1995 edition of the Chinese pharmacopoeia, states that the rhizome of ginseng should also be used.

1.2 Approaches for selecting projects

1.2.1 The current challenges to Chinese medicine processing research

For the research topic of Chinese medicine processing, first of all, we should carefully review the dynamic trend and challenges of the current research. This will broaden our thinking and enable us to find the major research goals. From published literature on Chinese medicine processing, you may find following.

1.2.1.1 For the same Chinese medicine, different processing research may draw totally different conclusions. For example, the active ingredients in frankincense that act as stimulants of blood circulation and/or analgesia. Some believe that the active ingredient is resin and therefore oil should be removed during processing for medicinal purposes, while others believe that the effective part of its analgesic effect is volatile oil. Either raw frankincense should be used or volatile oil shall be extracted for medication. Therefore, both the active components of frankincense and the effective processing method are yet to be validated.

1.2.1.2 Different opinions exist regarding the use of different adjuvants for processing the same Chinese medicine. For example, in the 2020 edition of the Chinese pharmacopoeia, it is recommended that the Corydalis rhizoma (Yanhusuo) be broiled or boiled in vinegar, because the total amount of alkaloids in the vinegar broiled Yanhusuo decoction is almost twice that of the wine broiled extract. However, it has been reported that both vinegar and wine broiled Yanhuso can improve the extraction of total alkaloids and tetrahydropalmatine in the water decoction and the analgesic effect of the wine broiled extract is second to vinegar broiling and wine steaming. It remains a research question, whether or not wine steaming can replace vinegar roasting in Yanhusuo processing.

1.2.1.3 There are different opinions on the processing procedures of the same Chinese medicine. For example, for the processing of Paeoniae radix, it is stipulated in the 2020 edition of the Chinese Pharmacopoeia that the peony should be washed after harvest, the head, tail and fine roots should be removed and bark should be peeled after boiling in water. The peeled peony root should then be boiled again and dried before storage. However, it was reported that the content of paeoniflorin in the original unprocessed fresh peony roots was 3.02%, which decreased to 1.49% after the removal of the bark, and it is therefore suggested that the bark not be removed. On the other hand, it has also been reported that the bark of Paeoniae radix contains not only the same chemical components as the inner root of Paeoniae radix, but also other unique chemical components. Therefore, it may be argued that the removal of the peony outer layer is still a valid procedure, as it will reduce a proportion of the non-medicinal parts. Based on these contrary arguments, the processing of the bark of Paeoniae radix still remains as a topic of investigation.

1.2.1.4 The lack of objective criteria for the degree of processing. Currently, there is no objective criterion for processing Chinese medicine and most practitioners still rely on traditional experience. The methods of Rehmanniae radix praeparata processing, for example, include simple steaming with water or wine-added steaming. The latter can be done in a steamer or a stew pot or through nine-steaming-nine-sun drying, until it turns sticky and brightly dark black. In the practical production of Rehmanniae radix praeparata, it is difficult to master its processing consistently. The content of catalpol in Rehmanniae radix praeparata is reported to be related to the appearance of its black color. Catalpol can be used for lowering blood sugar, diuresis, and laxness. Therefore, the experience-based judgement in combination with contents of catalpol and color change may be developed as the quality control index of the processing of Rehmanniae radix praeparata.

1.2.1.5 Inconsistency between processing theory of traditional Chinese medicine and modern experiment data. Traditional processing theory shall be ideally verified and developed with modern experiment methodologies. In both the Compendium of Material Medica (Depei Bencao) and the Chinese Pharmacopoeia, Alismatis rhizoma was recorded as a diuretic agent that should be prepared in salt water. However, experiment results showed that raw Alismatis rhizoma, rice wine stir-fried, and bran fried Alismatis rhizoma, all have a diuretic effect, whereas salt stir-fried products do not. Therefore, both the salt-mediated preparation of Alismatis rhizoma and its effective diuretic components requires further scientific validation.

1.2.1.6 Careful consideration has to be given to the major components as well as the trace elements in Chinese medicine. Experiment data showed that the majority of Halite Violaceous (purple salt ammoniac) from vinegar extraction is relatively pure sodium chloride (>98%), and this raises the question, whether or not salt can be used to replace Halite Violaceous for medical treatment. In ancient Chinese medicine Halite Violaceous was considered to be capable of rusting metals and stone, and damaging the intestine and stomach.The aim of processing is to remove the toxic components and discard the dust particles. Modern research suggests that Halite Violaceous may also be used for the treatment of cancer, as its product has the inhibitory effect on S_{180} sarcoma in mice, however, sodium chloride as the major component of the Halite Violaceous, has no such effect. Therefore, it is believed that the active anticancer ingredients in Halite Violaceous are likely to be trace ions, which need to be elucidated.

1.2.1.7 Traditional Chinese processing may need to be optimized with scientific analysis, rather than simply following ancient processing methods without modern scientific validation. For example, Aconitum carmichaelii and Aconiti lateralis radix praeparata are from the same plant, but their processing methods are quite different. In all previous versions of the Chinese Pharmacopoeia, it is documented that after harvesting Aconiti lateralis radix praeparata should be processed into a salty product, black or white slices. Salty products needs to de-salted before use. It was reported that 81.30% of total alkaloid would be lost after complicated processing of Aconiti lateralis radix praeparata by washing, soaking in gall, boiling, peeling, slicing, drifting, steaming, baking, etc. The purpose of processing Aconitum carmichaelii and Aconiti lateralis radix praeparata is to reduce their toxicity via hydrolysis or the decomposition of toxic diester type aconitine. There is no proportional relationship between total alkaloid and the toxicity of these toxic medicines. Therefore the following research hypothesis is presented, if the excessive loss of total alkaloid during the soaking process is reduced with an alternative pressure steaming method, the diester type aconitine may be converted into low toxic benzoyl monoester type aconitine and nearly non-toxic aconine.

1.2.2 Selecting projects from special known components in Chinese medicine

For Chinese medicines that have well defined special compositions and properties, qualitative and quantitative methods may be developed to further analyze their key composition before and after processing. For example, recent studies have shown that in addition to gardenoside, Gardeniae fructus also contains ursolic acid. Ursolic acid has the obvious effects of reducing anxiety, promoting sleep and reducing fever, and it is the active ingredient in Gardeniae fructus for antipyretic and cooling effects. Therefore, HPLC chromatography may be used to determine the content of gardenoside and ursolic acid in different processed products of Gardeniae fructus.

1.2.3 Selecting projects from efficacy or toxic side effects of Chinese medicine

The main purpose of Chinese medicine processing is to enhance the therapeutic effects and to lower side effects. The criteria for measuring the therapeutic effects and toxicity in line with Chinese medicine theory should be investigated. For example, Astragali radix was considered to be an effective Chinese medicine for treating carbuncle-abscess since Shennong's Classic of Materia Medica, and was used in the prescriptions of QianjinNeituo Powder and TuoliXiaodu Powder for internal abscess drainage. Japanese scientist Kubo demonstrated that Astragali radix has a strong anti-bacterial effect, which may be mediated by L–3–hydroxy–9–methoxy pterocarpin. Therefore the bacteriostasis may be used as an indicator for ulcer healing and muscle generation. In fact, quite a large number of Chinese medicines have the ability to boost the body's defense system thereby increasing disease resistance.

Toxicity of Chinese medicine can generally be divided into two types. One type is that the toxic and therapeutic components are different, and Chinese medicine processing is required to remove the toxic ingredients, such as crotin in Crotonis fructus, ricin in the Ricini semen, *etc*. Another type is that the toxic and therapeutic ingredients are the same components, and Chinese medicine processing is required to extract the key ingredient and to convert it into a low toxic substance. This includes brucine and strychnine in Strychni semen, aconitine in Aconitum carmichaelii and Aconiti lateralis radix praeparata, and cantharidin in Mylabris, *etc*. For those Chinese medicines whose toxic ingredients and active ingredients are unclear, we can adopt the main indexes of pharmacodynamics and toxicology to compare the products from various processing products.

1.2.4 From the theory and technology of compatibility of Chinese medicine

Compatibility is one of the characteristics of Chinese medicine, through which Chinese medicine can be synergized or detoxified. With the theory and experience of Chinese medicine compatibility, we can create new Chinese medicine products. For example, National Standards for the Processing of Chinese Medicine (1988 edition) contained Calamina processed with Sanhuang decoction, which was not only the traditional processed product, but also provided ideas to create new processed products. Research on a Chinese medicine formula composed of Rhizoma coptidis, Cortex phellodendri, Radix et rhizoma rhei and Radix glycyrrhizae found that in the process of metabolism of staphylococcus aureus, Cortex phellodendri had a strong inhibitory effect on the synthesis of bacterial RNA, Radix et rhizoma rhei had the strongest inhibitory effect on lactate dehydrogenase production in bacteria, while Rhizoma coptidis strongly inhibited bacterial respiration and nucleic acid synthesis. It was deduced that Calamina processed with the Sanhuang decoction could affect bacterial metabolism via a variety of pathways, and that the Sanhuang decoction could synergize the activity of Calamina by promoting tissue regeneration and anti-inflammation. Again, for example, Rhizoma coptidis processed with Fructus euodiae decoction is the application of "Zuojin pills" compatibility theory in the processing.

1.2.5 Seeking projects from ancient medical classics

Reading ancient books on Chinese medicine is not only a necessary way to gather information on the history of processing Chinese medicine, but also an important approach towards selecting a project on Chinese medicine processing. Reading may provide inspiration and enable you to comprehensively develop and put forward your own project. For example, since ancient times, crude Rhizoma pinelliae is believed to be toxic and have properties that can "irritate your throat" and "make you vomit" needs to be soaked in water for a long time for detoxification. Xuemin Zhao in Qing dynasty has pointed out in The Supplement to the Compendium of Materia Medica, "the Rhizoma pinelliae sold in drug store is only processed by soaking in water, when its lixivium is discarded, it lost all its nature, and then taking it is just like eating dross of Rhizoma pinelliae, which hasn't any benefit." We can also conclude from experiment results that toxic substances in Rhizoma pinelliae are insoluble or poorly soluble in water, so soaking in water for short term can't get it detoxified, but long term soaking in water will lead to 88.1% loss of its soluble components, 87.5% loss of its liposoluble components, 76.6% loss of chloroform and methanol soluble components, 50% loss of alkaloids. There is also a report shows that Rhizoma pinelliae can be simply detoxified by treating under high temperature (115°C for 150 minutes or 121°C for 100 minutes) and high pressure (132~152 kPa/cm^2 for 2 hours). Since the active and toxic components of Rhizoma pinelliae are still unclear, it is worth further studying whether or not processing Rhizoma pinelliae by soaking it in water can be replaced with high pressure and high temperature processing.

1.2.6 Introduce theory and technology of other disciplines to Chinese medicine processing

We can apply chemistry, pharmacology, microbiology, immunology, biochemistry, physics and other modern science and technology to carry out research on the principle, method and techniques of Chinese medicine processing. For example, we can determine paeoniflorin, paeonol and benzoic acid in five processed products of Radix paeoniae by using thin-layer chromatography (TLC), ultraviolet spectrophotometry (UV), and the high performance liquid chromatography (HPLC). We can establish dynamics equations of changes of anthraquinones in Radix polygonimultiflori over the time of steaming by using chemical dynamics method. We can explore effect of Radix et rhizoma rhei on serum antigen and antibody response and antibody formation with immunological methods. We can also measure the activities of trypsin, pepsin, pancreatic lipase, and pancreatic amylase in four processed products of Radix et rhizoma rhei with enzyme theory and technology. All of the above are gratifying achievements.

2. Experiment design

2.1 Design method

2.1.1 The starting point for designing the clinical efficacy of TCM

The effectiveness of traditional Chinese medicine can be demonstrated by its long-term clinical use and practice. Research and understanding concerning the uses of traditional Chinese medicine must not be restricted to the study of a certain chemical component or a certain pharmacological model that only focuses upon pure chemical components and neglects the characteristics of the medicine. For example, the traditional Chinese medicine Sijiqing has the effect of clearing heat and detoxification internally, but has no antibacterial effect in vitro. Therefore, the indicators that are used to measure the effectiveness or toxicity and side effects of traditional Chinese medicine are worth exploring in order to conform to the theory of traditional Chinese medicine. Another example is the anti-infective effect of the Chinese medicine, Qingrejiedu, which is often used not because it has a direct antimicrobial effect, but rather due to its immunoregulatory effects. As another example, malt, medicated leaven, hawthorn, the membrane of a chicken's gizzard and other abductive dispersing medicine are traditionally fried until they are burnt before being used as medicine. Their medicinal use would be very limited if their enzymatic properties alone were to be used to explain their digestion promoting effects. This is, because amylase, protease and other enzymes are destroyed after heating and frying, or even if the medicines are added to the decoction. Even if the enzymes are not completely destroyed during processing, the amylase (the most suitable pH is 6.8) will be inactivated by the action of gastric acid after oral administration. Some drugs have a bitter taste after being fried to the scorch. Slight bitterness can have a mild stimulating effect on the apex of the tongue and the gastrointestinal mucosa. The reflex function can correct gastrointestinal weakness and improve digestive function. It is not a complete study if the effects of traditional Chinese medicine processing with chemical ingredients or pharmacological indicators alone are used to evaluate outcomes. It is necessary to design appropriate component indicators and pharmacological experiment models based on the clinical efficacy of traditional Chinese medicine.

2.1.2 Research on the principle of traditional Chinese medicine processing based on the model of "Symptom"

Syndrome differentiation is a characteristic of traditional Chinese medicine. Syndromes are summarized based on the overall macroscopic presentation of symptoms in patients. A disease may present different symptoms that need to be treated differently, while different diseases may present the same symptoms that need to be treated in the same way by the same method. At present, most of the research on the pharmacology of traditional Chinese medicine is based on the symptoms. Therefore, some research results are not acceptable to Chinese medicine practitioners. For example, the "Hot plate method in mouse" or "mouse acetic acid writhing method" is commonly used for analgesia experiments. Therefore, medicines that are used to improve blood circulation, which also act as analgesics, such as corydalis tuber (regulating vital energy), radix aucklandiae (dispel pathogenic cold), cinnamon (dispel the wind), angelica tuhuo (decreasing swelling) or pain relievers such as paris polyphylla smith may not be suitable in their use. As another example, most carbonized drugs are used to stop bleeding. Therefore, it is not comprehensive to study the carbonized drugs with bleeding and blood clotting time as indicators. Because carbonized drugs have other functions, even if there is bleeding, there may be different causes for the bleeding. There is bleeding due to blood-heat, bleeding due to blood stasis, bleeding due to the inability of the spleen to regulate the blood, and bleeding due to the hyperactivity of yang owing to yin deficiency, as well as traumatic bleeding, gastrointestinal bleeding, respiratory tract bleeding, etc.

Clinical studies indicate that the sympathetic nerve-adrenal system function activity in patients with heat syndrome is enhanced, while it is decreased in patients with cold syndrome. Research indicates that feeding rats drugs of cold and cool nature (Coptis chinensis, Scutellaria baicalensis, Cortex phellodendri, etc.) can also reduce the sympathetic nerve-adrenal system functional activity in the long-term, resulting in a "cold syndrome" model. While feeding rats drugs of a warm-heat nature (mankshood, rhizoma zingiberis, cinnamon, etc.) enhances the functional activity of the system, resulting in a "heat syndrome" model. Nibo Kubo et al, developed an animal model with sun disease to observe the curative effects of a cinnamon twig decoction. In order to observe the anti-allergic effect of a small qinglong decoction, another model of sun disease was also developed. Such animal models have broadened our thinking and provide a reference for our research on the processing of traditional Chinese medicine.

2.1.3 Incorporate traditional Chinese medicine processing into prescriptions for research

The prescription is an optimal treatment system for adjusting the balance of processes in the body. It is also a major feature of clinical medicine in TCM. The composition of a prescription can produce medicines that may play synergistic, detoxifying or alleviating roles and may even lead to the discovery of new drug effects. The results of research on a single Chinese medicine are often not completely consistent with the results from experiments using a prescription that has the same medicine. Some experiments may even have the opposite results. This is one of the reasons why some results from experiments on processed traditional Chinese medicine are not easy to popularize and apply.

The processing of Radix paeoniae alba is incorporated into a paeoniae and licorice decoction for research, and some problems have been clarified. The paeonol is not contained in the paeoniae and licorice decoction, which comprises of 5 kinds of Radix paeoniae alba. Its content of paeoniflorin is significantly higher than that of the crude Radix paeoniae alba decoction, except for the paeoniae and licorice decoction processed with sauteed alcohol, indicating that licorice could increase the amount of paeoniflorin decoction in the recipe. The traditional Chinese herbal medicines crude Radix paeoniae alba or its fried, stir-fried products and bran stir-fried products have a high content of paeoniflorin. There is no significant difference between the two stir-fried products. However, the content of benzoic acid in paeoniae and licorice decoction of bran-fried Baizhi is the lowest, so it seems more suitable for patients with a weak spleen and stomach. The various processed products of Radix paeoniae alba will not reduce the decoction of glycyrrhetic acid in paeoniae and licorice decoction. The content of tannin in raw white scallion is the lowest, and the tannin content in the mixed decoction of licorice and Radix paeoniae alba is significantly lower than the combined value of decoction for respective processing. And because the content of tannin inpaeoniae and licorice decoction is not parallel to its anti-inflammatory effect. Therefore, paeoniae and licorice decoction can be fried together.

2.2 Design notice

2.2.1 Adhere to the principles of balanced control, randomization and repetition

To improve research efficiency and ensure the correctness and reliability of scientific research results, the principles of balanced control, randomization, and repetition should be adhered to in the design of experiments. The design of the control should be based on the principle of "uniform comparison", that is, in addition to the explored factors, the various conditions of the study group and the control group must be as same as possible to compare. In the literature, a comparison of blood and coagulation time with 10g of crude drug and 10g of carbonized drugs is made to show whether the hemostatic effect of the drug is enhanced or weakened after making carbonized drugs. Because of 10g of crude drug cannot be obtained 10g of carbonized drugs after carbonized production. At present, it is common to use various methods or different auxiliary materials to process various processed products. Instead of sampling according to the yield and equilibrium moisture of various processed products, the sampling volume of various processed products is equal to the original drug in the comparison, which is not a concerted consistent comparison.

Randomization is to divide the research object into several groups, so that the chances of being divided into the research group and the control group are equal, so as to minimize the systematic error. The practice that violates the principle of randomization exists in processing research. For example, after the sample is crushed, it passes through only one sieve, without the specified upper and lower limits, and no randomization is performed when sampling. The first captured animals (inactive) are included as one group, and the later captured (active) animals are included as another group, experiment observation order is not randomized, etc.

It is not easy to achieve randomization, and researchers need to do their best. This is the responsibility of the researcher and also reflects the research ethics of the researcher. Some research results can't be replicated by others. Although there can be many reasons, a common reason to a large extent is that there is insufficient adherence to the principle of randomization.

Duplication is one of the important measures to ensure the reliability of scientific research results. Repetition has two levels of meanings, one is that the experiment process is repeated many times, the other is that the methods and results proposed in the design can be repeated by others. Because scientific truth is not afraid of repetition at any time. It was reported in 1963 that rutin was greatly lost after carbonized frying of sophora flower, but the tannin was increased by 4 times. It was believed that the hemostatic effect of sophora flower after carbonized frying was enhanced, which may be caused by the increase in tannin. Since then, although there have been reports that tannins were decreased instead of increased after carbonized frying, further research proved that the previous report was correct, and it was observed that pure rutin can indeed be transformed into tannins when heated. The conversion is closely related to the heating temperature and time. It is not easy to obtain reproducible results in processing research. Because it is closely related to the heat control, processing time, the size of the pieces, the extraction conditions of the sample liquid, and the experiment operation technology. It is not easy to deny the concocted theories and techniques of predecessors for thousands of years based on one or two experiment reports.

2.2.2 Correctly treat and choose mathematical statistics methods

To use statistical processing for data collected in scientific research or not?, There were two different views in the past: one view believes that mathematical statistics are almighty and imysterious, while the other view is more skeptical and believes that mathematical statistics are a tool used to artificially prove a point of view. These are one-sided points of view. The appropriate and correct application of mathematical statistics methods can make the data closer to the facts and is necessary to understand the nature of things. For example, someone applied a medicine to treat 20 cases of tinea manuum and pedis disease, and it was concluded that the cure rate was 50% with 10 patients being cured. This is obviously not credible. It can be known through mathematical statistics processing that the actual possible range of 10/20 is 27% to 73% ($P = 0.05$), not necessarily 50%.

It can be seen that it is necessary to properly apply mathematical statistics in processing research. However, it must be pointed out that the application of mathematical statistics can only scientifically process the obtained data. It cannot prove whether the data source is correct. Mathematical statistics cannot replace scientific thinking, nor can it replace analysis of dialectical materialism.

Measurements or counts from concocted research often requires statistical processing. The hypothesis testing method selected should meet its application conditions. The *t*-test is commonly used for comparison of measurement data, and the X^2 test is commonly used for comparison of count data. For the same measurement data, the paired design and the completely random design (group comparison) *t*-test methods are also different. For example, the comparison of experiment indicators before and after the processing of a certain medicinal material should be paired data comparison. If the *t*-test method is used for the group comparison of processing, it will not only waste information, but also may lead to wrong conclusions. A large sample for *u*-test cannot be used to replace a small sample for *t*-test, and a general *t*-test cannot be used to replace the test with uneven variance.

第二章 中药炮制验证性实验

PPT

实验一 净制、切制

实验目的

1. **掌握** 中药材净制、饮片切制的基本操作方法，中药饮片类型和干燥方法。

2. **了解** 中药材净制、饮片切制的目的和意义。

实验原理

1. **净制的作用** ①除去杂质，便于临床调配与制剂。②分离药用部位，更好发挥药效。③大小分档，便于切制和炮炙。④除去非药用部位，保证用药剂量的准确。

2. **饮片切制的作用** ①便于有效成分煎出。②利于炮炙。③利于调配和制剂。④便于鉴别。⑤利于贮存。

实验内容

1. **净选** 采用挑选、筛选、风选、水选、摘、揉、擦、刷、刮、剪切等方法，去除杂质，除非药用部位等。

2. **软化** 根据实验条件和中药材特性可采用下列不同方法：①常用水处理的方法，主要有淋法、洗法、泡法、漂法、润法等；②湿热软化法，主要有减压加蒸汽润药法、减压浸渍法、直接蒸润法、烘烤法等。

3. **切制** 采用手工切制和机器切制的方法，根据不同药材性质，分别切制成极薄片、薄片、厚片、丝、段、块等。

4. **干燥** 采用控温电热烘箱干燥，温度控制在50~80℃，并定时翻动至全部干燥，取出放凉。

实验器具和材料

1. **实验器具** 片刀、切药刀（铡刀）、压板、铁夹、切药机、盆、竹匾、竹把、刀具、剪刀、刷子、筛子、大中小搪瓷盘（具盖）、烘箱、真空加温润药机、气相置换真空润药机、蒸锅等。

2. **实验材料** 当归、槟榔、白芍、川芎、丹参、甘草、大黄、黄芪、白术、党参、麻黄、荆芥、陈皮、瓜蒌皮、阿胶。

实验方法

1. **当归** 取原药材适量，除去杂质，洗净，稍润，切薄片，低温干燥，放凉，筛去碎屑。

2. **槟榔** 取原药材适量，除去杂质，洗净，浸润软化，润透，切薄片，干燥，放凉，筛去碎屑。

3. **白芍** 取原药材适量，除去杂质，大小分档，洗净，浸、润软化，润透，切薄片，干燥，放凉。筛去碎屑。

4. **川芎** 取原药材适量，除去杂质，大小分档，洗净，浸、润软化，润透，切薄片，干燥，放凉，筛去碎屑。

5. **丹参** 取原药材适量，除去杂质及残茎，洗净，润透，切厚片，干燥，放凉，筛去碎屑。

6. **甘草** 取原药材适量，除去杂质，洗净，润透，切厚片，干燥，放凉，筛去碎屑。

7. **大黄** 取原药材适量，除去杂质，大小分档，洗净，浸、润软化，润透，切厚片，低温干燥，放凉，筛去碎屑。

8. **黄芪** 取原药材适量，除去杂质，洗净，润透，切斜片，干燥，放凉，筛去碎屑。

9. **白术** 取原药材适量，除去杂质，洗净，润透，切直片，干燥，放凉，筛去碎屑。

10. **党参** 取原药材适量，除去杂质，洗净，润透，切段，干燥，放凉，筛去碎屑。

11. **麻黄** 取原药材适量，除去残根、木质茎及杂质，抢水洗净，稍润，切段，干燥，放凉，筛去碎屑。

12. **荆芥** 取原药材适量，除去杂质，抢水洗净，稍润，切段，干燥，放凉，筛去碎屑。

13. **陈皮** 取原药材适量，除去杂质，喷淋清水，润透，切细丝，低温干燥，放凉，筛去碎屑。

14. **瓜蒌皮** 取原药材适量，除去杂质，洗净，稍润，切宽丝，干燥，放凉，筛去碎屑。

15. **阿胶** 取阿胶块适量，烘软，趁热切成小丁。

实验结果

1. **当归** 类圆形、椭圆形或不规则薄片。外表皮黄棕色至棕褐色。切面黄白色或淡棕黄色，平坦，有裂隙，中间有浅棕色的形成层环，并有多数棕色的油点，香气浓郁，味甘、辛、微苦。

2. **槟榔** 类圆形薄片。切面可见棕色种皮与白色胚乳相间的大理石样花纹。气微，味涩、微苦。

3. **白芍** 类圆形的薄片。表面淡棕红色或类白色，平滑。切面类白色或微带棕红色，形成层环明显，可见稍隆起的筋脉纹呈放射状排列。气微，味微苦、酸。

4. **川芎** 不规则厚片。外表皮黄褐色，有皱缩纹。切面黄白色或灰黄色，具有明显波状环纹或多角形纹理，散生黄棕色油点，质坚实。气浓香，味苦、辛，微甜。

5. **丹参** 类圆形或椭圆形的厚片。外表皮棕红色或暗棕红色，粗糙，具纵皱纹。切面有裂隙或略平整而致密，有的呈角质样，皮部棕红色，木部灰黄色或紫褐色，有黄白色放射状纹理。气微，味微苦涩。

6. **甘草** 类圆形或椭圆形厚片。表面黄白色，中间有明显的棕色形成层环纹及射线，传统称为“菊花心”，纤维粉性；周边棕红色、棕色或灰棕色，粗糙，具纵皱纹。气微，味甜微苦。

7. **大黄** 不规则厚片或块。黄棕色或黄褐色，中心有纹理，微显朱砂点，习称“锦纹”。质轻，气清香，味苦而微涩。

8. **黄芪** 类圆形或椭圆形厚片。表面黄白色，外层有曲折裂隙，内层有棕色环纹及放射状纹理，中心深黄色，纤维性强，有粉性，周边黄色或浅棕色。气微，味微甜，嚼之有豆腥气味。

9. 白术 不规则厚片。表面灰黄色或灰棕色，切面黄白色至淡棕色，散生棕黄色的点状油室，木部具放射状纹理，烘干者切面角质样，色较深或有裂隙。气清香，味甘、微辛，嚼之略带黏性。

10. 党参 类圆形的厚片。外表皮灰黄色至黄棕色，切面皮部淡黄色至淡棕色，木部淡黄色，有裂隙或放射状纹理。有特殊香气，味微甜。

11. 麻黄 圆柱形短节段。表面黄绿色，粗糙，有细纵棱线。质轻，有韧性，断面中心显红黄色，粉性。气微香，味苦涩。

12. 荆芥 不规则的段。茎呈方柱形，表面淡黄绿色或淡紫红色，被短柔毛，切面类白色，叶多已脱落，穗状轮伞花序。气芳香，味微涩而辛凉。

13. 陈皮 不规则丝状或条状。外表面橙红色或红棕色，有细皱纹和凹下的点状油室；内表面浅黄白色，粗糙，附黄白色或黄棕色筋络状维管。气香，味辛，苦。

14. 瓜蒌皮 丝状片。外表面橙黄色或红黄色，有光泽；内表面淡黄白色，质较软。味淡微酸。

15. 阿胶 呈黑褐色，具光泽，断面光亮，对光照视呈棕色，半透明。质硬脆。气微腥，味微甘。

注意事项

（1）在药材水选时，应严格掌握时间，对其有效成分易溶于水的药材，一般采用“抢水洗”法(快速洗涤药材，缩短药材与水接触时间)，以免损失药效，并及时干燥，防止霉变后降低疗效。根据药材性质，水选可分为洗净、淘洗、浸漂三种方法。

（2）药材软化前，应大小分档，要以少泡多润、药透水尽为软化原则，防止药材“伤水”和成分流失。

（3）软化时注意药材体积、质地、季节等因素的影响：一般体积粗大、质地坚实的药材，冬春季节气温较低时，浸、润时间宜长些；体积细小、质轻者，夏秋季节气温较高时，浸、润时间宜短些。应勤检查，发现问题及时处理。

（4）机器切制应注意检查机器，严格操作程序操作。手工切制时，操作要规范，注意操作安全。

（5）人工干燥应控制好干燥温度和时间，一般饮片以不超过 80℃为宜，含芳香挥发性成分的饮片以不超过 50℃为宜。已干燥的饮片需放凉后再贮存。

思考题

1. 简述常用清除杂质的方法。
2. 简述切制前常用的软化处理方法及适宜加工的药材类型。
3. 简述中药材切制成饮片的目的。
4. 简述中药饮片的切制方法及特点。
5. 简述中药材浸泡对饮片切制的影响。

Chapter 2 Validation Experiment of Chinese Medicine Processing

Experiment 1 Cleaning and cutting

Aims

1.1 To master the basic operation of cleaning of raw Chinese medicines and cutting of decoction pieces, the types and the drying methods of Yinpian.

1.2 To understand the purposes and significance of cleaning of raw Chinese medicines and cutting of Yinpian.

Principles

2.1 The function of cleaning

Remove impurities to be convenient for clinical using and preparations. Separate the different parts of medicines for better effect. Classify crude drugs by size to be easy to cut and process. Remove non-medicinal parts to ensure the accuracy of dosage.

2.2 The function of cutting

Easy to decoct out the active ingredients. Conducive to processing. Beneficial to formulation and preparation. Conductive to dentificate. Convenient for storage.

Contents

3.1 Cleaning selection

It is using selection, sifting, winnowing, washing, picking, kneading, rubbing, brushing, scraping, shearing and other methods to remove impurities and non-medicinal parts.

3.2 Softening

According to the experimental conditions and the characteristics of raw Chinese medicines, the following different methods can be used. The common method of softening are mainly flushing, washing, soaking, rinsing, moistening and so on. The main methods of wet-heat softening include infiltration with decompressed steaming, decompressed maceration, infiltration with simple steaming and baking, etc.

3.3 Cutting

According to the properties of different raw Chinese medicines, manual cutting and machine cutting are used for cutting into extremely thin slices, thin slices, thick slices, sliver, segments, blocks and so on.

3.4 Drying

A temperature-controlled electric oven can be used for drying, the temperature should be controlled at 50~80℃, and the Yinpian should be turned regularly until they are completely dried,remove the drugs, and allow to cool.

Materials

4.1 Experimental apparatuses

Slicing knife, fodder chopper, pressing plate, iron clamp, slicing machine, basin, bamboo basket, scissors, brush, filter, small and medium enamel plate with cover, oven, decompressed steam moistening machine, gas phase replacement infiltration chambers, steamer, etc.

4.2 Experimental materials

Angelicae Sinensis Radix, Arecaesemen, Paeoniae Radix Alba, ChuanXiong Rhizoma, Salviae Miltiorrhizae Radix et Rhizoma, Glycyrrhizae Radix et Rhizoma, Rhei Radix et Rhizoma, Astragali Radix, Atractylodis Macrocephalae Rhizoma, Codonopsis Radix, Ephedrae Herba, Schizonepetae Herba, Citri Reticulatae Pericarpium, Trichosanthis Pericarpium,Asini corii colla.

Methods

5.1 Angelicae Sinensis Radix

Take appropriate amount of the crude Chinese medicines, remove the impurities, wash them, and moisten slightly, then cut them into thin slices and dry at low temperature,allow to cool and sift detritus.

5.2 Arecaesemen

Take appropriate amount of the crude Chinese medicines, remove the impurities, wash them, macerate and moisten them until they are completely soft, then cut them into thin slices and dry, allow to cool and sift detritus.

5.3 Paeoniae Radix Alba

Take appropriate amount of the crude Chinese medicines, remove the impurities, classify crude drugs by size, wash them, macerate moisten them until they are completely soft, then cut them into thin slices and dry, allow to cool and sift detritus.

5.4 ChuanXiong Rhizoma

Take appropriate amount of the crude Chinese medicines, remove the impurities, classify crude drugs by size, wash them, macerate and moisten them until they are completely soft, then cut them into thin slices and dry, allow to cool and sift detritus.

5.5 Salviae Miltiorrhizae Radix et Rhizoma

Take appropriate amount of the crude Chinese medicines, remove the impurities and remnant stems, wash them, and moisten them until they are completely soft, then cut them into thick slices and dry, allow to cool and sift detritus.

5.6 Glycyrrhizae Radix et Rhizoma

Take appropriate amount of the crude Chinese medicines, remove the impurities, wash them, and moisten them until they are completely soft, then cut them into thick slices and dry, allow to cool and sift detritus.

5.7 Rhei Radix et Rhizoma

Take appropriate amount of the crude Chinese medicines, remove the impurities and classify crude drugs by size, wash them, and moisten them until they are completely soft, then cut them into thick slices and dry, allow to cool and sift detritus.

5.8 Astragali Radix

Take appropriate amount of the crude Chinese medicines, remove the impurities, wash them, and moisten them until they are completely soft, then cut them into oblique slices and dry, allow to cool and sift detritus.

5.9 Atractylodis Macrocephalae Rhizoma

Take appropriate amount of the crude Chinese medicines, remove the impurities, wash them, and moisten them until they are completely soft, then cut them into vertical slices and dry, allow to cool and sift detritus.

5.10 Codonopsis Radix

Take appropriate amount of the crude Chinese medicines, remove the impurities, wash them, and moisten them until they are completely soft, then cut them into segments and dry, allow to cool and sift detritus.

5.11 Ephedrae Herba

Take appropriate amount of the crude Chinese medicines, remove the remnant roots, woody stems and impurities, wash quickly, and moisten them slightly, then cut them into segments and dry, allow to cool and sift detritus.

5.12 Schizonepetae Herba

Take appropriate amount of the crude Chinese medicines, remove the impurities, wash quickly, and moisten them slightly, then cut them into segments and dry, allow to cool and sift detritus.

5.13 Citri Reticulatae Pericarpium

Take appropriate amount of the crude Chinese medicines, remove the impurities, spray appropriate amount of water on them and moisten them until they are completely soft, then cut them into marrow slivers and dry them at low temperature, allow to cool and sift detritus.

5.14 Trichosanthis Pericarpium

Take appropriate amount of the crude Chinese medicines, remove the impurities, wash them, and moisten them slightly, then cut them into broad slivers and dry, allow to cool and sift detritus.

5.15 Asini corii colla

Take appropriate amount of donkey-hide Glue picecs, bake them until they are soft and cut into small cubes while hot.

Results

6.1 Angelicae Sinensis Radix

They are like round, oval or irregular thin slices. The appearance is yellow-brown to brown. The cut surface is yellowish-white or light brownish yellow and flat with cracks and a light brown layered ring in the middle, and there are some brown oily points are rich aroma. The flavour is sweet, acrid and slightly bitter.

6.2 Arecae semen

They are a kind of round thin slices. Marble pattern with brown seed coat and white endosperm can be seen on the cut surface. The smell is slight and the flavour is puckery and slightly bitter.

6.3 Paeoniae Radix Alba

They are round thin slices. The surface is smoothy with light brown-red or white color. The cut surface is white or reddish brown, and the cambium ring is obvious. It can be seen the slightly raised veins are arranged radially. The smell is slight and the flavour is slightly bitter and sour.

6.4 ChuanXiong Rhizoma

They are irregular thick slices. The outer skin is yellow-brown with wrinkles. The cut surface is yellow-white or gray-yellow with obvious wavy ring or polygonal texture with scattered yellow-brown oil spots. It is hard. The smell is strong and the flavour is bitter, acrid and slightly sweet.

6.5 Salviae Miltiorrhizae Radix et Rhizoma

They are round or oval thick slices. The outer surface is rough and brownish red or dark brownish red with longitudinal wrinkles. The cut surface is cracked or slightly flat and dense and some cut surface is hard and glossy, and the cortex is brownish red and the xylem is grayish yellow or purple brown with yellow white radial texture. The smell is slight and the favour is slightly bitter and astringent.

6.6 Glycyrrhizae Radix et Rhizoma

They are a round or oval thick slices. The surface is yellow white, and there are obvious brown cambium rings and rays in the middle. Traditionally, it is called "chrysanthemum heart" , and the fiber is powdery. The periphery is brownish red, brown or grayish brown, and rough with longitudinal wrinkles. The smell is slight and the flavour is sweet and slightly bitter.

6.7 Rhei Radix et Rhizoma

They are irregular thick slices or pieces with yellowish brown or yellowish brown with texture in the center, slightly showing cinnabar dots, commonly known as "brocade pattern" . The texture is light. The smell is fragrant and the flavour is bitter and slightly astringent.

6.8 Astragali Radix

They are round or oval thick slices. The surface is yellowish white. There are some zigzag cracks in outer layer and brown ring patterns and radial texture in the inlayer, and the center is dark yellow with rich and powdery fiber, and its periphery is yellow or light brown. The smell is slight and the flavour is slightly sweet with soy smell.

6.9 Atractylodis Macrocephalae Rhizoma

They are irregular thick slices. The surface is grayish yellow or grayish brown and the section is yellowish white to light brown with scattered brownish yellow spot oil chamber. There are some radial texture in xylem. The dried one's cutting surface is hard and glossy and the color is deeper or with cracks. The smell is fragrant and the flavour is sweet and slightly acrid. It is slightly sticky with chewing.

6.10 Codonopsis Radix

They are round thick slices. The appearance is grayish yellow to yellowish brown. It is pale yellow to light brown at the edge of the cutting surface and the xylem is yellowish with cracks or radial texture. The smell is special and the flavour is slightly sweet.

6.11 Ephedrae Herba

They are cylindrical short segments. The surface is yellowish green and rough with fine vertical ridges. The texture is light and tough and it is reddish yellow in the center of fraction surface and powdery. The smell is slight and the flavour is bitter and astringent.

6.12 Schizonepetae Herba

It is irregular segments. The stem is square columnar and the surface is pale yellowish green or lavender-red with pubescent. The cutting surface is white. Most leaves fallen off. It is spicate cyme. The smell is fragrant and the flavour is slightly astringent , acrid and cool.

6.13 Citri Reticulatae Pericarpium

They are irregular slivers and strips. The outer surface is orange red or reddish brown with fine wrinkles and sunken dot oil chambers. The inner surface is yellow white and rough with yellow white or yellow brown tendon-like vascular. The smell is fragrant and the flavour is acrid and bitter.

6.14 Trichosanthis Pericarpium

They are slivers. The outer surface is orange yellow or red yellow and shiny. The inner surface is pale yellow white, it has soft texture. The flavour is light and slightly sour.

6.15 Asini corii colla

They are dark brown with luster and the fraction surface is bright. It is brown and translucent when exposed to light. The texture is hard and crisp. The smell is slightly fishy and the flavour is slightly sweet.

Notes

7.1 During washing of raw Chinese medicines, it should be strict to control the time and wash the raw Chinese medicines quickly to shorten the washing time, so as to avoid losing the efficacy, then dry them in time to prevent mildewing and reducing efficacy. According to the nature of raw Chinese medicines, it is usually divided into three methods, washing, elutriation and rinsing.

7.2 To classify crude drugs by size before softening. The principle of softening is less soaking and more moisteming to prevent losing the ingredients of raw Chinese medicines.

7.3 Pay attention to the influence of the sizes, the texture and the seasons of raw Chinese medicines and other factors when softening. Generally, it will take long time to soften the raw Chinese medicines which are large, hard texture when they are softened at the low temperature in winter and spring. On the contrary, it will takes short time to soften the raw Chinese medicines which is small, soft texture when they are softened at a higher temperature in summer and fall. Check frequently and deal with problems in time.

7.4 Machine cutting should pay attention to check the machine and strictly operate the procedures. When cutting by hand, the operation should be standardized and pay attention to the safety of operation.

7.5 The drying temperature and time of artificial drying should be well controlled. Generally, the temperature should not exceed 80℃, and the temperature of slices containing aromatic volatile components should not exceed 50℃. The dried slices should be cooled before storage.

Questions

8.1 Briefly describe the common methods for removing impurities.

8.2 Briefly describe the softening methods commonly used before cutting and the types of raw Chinese medicines suitable for processing.

8.3 Briefly describe the purposes of raw Chinese medicines cutting into decoction pieces.

8.4 Briefly describe the cutting methods and characteristics of decoction pieces.

8.5 Briefly describe the effects of soaking raw Chinese medicines on the cutting of slices.

PPT

实验二　清炒法

实验目的

1. **掌握**　炒黄、炒焦、炒炭的基本操作方法、注意事项及成品质量。
2. **了解**　清炒法的目的和意义。

实验原理

1. **增强疗效**　如酸枣仁、王不留行、焦麦芽。
2. **降低毒性或副作用**　如牵牛子、莱菔子。
3. **缓和药性**　如葶苈子、川楝子。
4. **增强或产生止血作用**　如大蓟、荆芥。
5. **保存疗效，利于贮存**　如槐米、芥子。

实验内容

1. **炒黄**　酸枣仁、王不留行、芥子、苏子、莱菔子、牵牛子、苍耳子、白果仁。
2. **炒焦**　山楂、槟榔、麦芽、栀子、神曲。
3. **炒炭**　蒲黄、地榆、槐米、荆芥、干姜、乌梅。

实验器具和材料

1. **实验器具**　炒锅、炒药铲、瓷盘或不锈钢盘、筛子、温度计、天平、喷壶等。

2. **实验材料**　酸枣仁、王不留行、芥子、苏子、莱菔子、牵牛子、苍耳子、白果仁、山楂、槟榔、麦芽、栀子、神曲、蒲黄、地榆、槐米、荆芥、干姜、乌梅。

实验方法

炒王不留行

炒莱菔子

1. 炒黄

（1）炒酸枣仁　取净酸枣仁适量，置热锅内，用文火炒至鼓起微有爆裂声，颜色微变深，断面淡黄色，并逸出香气时，出锅放凉，即得。

（2）炒王不留行　取净王不留行适量，置热锅内，用中火加热，不断翻炒至大部分爆成白花，迅速出锅放凉，即得。

（3）炒芥子　取净芥子适量，置热锅内，用文火加热，炒至颜色加深，有爆鸣声，断面浅黄色，有香气逸出时即可，取出放凉，即得。

（4）炒苏子　取净苏子适量，置热锅内，用文火加热，炒至表面颜色加深，断面浅黄色，有香气逸出时即可，取出放凉，即得。

（5）炒莱菔子　取净莱菔子适量，置热锅内，用文火加热，炒至鼓起，爆鸣声减弱，手捻易碎，断面浅黄色，有香气逸出时即可，取出放凉，即得。

（6）炒牵牛子　取净牵牛子适量，置热锅内，用中火加热，炒至稍鼓起，爆裂声减弱时，取出放凉，即得。

（7）炒苍耳子　取净苍耳子适量，置热锅内，用中火加热，炒至黄褐色时，取出，放凉，去刺，筛净，放凉，即得。

（8）炒白果仁　取净白果仁适量，置热锅内，用文火加热，炒至深黄色，并有香气逸出时，取出放凉，即得。

2. 炒焦

（1）焦山楂　取净山楂适量，置热锅内，用中火加热，不断翻炒至表面焦褐色、内部焦黄色、有焦香气溢出时，取出放凉，筛去碎屑，即得。

（2）焦槟榔　取净槟榔片适量，置热锅内，用中火加热，不断翻炒至焦黄色、具焦斑，取出放凉，筛去碎屑，即得。

（3）焦麦芽　取净麦芽适量，置热锅内，用中火加热，不断翻动，炒至表面焦褐色、鼓起，并有焦香气时，取出放凉，筛去碎屑，即得。

（4）焦栀子　取净栀子适量，碾碎，置热锅内，用中火炒至焦黄色，具焦香气，取出放凉，筛去灰屑，即得。

（5）焦神曲　取净神曲适量，置热锅内，用文火加热，不断翻动，炒至表面呈焦褐色、内部微黄色、有焦香气时，取出放凉，筛去碎屑，即得。

3. 炒炭

（1）蒲黄炭　取净蒲黄适量，置热锅内，用中火加热，不断翻炒至焦褐色，喷淋少量清水，灭尽火星，略炒干，取出，摊晾，干燥，即得。

（2）地榆炭　取净地榆片适量，置热锅内，用武火加热，不断翻炒至外表焦黑色、内部棕褐色，喷淋清水灭尽火星，略炒至干，取出放凉，筛去碎屑，即得。

炒地榆炭

（3）槐米炭　取净槐米适量，置热锅内，用中火加热，不断翻炒至黑褐色，发现火星时，可喷淋适量清水熄灭，炒干，取出放凉，筛去灰屑，即得。

（4）荆芥炭　取净荆芥段适量，置热锅内，用武火加热，不断翻炒至黑褐色，喷淋少许清水，灭尽火星，略炒干，取出，摊晾，干燥，筛去灰屑，即得。

（5）姜炭　取干姜块适量，置炒制容器内，用武火加热，炒至表面黑色、内部棕褐色，喷淋少许清水，灭尽火星，文火炒干，取出，放凉，筛去碎屑，即得。

（6）乌梅炭　取净乌梅或乌梅肉适量，置炒制容器内，用武火加热，不断翻动，至皮肉发泡、表面焦黑色，取出，放凉，筛去碎屑。

实验结果

1. 炒黄

（1）炒酸枣仁　形如酸枣仁，表面微鼓起，微具焦斑，略有焦香气，味淡。

（2）炒王不留行　类球形爆花状，表面白色，质松脆。

（3）炒芥子　形如芥子，表面淡黄色至深黄色（炒白芥子）或深黄色至棕褐色（炒黄芥子），偶有焦斑，有香辣气。

（4）炒苏子　形如紫苏子，表面灰褐色，有细裂口，有焦香气。

（5）炒莱菔子　形如莱菔子，表面微鼓起，色泽加深，质酥脆，气微香。

（6）炒牵牛子　形如牵牛子，表面黑褐色或黄棕色，稍鼓起，微具香气。

（7）炒苍耳子　形如苍耳子，表面黄褐色，有刺痕，微有香气。

（8）炒白果仁　形如白果仁，表面黄色，有火色斑点，气香。

2. 炒焦

（1）焦山楂　表面焦褐色，内部黄褐色，有焦香气。

（2）焦槟榔　形如槟榔，表面焦黄色。

（3）焦麦芽　形如麦芽，表面焦褐色，有焦斑，有焦香气，味微苦。

（4）焦栀子　形如栀子或碎块状，表面焦褐色或焦黑色，味微酸而苦。

（5）焦神曲　表面焦黄色，内为微黄色，有焦香气。

3. 炒炭

（1）蒲黄炭　形如蒲黄，表面棕褐色或黑褐色，具焦香气，味微苦、涩。

（2）地榆炭　形如地榆片，表面焦黑色，内部棕褐色，具焦香气，味微苦涩。

（3）槐米炭　形如槐米，表面焦褐色，质轻，味涩。

（4）荆芥炭　表面黑褐色，内部焦褐色，略具焦香气，味苦而辛。

（5）姜炭　表面焦黑色，内部棕褐色，体轻，质松脆，味微苦，微辣。

（6）乌梅炭　皮肉鼓起，表面呈焦黑色，味酸略有苦味。

注意事项

1. 炒前药物应大小分档，分次炒制，避免炒制生熟不均。

2. 炒时应选择适当火力，并控制加热时间，炒黄一般用文火，炒焦一般用中火，炒炭一般用武火。

3. 操作时，先预热锅，勤翻动，避免生熟不匀的现象。

4. 炒黄的中药要防止焦化，炒焦的中药要防止炭化，炒炭的中药要防止灰化。

5. 炒炭需存性，火候适当，产生火星喷少量清水，质地坚实者宜用武火，质地疏松者可用中火。

6. 炒焦、炒炭要注意防火，需冷透后收贮，炭药宜用耐火容器盛装，防止复燃。

思考题

1. 简述炒黄、炒焦、炒炭三种炒制方法的异同点及注意事项。
2. 简述炒黄、炒焦、炒炭的火候判断标准。
3. 简述火力与火候的含义与要点。
4. 简述实验中各药物炮制作用。

Experiment 2 Simple stir-baking

Aims

1.1 To master the basic operation, notes and the finished product quality of stir-baking until yellowish, stir-baking until burnt-brown or burnet-black, carbonizing by stir-baking.

1.2 To understand the aims and significance of simple stir-baking.

Principles

2.1 To enhance curative effect

For example, Ziziphi Spinosae Semen, Vaccariae Semen , Coke Hordei Fructus Germinatus.

2.2 To reduce toxicity or side effects

For example, Pharbitidis Semen, Raphani Semen.

2.3 Mitigate drug effect

For example, Descurainiae semen lepidii semen, Toosendan Fructus.

2.4 To enhance or produce hemostatic effects

For example, Cirsii Japonici Herba , Schizonepetae Herba.

2.5 To preserve efficacy, conducive to storage

For example, Sophoraeflos Immaturu ,Sinapis semen.

Contents

3.1 Stir-baking until yellowish

Ziziphi Spinosae Semen, Vaccariae Semen, Sinapis semen, Perillae Fructus, Raphani Semen, Pharbitidis Semen, Xanthii Fructus, Ginkgo Semrn.

3.2 Stir-baking until burnt-brown or burnt-black

Crataegi Fructus, Arecaesemen, Hordei Fructus Germinatus, Gardeniae Fructus, Massa Fermentata.

3.3 Stir-baking until carbonized

Typhaepollen, Sanguisorbae Radix, Sophoraeflos Immaturus, Schizonepetae Herba, Zingiberis Rhizoma, Mume Fructus.

Materials

4.1 Experimental apparatuses

Pot, shovel, filter, porcelain or stainless steel plate, thermometer, balance, etc.

4.2 Experimental materials

Ziziphi Spinosae Semen, Vaccariae Semen, Sinapis semen, Perillae Fructus, Raphani Semen, Pharbitidis Semen, Xanthii Fructus, Ginkgo Semrn, Crataegi Fructus, Arecaesemen, Hordei Fructus Germinatus, Gardeniae Fructus, Massa Fermentata, Typhaepollen, Sanguisorbae Radix, Sophoraeflos

Immaturus, Schizonepetae Herba, Zingiberis Rhizoma, Mume Fructus.

Methods

5.1 Stir-baking until yellowish

5.1.1 Stir-baking Ziziphi Spinosae Semen

Put the appropriate amount of clean Ziziphi Spinosae Semen into a hot pot and heat on a gentle fire until the surfaces expanded with a slight crackle, and the fracture surface is light yellow with aroma, then take them out and allow to cool.

5.1.2 Stir-baking Vaccariae Semen

Put the appropriate amount of clean Vaccariae Semen into a hot pot and heat on a medium fire until most of them burst into popcorn, then quickly take them out and allow to cool.

5.1.3 Stir-baking Sinapis semen

Put the appropriate amount of clean Sinapis semen into a hot pot and heat on a gentle fire until the color of the surfaces deepen, and the fracture surface is light yellow, with crackle and aroma, then take them out and allow to cool.

5.1.4 Stir-baking Perillae Fructus

Put the appropriate amount of clean Perillae Fructus into a hot pot and heat on a gentle fire until the color of the surfaces deepen, and the fracture surface is light yellow with aroma, then take them out and allow to cool.

5.1.5 Stir-bakeing Raphani Semen

Put the appropriate amount of clean Raphani Semen into a hot pot and heat on a gentle fire until the surface expanded, the crackle is weakened, it's easy to break by hand, and the fracture surface is light yellow with aroma, then take them out and allow to cool.

5.1.6 Stir-baking Pharbitidis Semen

Put the appropriate amount of clean Pharbitidis Semen into a hot pot and heat on a medium fire until the surfaces expanded slightly, and the crackle is weakened, then take them out and allow to cool.

5.1.7 Stir-baking Xanthii Fructus

Put the appropriate amount of clean Xanthii Fructus into a hot pot and stir-fry them on a medium fire until the surfaces become yellow brown, take them out, allow to cool, remove the thorns and sift them cleanly.

5.1.8 Stir-frying Ginkgo Semrn

Put the appropriate amount of clean Ginkgo Semrn into a hot pot and heat on a gentle fire until the surfaces become deep yellow with aroma, then take them out and allow to cool.

5.2 Stir-baking until burnt-brown or burnt-black

5.2.1 Stir-baking Crataegi Fructus until burnt-brown

Put the appropriate amount of clean crude Chinese medicines into a hot pot and heat on a medium fire till the surfaces become burnt brown and the inside is burnt yellow with burnt aroma, then take them out, allow to cool and sift the detritus.

5.2.2 Stir-baking Arecaesemen until burnt-brown

Put the appropriate amount of clean slices into a hot pot and heat on a medium fire till the surfaces become burnt yellow with burnt spots, then take them out, allow to cool and sift the detritus.

5.2.3 Stir-baking Hordei Fructus Germinatus until burnt-brown

Put the appropriate amount of clean Hordei Fructus Germinatus into a hot pot and heat on a medium fire till the surfaces become brown, the drugs expanded crisply and have a burning aroma, then take them out, allow to cool and sift the detritus.

5.2.4 Stir-baking Gardeniae Fructus until burnt-brown

Put the appropriate amount of clean Gardeniae Fructus into a hot pot and heat on a medium fire till the surfaces become burnt yellow with burnt aroma, then take them out, allow to cool and sift the dust and detritus.

5.2.5 Stir-baking Massa Fermentata until burnt-brown

Put the appropriate amount of clean Massa Fermentata into a hot pot and heat on a gentle fire till the surfaces become burnt brown and the inner parts become light yellow with burnt aroma, then take them out, allow to cool and sift the detritus.

5.3 Carbonizing by stir-baking

5.3.1 Stir-baking Typhaepollen until carbonized

Put the appropriate amount of clean Typhaepollen into a hot pot and heat on a medium fire till the surface becomes burnt brown. Spray a little water to extinguish the sparks. heat slight dry, take them out, spread and cool and dry.

5.3.2 Stir-baking Sanguisorbae Radix until carbonized

Put the appropriate amount of clean Sanguisorbae Radix into a hot pot and heat on a strong fire until the surfaces become brownish-black , and the inner parts become dark brown. Spray a little water to extinguish any spark. Take them out, allow to cool and sift the detritus.

5.3.3 Stir-baking Sophoraeflos Immaturus until carbonized

Put the appropriate amount of clean Sophoraeflos Immaturus into a hot pot and heat on a medium fire till the surfaces become black brown, spray a little water to extinguish the sparks. Heat slight dry, take them out,allow to cool and sift the detritus.

5.3.4 Stir-baking Schizonepetae Herba until carbonized

Put the appropriate amount of clean Schizonepetae Herba into a hot pot and heat on a strong fire till the surfaces become black brown, spray a little water to extinguish the sparks, heat slight dry, take them out, spread and cool and dry, and sift the detritus.

5.3.5 Stir-baking Zingiberis Rhizoma until carbonized

Put the appropriate amount of Zingiberis Rhizoma into the frying container and heat on a gentle fire till the surfaces become black and the inner parts become brown, spray a little water to extinguish the sparks, heat slight dry, take them out, allow to cool and sift the detritus.

5.3.6 Stir-baking Mume Fructus until carbonized

Put the appropriate amount of Mume Fructus or flesh into the container and heat on a strong fire till the surfaces become burnt black, and the flesh expanded, then take them out, allow to cool, sift the detritus.

Results

6.1 Stir-baking until yellowish

6.1.1 Stir-baking Ziziphi Spinosae Semen

It is shaped like Ziziphi Spinosae Semen. The surface expanded slightly with slight burnt spots. The smell is burnt aroma and the flavour is light.

6.1.2 Stir-baking Vaccariae Semen

It is shaped like spherical popcorn.The surface is white and the texture is loose and crisp.

6.1.3 Stir-baking Sinapis semen

It is shaped like Sinapis semen. The surface is light yellow or deep yellow or brown with occasional burnt spots. The flavour is spicy.

6.1.4 Stir-baking Perillae Fructus

It is shaped like Perillae Fructus. The surface is grayish brown with fine cracks and burnt aroma.

6.1.5 Stir-bakeing Raphani Semen

It is shaped like Raphani Semen. The surface slightly expanded and the color deepened and the texture is crisp.The smell is slight aroma.

6.1.6 Stir-baking Pharbitidis Semen

It is shaped like Pharbitidis Semen. The surface is black brown or yellow brown with slight expandged seed coat and slight aroma.

6.1.7 Stir-baking Xanthii Fructus

It is shaped like Xanthii Fructus. The surface is yellow brown with thorns. The smell is slight aroma.

6.1.8 Stir-frying Ginkgo Semrn

It is shaped like Ginkgo Semrn. The surface is yellow with fire-colored spots. The smell is aroma.

6.2 Stir-baking until burnt-brown or burnt-black

6.2.1 Stir-baking Crataegi Fructus until burnt-brown

The surface is burnt brown.The inner part is yellow brown with burnt aroma.

6.2.2 Stir-baking Arecaesemen until burnt-brown

It is shaped like Arecaesemen. The surface is burnt yellow.

6.2.3 Stir-baking Hordei Fructus Germinatus until burnt-brown

It is shaped like Hordei Fructus Germinatus. The surface is burnt brown with burnt spots and burnt aroma. The flavouris slight bitter.

6.2.4 Stir-baking Gardeniae Fructus until burnt-brown

It is shaped like Gardeniae Fructus or pieces. The surface is burnt brown or burnt black.The flavour is slight sour and bitter.

6.2.5 Stir-baking Massa Fermentata until burnt-brown

The surface is burnt yellow and the inner part is light yellow with burnt aroma.

6.3 Carbonizing by stir-baking

6.3.1 Stir-baking Typhaepollen until carbonized

It is shaped like Typhaepollen. The surface is brown or black brown with burnt aroma. The flavour is slight bitter and astringent.

6.3.2 Stir-baking Sanguisorbae Radix until carbonized

It is shaped like Sanguisorbae Radix. The surface is burnt black and the inner part is black brown with burnt aroma. The flavour is slight bitter and astringent.

6.3.3 Stir-baking Sophoraeflos Immaturus until carbonized

It is shaped like Sophoraeflos Immaturus. The surface is burnt brown.The texture is light and the flavour is astringent.

6.3.4 Stir-baking Schizonepetae Herba until carbonized

The surface is black brown and the inner part is burnt brown with burnt aroma. The flavour is slight bitter and acrid.

6.3.5 Stir-baking Schizonepetae Herba until carbonized

The surface is burnt black and the inner part is black brown.The texture is loose and crisp. The flavour is slight bitter and spicy.

6.3.6 Stir-baking Mume Fructus until carbonized

The surface is burnt black with the expanded flesh. The flavour is slight sour and bitter.

Notes

7.1 Before stir-baking, the raw Chinese medicines should be classify crude drugs by size, and stir-bake them separately. This is can avoid stir-bakeing unevenly.

7.2 Proper firepower should be selected and heating time should be well controlled when stir-baking. Generally, gentle fire is used for stir-baking until yellowish, medium fire is used for stir-baking until burnt brown or burnt black, and strong fire is used for carbonizing by stir-baking.

7.3 During operation, preheat a hot pot firstly and stir it frequently to avoid the unevenness of stir-frying.

7.4 The Chinese medicines which are needed stir-baked till yellow should be prevented from becoming burnt brown or burnt black, the Chinese medicines which are needed stir-bake till burnt brow or burnt black should be prevented from carbonizing, and the Chinese medicines which are needed carbonized should be prevented from ashing.

7.5 The carbonized Chinese medicines should retain the properties, the fire is appropriate. Spray a little water to extinguish the sparks. Hard-textured drugs are suitable for being processed on a strong fire and loose-textured drugs are suitable for being processed on a medium fire.

7.6 Attention shall be paid to fire prevention when stir-bake until burnt brown or burnt black or carbonized. The processed Chinese medicines shall be stored after being cooled thoroughly. The carbonized drugs shall be filled in fire-resistant containers to prevent reignition.

Questions

8.1 Briefly describe the precautions, similarities and differences of the three methods of stir-baking until yellowish, burnt brown or burnt black, carbonized.

8.2 Briefly describe the judgmental criterions of firepower of stir-baking until yellowish, burnt brown or burnt black, carbonized.

8.3 Briefly describe the meanings and key points of firepower and the heat setting.

8.4 Briefly describe the processing effects of the raw Chinese medicines in the experiment.

PPT

实验三　加固体辅料炒

实验目的

1. **掌握**　麸炒、米炒、砂炒、土炒、蛤粉炒、滑石粉炒的操作方法、注意事项及成品质量。

2. **了解**　加固体辅料炒的目的和意义。

实验原理

1. **麸炒的作用**　①增强疗效，如山药、白术。②缓和药性，如枳实、苍术。③矫臭矫味，如僵蚕。

2. **米炒的作用**　①增强健脾止泻作用，如党参。②降低毒性和刺激性，如斑蝥、红娘子。③矫正不良气味，指示炮制程度，如斑蝥。

3. **土炒的作用**　增强补脾止泻的作用，如山药、白术。

4. **砂炒的作用**　①增强疗效，便于调剂和制剂，如狗脊、穿山甲、鳖甲。②降低毒性，如马钱子。③便于去毛，如骨碎补。④矫臭矫味，如鸡内金。

5. **蛤粉炒的作用**　①使药物质地酥脆，便于制剂和调剂，如阿胶、鹿角胶。②降低药物的滋腻之性，矫正不良气味，如阿胶、鹿角胶。③增强功效，如阿胶。

6. **滑石粉炒的作用**　①使药物质地酥脆，便于粉碎和煎煮，如水蛭。②降低毒性及矫正不良气味，如水蛭、刺猬皮。

实验内容

1. **麸炒**　白术、枳壳、苍术、僵蚕。

2. **米炒**　斑蝥、党参。

3. **土炒**　山药。

4. **砂炒**　马钱子、穿山甲、鸡内金、鳖甲。

5. **蛤粉炒**　阿胶。

6. **滑石粉炒**　刺猬皮、水蛭。

实验器具和材料

1. **实验器具**　炒锅、炒药铲、瓷盘或不锈钢盘、筛子、温度计、天平等。

2. **实验材料**　白术、枳壳、苍术、僵蚕，斑蝥、党参、山药、马钱子、穿山甲、鸡内金、鳖甲、阿胶、刺猬皮、水蛭。

实验方法

1. **麸炒**

（1）白术　先将麦麸撒于热锅内，用中火加热，至冒烟时，投入一定量的白术片，翻炒至表面深黄色，有香气逸出时，取出，筛去麸皮，放凉，即得。每 100kg 白术片，用麦麸 10kg。

（2）枳壳　先将麦麸撒于热锅内，用中火加热，至冒烟时投入一定量的枳壳片，迅速翻动，炒至枳壳表面深黄色时，取出。筛去麸皮，放凉，即得。每 100kg 枳壳片，用麦麸 10kg。

（3）苍术　先将麦麸撒于热锅内，用中火加热，至冒烟时，投入一定量的苍术片，翻炒至表面深黄色，取出。筛去麸皮，放凉，即得。每 100kg 苍术片，用麦麸 10kg。

（4）僵蚕　先将麦麸撒于热锅内，用中火加热，至冒烟时，投入一定量的净僵蚕，翻炒至表面黄色，取出。筛去麸皮，放凉，即得。每 100kg 僵蚕，用麦麸 10kg。

2. 米炒

（1）斑蝥　取一定量的净斑蝥与米置热锅内，用中火加热，翻炒至米呈黄褐色，取出。筛去米粒，放凉。或取湿米置炒制容器内，使其均匀地平铺一层，用中火加热至米黏住锅底并起烟时，投入一定量的净斑蝥，在米上轻轻翻动，炒至斑蝥变色、米的上表面黄褐色时，取出，筛去焦米，放凉。每 100kg 斑蝥，用大米 20kg。

（2）党参　将大米置热锅内，用中火加热，至大米冒烟时，投入一定量的党参片，翻炒至大米呈焦褐色，党参呈老黄色时，取出。筛去米、放凉。称重。每 100kg 党参片（段），用大米 20kg。

米炒党参

3. 土炒

山药　先将伏龙肝粉（或赤石脂粉）置热锅内，用中火加热，至土粉轻松灵活状态时，投入一定量的山药片，不断翻炒，至山药挂土色，表面显土黄色，并透出山药之固有香气时，取出。筛去土，放凉。称重。每 100kg 山药，用土粉 30kg。

4. 砂炒

（1）马钱子　将净砂置热锅内，用武火加热，至滑利容易翻动时，投入一定量的马钱子，不断翻炒，至外表呈棕褐色或深褐色、内部红褐色、鼓起小泡时，取出。筛去砂，放凉。称重。

（2）穿山甲　将净砂置热锅内，用武火加热，至滑利容易翻动时，倒入一定量的大小一致的穿山甲片，不断翻炒，至鼓起、表面呈金黄色、边缘向内卷曲时，取出。筛去砂子，及时倒入醋中，搅拌，稍浸，捞出，干燥。称重。每 100kg 穿山甲，用米醋 30kg。

（3）鸡内金　将净砂置热锅内，用中火加热，至滑利容易翻动时，倒入一定量的大小一致的鸡内金，不断翻炒，至鼓起、卷曲、表面金黄色时，立即取出。筛去砂，放凉。称重。

（4）鳖甲　将净砂置热锅内，用武火加热，至滑利容易翻动时，倒入一定量的大小一致的鳖甲片，不断翻炒，至酥脆、表面呈深黄色，取出。筛去砂子，及时倒入醋中，搅拌，稍浸，捞出，干燥。称重。每 100kg 鳖甲，用米醋 20kg。

砂炒醋淬鳖鱼

5. 蛤粉炒

阿胶　先将胶块烘软，切成小胶丁备用。取蛤粉置热锅内，用中火加热至灵活状态，放入一定量的阿胶丁，不断翻埋，烫至阿胶丁鼓起呈圆球形，内无溏心，颜色由乌黑转为深黄色，表面附着一层薄薄的蛤粉时，迅速取出。筛去蛤粉，放凉。称重。每 100kg 阿胶，用蛤粉 40kg。

蛤粉炒阿胶

6. 滑石粉炒

（1）刺猬皮　先将滑石粉置热锅内，用中火加热至灵活状态，投入一定量的净刺猬皮块，炒至焦黄色、鼓起、皮卷曲、刺尖秃时取出。筛去滑石粉，放凉。称重。每 100kg 刺猬皮，用滑石粉 40kg。

（2）水蛭　先将滑石粉置热锅，用中火加热至灵活状态，倒入一定量的净水蛭段，勤翻炒至微鼓起，呈黄棕色时取出。筛去滑石粉，放凉。称重。每 100kg 水蛭，用滑石粉 40kg。

实验结果

1. 麸炒

（1）白术　形如白术，表面黄棕色，偶见焦斑，略有焦香气。

（2）枳壳　形如枳壳片。表色较深，偶有焦斑。

（3）苍术　表面深黄色，散有多数棕褐色油室。有焦香气。

（4）僵蚕　表面黄色，偶有焦黄斑，腥气减弱。

2. 米炒

（1）斑蝥　形同斑蝥，微挂火色，显光泽，臭味轻微。

（2）党参　表面深黄色，偶有焦斑。

3. 土炒

山药　本品表面轻挂薄土，呈土黄色，无焦黑斑和焦苦味。具土香气。

4. 砂炒

（1）马钱子　本品表面呈深褐色或棕褐色，击之易碎，其内面鼓起小泡。具苦香味。

（2）穿山甲　本品膨胀鼓起，边缘向内卷曲，表面金黄色，质脆。略有醋气。

（3）鸡内金　本品膨胀鼓起，表面金黄色，质脆，具焦香气。

（4）鳖甲　本品深黄色，质酥脆，略具醋气。

5. 蛤粉炒

阿胶　本品呈类圆球形，质松泡，外表灰白色或灰褐色，内部呈蜂窝状，气微香，味微甘。

6. 滑石粉炒

（1）刺猬皮　质地发泡，鼓起，黄色，刺体膨胀，刺尖秃，易折断，边缘皮毛脱落，呈焦黄色，皮部边缘向内卷曲，微有腥臭气味。

（2）水蛭　不规则扁块状或扁圆柱形，略鼓起，表面棕黄色至黑褐色，附有少量白色滑石粉。断面松泡，灰白色至焦黄色。气微腥。

注意事项

1. 麸炒、土炒、米炒、蛤粉炒、滑石粉炒一般用中火，砂炒一般用武火。操作时翻动要勤，成品出锅要快，并立即筛去辅料。有需醋浸淬的药物，应趁热浸淬、干燥。

2. 麸炒药物火力可稍大，麦麸要均匀撒布热锅中，待起烟投药。借麸皮之烟熏使药物变色，但火力过大，则麸皮迅速焦黑，不产生浓烟而达不到麸炒的目的。土炒、蛤粉炒、滑石粉炒、砂炒时，应先将辅料加热至灵活状态再投入药物翻炒。

3. 米炒火力不宜过大，温度过高使饮片烫焦，影响质量。

4. 阿胶丁一般边长以 8~10mm 为宜，大了不易透心，会成溏心，过小易被烫焦，二者均影响质量。

5. 炒过毒剧药物的辅料，不得再用于炒制其他药物，也不得乱倒。

6. 炮制斑蝥时，应注意劳动保护，操作人员应戴眼镜、口罩，以保护眼、鼻黏膜免受其损伤。工作完毕，用冷水清洗裸露部分，不宜用热水洗。炒制后的焦米要及时妥善处理，以免人畜误食，发生中毒。

思考题

1. 简述加固体辅料炒的炮制目的。
2. 简述加辅料炒温度对药物有何影响。
3. 简述砂烫与土炒的区别。
4. 简述实验中各药物的炮制作用。

Experiment 3 Stir-baking with solid excipients

Aims

1.1 To master the operation methods, precautions and product quality of stir-baking with bran, rice, sand, soil, powdered clam-shell and talc.

1.2 To understand the purpose and significance of stir-baking with solid excipients.

Principles

2.1 The role of stir-baking with bran

A. To enhance the curative effect, such as Dioscoreae Rhizoma and Atractylodis Macrocephalae Rhizoma, etc. B. To mitigate drug effect, such as Aurantii Fructus Immaturus and Atractylodis Rhizoma, etc. C. To neutralize the bad odor, such as Bombyx Batryticatus, etc.

2.2 The role of stir-baking with rice

A. To enhance the tonifying spleen and anti-diarrheal function, such as Codonopsis Radix, etc. B. To reduce toxicity and irritation, such as Mylabris and Huechys, etc. C. To correct the bad smell and indicate the degree of processing, such as Mylabris, etc.

2.3 The role of stir-baking with soil

To enhance the tonifying spleen and anti-diarrheal function, such as Dioscoreae Rhizoma and Atractylodis Macrocephalae Rhizoma, etc.

2.4 The role of stir-baking with sand

A. To enhance the curative effect and be convenient for dispensing and preparing, such as Cibotii Rhizoma, Manis Squama and Trionycis Carapax, etc. B. To reduce toxicity, such as Strychni Semen, etc. C. To easy to remove down the fluff, such as Drynariae Rhizoma, etc. D. To neutralize the bad odor, such as Galli Gigerii Endothelium Corneum, etc.

2.5 The role of stir-baking with powdered clam-shell

A. To make the drugs expanded crisply and be convenient for dispensing and preparing, such as Asini Corii Colla and Cervi Cornus Colla, etc. B. To reduce the greasy nature of drugs and correct the bad smell, such as Asini Corii Colla and Cervi Cornus Colla, etc. C. To enhance the curative effect, such as Asini Corii Colla, etc.

2.6 The role of stir-baking with talc

A. To make the drugs expanded crisply and easy to smash and boil, such as Hirudo, etc. B. To reduce toxicity and correct the bad smell, such as Hirudo and Cutis Erinacei, etc.

Contents

3.1 Stir-baking with bran

Atractylodis Macrocephalae Rhizoma, Aurantii Fructus, Atractylodis Rhizoma, Bombyx Batryticatus.

3.2 Stir-baking with rice

Mylabris, Codonopsis Radix.

3.3 Stir-baking with soil

Dioscoreae Rhizoma.

3.4 Stir-baking with sand

Strychni Semen, Manis Squama, Galli Gigerii Endothelium Corneum, Trionycis Carapax.

3.5 Stir-baking with powdered clam-shell

Asini Corii Colla.

3.6 Stir-baking with talc

Cutis Erinacei, Hirudo.

Materials

4.1 Experimental apparatuses

Wok, truner, enameled tray/stainless steel tray, sieve, thermometer, electronic scale, etc.

4.2 Experimental materials

Atractylodis Macrocephalae Rhizoma, Aurantii Fructus, Atractylodis Rhizoma, Bombyx Batryticatus, Mylabris, Codonopsis Radix, Dioscoreae Rhizoma, Strychni Semen, Manis Squama, Galli Gigerii Endothelium Corneum, Trionycis Carapax, Asini Corii Colla, Cutis Erinacei, Hirudo.

Methods

5.1 Stir-baking with bran

5.1.1 Atractylodis Macrocephalae Rhizoma

Put bran in a hot pot and heat on a medium fire until the bran smokes. Put the clean crude drugs into the pot, stir quickly until the surface of crude drugs turns deep yellow, take them out, remove the bran by sifting, and allow to cool. Use 10kg of bran for each 100kg of the slices of Atractylodis Macrocephalae Rhizoma.

5.1.2 Aurantii Fructus

Put bran in a hot pot and heat on a medium fire until the bran smokes. Put the clean crude drugs into the pot, stir quickly until the surface of crude drugs turns deep yellow, take them out, remove the bran by sifting, and allow to cool. Use 10kg of bran for each 100kg of the slices of Aurantii Fructus.

5.1.3 Atractylodis Rhizoma

Put bran in a hot pot and heat on a medium fire until the bran smokes. Put the clean crude drugs into the pot, stir quickly until the surface of crude drugs turns deep yellow, take them out, remove the bran by sifting, and allow to cool. Use 10kg of bran for each 100kg of the slices of Atractylodis Rhizoma.

5.1.4 Bombyx Batryticatus

Put bran in a hot pot and heat on a medium fire until the bran smokes. Put the clean crude drugs into the pot, stir quickly until the surface of crude drugs turns deep yellow, take them out, remove the bran by sifting, and allow to cool. Use 10kg of bran for each 100kg of the slices of Bombyx Batryticatus.

5.2 Stir-baking with rice

5.2.1 Mylabris

Put the clean crude drugs and rice in a hot pot, heat on a medium fire, stir quickly until the surface of rice turns tan, take them out, remove the rice by sifting, and allow to cool. Another way, put the wet rice in a hot pot and heat on a medium fire until the rice sticks to the bottom of the pan and starts to smoke. Put the clean crude drugs on the rice, stir lightly until the color of crude drugs changes and the upper surface turns tawny, take them out, remove the bran by sifting, and allow to cool. Use 20kg of rice for each 100kg of the clean Mylabris.

5.2.2 Codonopsis Radix

Put the rice in a hot pot and heat on a medium fire until the rice smokes. Add the slices of Codonopsis Radix, stir quickly until the surface of crude drugs turns deep yellow and the rice turns tan, take them out, remove the rice by sifting, and allow to cool. Use 20kg of rice for each 100kg of the slices (or sections) of Codonopsis Radix.

5.3 Stir-baking with soil

Dioscoreae Rhizoma

Put fulong liver powder (or red stone powder) in a hot pot and heat on a medium fire, add the slices of Dioscoreae Rhizoma while the soil powder is dry and loose, stir quickly until the Dioscoreae Rhizomais stained with soil powder, the surface is yellowish, and the inherent aroma is revealed, take out. Remove the soil by sifting, allow to cool and weigh. Use 30kg of the soil powder for each 100kg of the slices of Dioscoreae Rhizoma.

5.4 Stir-baking with sand

5.4.1 Strychni Semen

Put clean sand in a hot pot, heat on a strong fire until the sand can move smoothly in the pot, add the Strychni Semen, and keep baking until the surface becomes brown or dark brown, the internal is reddish brown and vesicles were bulging, take the drug out. Remove the sand by sifting, allow to cool and weigh.

5.4.2 Manis Squama

Put clean sand in a hot pot, heat on a strong fire until the sand can move smoothly in the pot, add Manis Squama with the same size, and keep baking until the drugs expanded crisply, the surface is golden yellow and the edges curl inward, take the drug out and remove sand by sifting, then, put the drugs into vinegar, stir, dip slightly, take out, dry and weigh. Use 30kg of the rice vinegar for each 100kg of the Manis Squama.

5.4.3 Galli Gigerii Endothelium Corneum

Put clean sand in a hot pot, heat on a strong fire until the sand can move smoothly in the pot, add Galli Gigerii Endothelium Corneum with the same size, stir frequently until the drugs expanded crisply, curled, and the surface becomes golden yellow, take the drugs out. Remove the sand by sifting, allow to cool and weigh.

5.4.4 Trionycis Carapax

Put clean sand in a hot pot, heat on a strong fire until the sand can move smoothly in the pot, add Trionycis Carapax with the same size in the pot, stir frequently until the drugs expanded crisply and the surface becomes dark yellow, take the drug outand remove sand by sifting, then, put the drugs into rice vinegar, stir, dip slightly, take out ,dry and weigh. Use 20kg of the rice vinegar for each 100kg of the Trionycis Carapax.

5.5 Stir-baking with powdered clam-shell

Asini Corii Colla

First, soften the rubber blocks by heating and cut into small squares (about 1cm long) for use. Then, put a quantity of powdered clam-shell in a hot pot, heat on a medium fire until the powders can move smoothly in the pot. Add the Asini Corii Colla, keep stir-baking until the drugs bulge into a ball,the inner is not runny, the color changes from black to dark yellow and with a thin layer of clam powder on the surface, take the drugs out immediately. Remove the powdered clam-shell by sifting, allow to cool and weigh. Use 40kg of the clam-shell for each 100kg of the Asini Corii Colla.

5.6 Stir-baking with talc

5.6.1 Cutis Erinacei

Put a quantity of talc in a hot pot, and heat on a medium fire until the powders can move smoothly in the pot. Add the cleaned drugs, keep stir-baking until the stingers are curled and bald, and the surface is burnt yellow, take them out. Remove the talc by sifting, allow to cool and weigh. Use 40kg of the talc for each 100kg of the Cutis Erinacei.

5.6.2 Hirudo

Put a quantity of talc in a hot pot, and heat on a medium fire until the powders can move smoothly in the pot. Add the clean sections of Hirudo, keep stir-baking until the drugs slightly expanded and the surface becomes yellow-brown, take them out. Remove the talc by sifting, allow to cool and weigh. Use 40kg of the talc for each 100kg of the Hirudo.

Results

6.1 Stir-baking with bran

6.1.1 Atractylodis Macrocephalae Rhizoma

Similar to the slices in shape, the surface is yellowish-brown, burned spots occasionally visible. Slightly with burned aromatic odour.

6.1.2 Aurantii Fructus

Similar to the slices in shape, the surface color is deep, burned spots occasionally visible on the surface.

6.1.3 Atractylodis Rhizoma

The surface is dark yellow, many brown oil cavities are scattered, burned aromatic odour.

6.1.4 Bombyx Batryticatus

The surface is yellow, sometimes with charred spots, fishy odor reduced.

6.2 Stir-baking with rice

6.2.1 Mylabris

The shape is similar to the Mylabris, the surface is slightly heat colours, showing gloss, and the odour is slight.

6.2.2 Codonopsis Radix

The surface is dark yellow, occasionally with burnt stains.

6.3 Stir-baking with soil

Dioscoreae Rhizoma

The surface of the slices is yellowish and covered with the thin soil,burned spots occasionally visible, slightly with burned aromatic odour.

6.4 Stir-baking with sand

6.4.1 Strychni Semen

The surface is brown or dark brown, the hardness is fragile, brown or dark endosperm visible in parallel sections. Taste extremely bitter.

6.4.2 Manis Squama

The whole inflated to curled, texture crisp and frangible, golden yellow. Possess vinegar odour.

6.4.3 Galli Gigerii Endothelium Corneum

The whole inflated to curled, texture crisp, golden yellow , charred-aromatic.

6.4.4 Trionycis Carapax

The surface is dark yellow, texture crisp, possess vinegar odour.

6.5 tir-baking with powdered clam-shell

Asini Corii Colla

Subround in shape externally brownish-yellow or pale white, covered with white powder. Texture light and crisp, easily broken. Cut surface hollowed or multiholed, pale yellow to brown. Odour is slight and taste slightly sweet.

6.6 Stir-baking with talc

6.6.1 Cutis Erinacei

Texture foaming, bulging, yellow, spiny body expansion, pointed bald, easy to break, the edge of the fur off, burnt yellow, skin edge curled inward, slightly fishy smell.

6.6.2 Hirudo

In irregular flattened pieces or cylinder, slightly expanded, externally brownish-yellow to blackish-brown, with a few white talc. Fracture loose, greyish-white to burned yellow. Odour is slightly fish smell.

Notes

7.1 A medium fire is commonly used during stir-baking with bran, rice, soil, powdered clam-shell and talc while a strong fire during stir-baking with sand. During the operation, it should be turned frequently, the finished product should be out of the pan quickly and the auxiliary materials should be sieved immediately. For drugs that require to be tempered with vinegar, dip the crude drugs into vinegar while hot and dry.

7.2 Stir-baking with bran can be heated by a bigger fire, spread the bran evenly over the hot pan. When the bran is smoking, pour in the crude drugs. Smoking is asked to discolor the drugs, but if the fire is too strong, the bran will turn black so fast that the smoke cann't be produced to achieve its purpose. Stir-baking with soil, stir-baking with powdered clam-shell , Stir-baking with talc and Stir-baking with sand must add the crude drugs until the powders can move smoothly in the pot.

7.3 The fire of stir-baking with rice should not be large because the high temperature will make slices scorch and affect the quality.

7.4 Generally, the side length of the Asini Corii Colla is 8~10mm. Otherwise, too big is to be soft-boiled, too small is to be burned, both affect the quality.

7.5 The accessories that have been fried with poisonous drugs shall not be used to bake other drugs, nor shall they be poured in disorder.

7.6 When processing Mylabris, labor protection should be paid attention to, operators should wear glasses, masks, to protect the eyes and the nose mucosa from damage. After the work is finished, the exposed part should be cleaned with cold water, not hot water; the burnt rice should be handled properly in time, in order to avoid human and animal ingestion, poisoning.

Questions

8.1 Briefly describe the purpose of stir-baking with solid adjuvants.

8.2 Briefly describe the effect of the temperature on the drug during the process of stir-baking with solid adjuvants.

8.3 Briefly describe the difference between sand and soil during the process of stir-baking with solid adjuvants.

8.4 Briefly describe the role of the processing on each drug in the experiment.

PPT

实验四　炙法

实验目的

1. **掌握**　酒炙、醋炙、盐炙、姜炙、蜜炙、油炙的操作方法、注意事项及成品质量。

2. **了解**　酒炙、醋炙、盐炙、姜炙、蜜炙、油炙的目的和意义。

实验原理

1. **酒炙的作用**　①改变药性，引药上行：如大黄、黄连、黄柏等。②增强活血通络作用：如当归、川芎等。③矫臭矫味：如乌梢蛇、蕲蛇、紫河车等。

2. **醋炙的作用**　①引药入肝，增强疗效：如乳香、没药、三棱、莪术等。②降低毒性，缓和药性：如京大戟、甘遂、芫花、商陆等。③矫臭矫味：如乳香、没药等。

3. **盐炙的作用**　①引药下行，增强疗效：如杜仲、巴戟天、益智仁、韭菜子等。②增强滋阴降火作用：如知母、黄柏等。③缓和药物辛燥之性：如补骨脂、益智仁等。

4. **姜炙的作用**　①缓和药物寒性，增强和胃止呕作用：如黄连，竹茹。②降低副作用，增强疗效：如厚朴。

5. **蜜炙的作用**　①增强润肺止咳的作用：如百部、冬花、紫菀。②增强补脾益气的作用：如黄芪、甘草、党参等。③缓和药性：如麻黄等。

6. **油炙的作用**　①增强疗效：如淫羊藿。②利于粉碎：如质地坚实的三七、蛤蚧。

实验内容

1. **酒炙**　当归、白芍、黄芩、续断、丹参、川芎。
2. **醋炙**　香附、延胡索、乳香、柴胡。
3. **盐炙**　杜仲、黄柏、车前子。
4. **姜炙**　厚朴、竹茹。
5. **蜜炙**　甘草、黄芪、百部、麻黄、百合。
6. **油炙**　淫羊藿、蛤蚧。

实验器具和材料

1. **实验器具**　炒锅、锅铲、煤气灶、搪瓷盘、电子秤、烧杯、量杯、玻璃棒等。

2. **实验材料**　黄酒、米醋、食盐、姜、蜂蜜、食用油；当归、白芍、丹参、黄芩、续断、川芎、香附、延胡索、乳香、柴胡、杜仲、黄柏、车前子、厚朴、竹茹、甘草、百合、百部、麻黄、黄芪、淫羊藿、蛤蚧。

实验方法

1. 酒炙法

（1）当归　取净当归饮片，加入定量黄酒拌匀，闷润至酒被吸尽，置热锅内，文火加热，炒至深黄色，取出，晾凉。每100kg当归片，用黄酒10kg。

（2）白芍　取净白芍饮片，加入定量黄酒拌匀，闷润至酒被吸尽，置热锅内，文火加热，炒至微黄色，取出，晾凉。每100kg白芍片，用黄酒10kg。

（3）黄芩　取净黄芩饮片，加入定量黄酒拌匀，闷润至酒被吸尽，置热锅内，文火加热，炒至深黄色，取出，晾凉。每100kg黄芩片，用黄酒10kg。

（4）续断　取净续断饮片，加入定量黄酒拌匀，闷润至酒被吸尽，置热锅内，文火加热，炒至微带黑色时，取出，晾凉。每100kg续断片，用黄酒10kg。

（5）丹参　取净丹参饮片，加入定量黄酒拌匀，闷润至酒被吸尽，置热锅内，文火加热，炒至黄褐色，取出，晾凉。每100kg丹参片，用黄酒10kg。

（6）川芎　取净川芎片，加入定量黄酒拌匀，闷润至酒被吸尽，置热锅内，文火加热，炒至表面带火色时，取出，晾凉。每100kg川芎片，用黄酒10kg。

2. 醋炙法

（1）香附　取净香附颗粒或片，加定量米醋拌匀，闷润至醋被吸尽，置热锅内，文火加热，炒至深黄色，取出，放凉。每100kg香附片，用米醋20kg。

（2）延胡索　取净延胡索片，加入定量米醋拌匀，闷润至醋被吸尽，置热锅内，文火加热，炒至深黄色，取出，放凉。每100kg延胡索片，用米醋20kg。

（3）乳香　取净乳香，置热锅内，文火加热，炒至冒烟，表面微熔，喷淋定量米醋，边喷边炒至表面显油亮光泽时，取出，摊开放凉。每100kg乳香，用米醋10kg。

（4）柴胡　取净柴胡片，加入定量米醋拌匀，闷润至醋被吸尽，置热锅内，文火加热，炒至色泽加深，取出，放凉。每100kg柴胡片，用米醋20kg。

3. 盐炙法

（1）杜仲　取杜仲丝或块，加盐水拌匀，闷透，置热锅内，用文火加热，炒至颜色加深、有焦斑、丝易断时，取出，晾凉。每100kg杜仲丝或块，用食盐2kg。

（2）黄柏　取黄柏丝或块，加盐水拌匀，闷透，置热锅内，用文火加热，炒至颜色变深、有焦斑时，取出，晾凉。每100kg黄柏丝或块，用食盐2kg。

（3）车前子　取净车前子，置热锅内，用文火加热，炒至略有爆裂声、微鼓起时，喷淋盐水，炒干，取出，晾凉。每100kg车前子，用食盐2kg。

4. 姜炙法

（1）厚朴　取厚朴丝，加姜汁拌匀，闷润至姜汁被吸尽，至热锅内，用文火加热，炒干，取出，晾凉。每100kg厚朴丝，用生姜10kg。姜汁可用煎汁（煎两次）或捣汁的方法制备。

（2）竹茹　取竹茹段或团，加姜汁拌匀，闷润至姜汁被吸尽，置热锅内，用文火加热，炒至微黄色、略有焦斑时，取出，晾凉。每100kg竹茹，用生姜10kg。姜汁可用煎汁（煎两次）或捣汁的方法制备。

5. 蜜炙法

（1）甘草　取炼蜜，加适量温开水稀释，淋入净甘草饮片中拌匀，闷润，置热锅内，用文火加热，炒至深黄色、不粘手时，取出，晾凉。每100kg甘草片，用炼蜜25kg。

（2）黄芪　取炼蜜，加适量温开水稀释，淋入净黄芪饮片中拌匀，闷润，置热锅内，用文火加热，炒至深黄色、不粘手时，取出，晾凉。每100kg黄芪片，用炼蜜25kg。

酒炙白芍

酒炙黄芩

醋炙乳香

盐炙杜仲

盐炙黄柏

盐炙车前子

姜炙厚朴

炙甘草

（3）百部　取炼蜜，加适量温开水稀释，淋入净百部饮片中拌匀，闷润，置热锅内，用文火加热，炒至不粘手时，取出，晾凉。每100kg百部片，用炼蜜12.5kg。

蜜炙百合

（4）麻黄　取炼蜜，加适量温开水稀释，淋入净麻黄饮片中拌匀，闷润，置热锅内，用文火加热，炒至不粘手时，取出，晾凉。每100kg麻黄，用炼蜜20kg。

（5）百合　取净百合，置热锅内，用文火加热，炒至颜色加深时，加入温开水稀释过的炼蜜，迅速翻炒均匀，炒至微黄色、不粘手时，取出，晾凉。每100kg百合，用炼蜜5kg。

6. 油炙法

油炙淫羊藿

（1）淫羊藿　取羊脂油置锅内加热熔化，加入淫羊藿丝，用文火加热，炒至油脂吸尽，均匀有光泽时，取出，晾凉。每100kg淫羊藿，用羊脂油（炼油）20kg。

（2）蛤蚧　取蛤蚧，涂以麻油，用无烟火烤至稍黄质脆，除去头爪及鳞片，切成小块。

实验结果

1. 酒炙

（1）当归　切面深黄色或浅棕黄色，略有焦斑。香气浓郁，并略有酒香气。

（2）白芍　成品表面微黄色或淡棕黄色，有的可见焦斑。微有酒香气。

（3）黄芩　成品形如黄芩片。略带焦斑，微有酒香气。

（4）续断　成品表面微黑色或灰褐色，略有酒香气。

（5）丹参　成品表面黄褐色，略有酒香气。

（6）川芎　成品表面色泽加深，偶见焦斑。

2. 醋炙

（1）香附　成品表面色泽较生品加深，略带焦斑，略有醋气。

（2）延胡索　成品表面呈深黄色，微具焦斑，略有醋气。

（3）乳香　成品表面深黄色，显油亮光泽，略有醋气。

（4）柴胡　成品表面色泽较生品加深，略有醋气。

3. 盐炙

（1）杜仲　成品表面色泽较生品加深，有焦斑，银白色橡胶丝减少，弹性减弱，略有咸味。

（2）黄柏　成品表面深黄色，略有焦斑，味微咸。

（3）车前子　成品色泽加深，形体略鼓起，微有咸味。

4. 姜炙

（1）厚朴　成品色泽加深，微带焦斑，稍具姜辣气味。

（2）竹茹　成品偶见黄色焦斑，微具姜辣气味。

5. 蜜炙

（1）甘草　成品呈老黄色，微有光泽，味甜，具焦香气。

（2）黄芪　成品表面呈深黄色，有光泽，味甜，具蜜香气。

（3）百部　成品表面呈深黄色或棕色，具黏性，偶有粘连块，味微甜。

（4）麻黄　成品表面呈深黄色，微显光泽，具蜜香气，味微甜。

（5）百合　成品表面黄色，偶见黄焦斑，略带黏性，味甜。

6. 油炙

（1）淫羊藿　成品呈黄绿色，有油光泽，具羊脂油气味。

（2）酥蛤蚧　成品表面稍黄，质较脆，具香酥气。

注意事项

1. 采用先拌辅料后炒药的方法时，辅料要与药物拌匀，闷润至被吸尽或渗透到药物组织内部后再进行炒制。

2. 酒炙药物闷润时，容器要加盖密闭，以防酒迅速挥发。

3. 溶解食盐时，水的用量一般以食盐量的 4~5 倍为宜。

4. 制备姜汁时，水的用量一般以最后所得姜汁与生姜量为 1∶1 为宜。

5. 蜜炙时间可稍长，尽量将水分除去，避免发霉；并注意放凉后密闭贮存。

6. 若液体辅料用量较少，不易与药物拌匀时，可先加适量开水稀释，以利拌匀润制药物。

7. 大部分药物应用文火炒制，勤加翻动，使药物受热均匀，炒至规定程度。

思考题

1. 简述各种炙法的异同点。

2. 简述实验中各药物炮制的作用。

3. 简述乳香等药物为何采用先炒药后加辅料的方法炮炙。

4. 简述蜜炙、姜炙、盐炙、羊油脂炙法所用辅料制备方法。

Experiment 4　Stir-baking with liquid excipients

Aims

1.1　To master the operation methods, precautions and product quality of the stir-baking with wine, vinegar, salt-water, ginger juice, honey and fat.

1.2　To understand the purpose and significance of the stir-baking with wine, vinegar, salt-water, ginger juice, honey and fat.

Principles

2.1　The purpose of stir-baking with wine

A. To change drug effect, such as Rhei Radix et Rhizoma, Coptidis Rhizoma and Phellodendri Chinensis Cortex, etc. B.To enhance blood circulation and dredge meridians, such as Angelicae Sinensis Radix and Chuanxiong Rhizoma, etc. C. To remove the bad odor of some drugs, such as Zaocys and Agkistrodon, etc.

2.2　The purpose of stir-baking with vinegar

A. To lead the effects of drugs to the liver meridian, so as to strengthen the effects, such as Olibanum, Myrrha, Sparganii Rhizoma and Curcumae Rhizoma, etc. B. To reduce the toxicity of drugs and moderate the properties of drugs, such as Euphorbiae Pekinensis Radix, Kansui Radix, Genkwa Flos and Phytolaccae Radix, etc. C. To remove the bad odor of some drugs, such as Olibanum and Myrrha, etc.

2.3　The purpose of stir-baking with salt-water

A. To conduct the effects of drugs to the kidney meridian and enhance the effects, such as Eucommiae Cortex, Morindae Officinalis Radix, Alpiniae Oxyphyllae Fructus and Allii Tuberosi Semen, etc. B. To strengthen the effects of nourishing yin deficiency and purge away fire, such as Anemarrhenae Rhizoma and Phellodendri Chinensis Cortex, etc. C. To moderate the properties of dryness in drugs, such as Psoraleae Fructus and Alpiniae Oxyphyllae Fructus, etc.

2.4　The purpose of stir-baking with ginger juice

A. To alleviate coldness of drugs, soothe the stomach to arrest vomit, such as Coptidis Rhizom and Bambusae Caulis in Taenias, etc. B. To reduce side effects and enhance efficacy, such as Magnoliae Officinalis Cortex, etc.

2.5　The purpose of stir-baking with honey

A. To strengthen the effect of moistening lung and stopping cough, such as Stemonae Radix, Farfarae flos, and Asteris Radix et Rhizima, etc. B. To enhance the effect of tonifying the spleen and invigorating *qi*, such as Astragali Radix, Glycyrrhizae Radix et Rhizoma and Codonopsis Radix, etc. C. To mitigate drug effect, such as Ephedrae Herba, etc.

2.6　The purpose of stir- baking with fat

A. To enhance efficacy, such as Epimedii Folium, etc. B. To good for crushing, such as the texture of solid Notoginseng and Gekko, etc.

Contents

3.1 Stir-baking with wine

Angelicae Sinensis Radix, Paeoniae Radix Alba, Scutellariae Radix, Dipsaci Radix, Salviae Miltiorrhizae Radix et Rhizoma, Chuanxiong Rhizoma.

3.2 Stir-baking with vinegar

Cyperi Rhizoma, Corvallis Rhizoma, Olibanum, Bupleuri Radix.

3.3 Stir-baking with salt-water

Eucommiae Cortex, Phellodendri Chinensis Cortex, Plantaginis Semen.

3.4 Stir-baking with ginger juice

Magnoliae Officinalis Cortex, Bambusae Caulis in Taenias.

3.5 Stir-baking with honey

Glycyrrhizae Radix et Rhizoma, Astragali Radix, Stemonae Radix, Ephedrae Herba, Lilii Bulbus.

3.6 Stir-baking with fat

Epimedii Folium, Gecko.

Materials

4.1 Experimental apparatuses

Wok, truner, electric stove, enameled tray, electronic scale, beaker, measuring glass and glass rod, etc.

4.2 Experimental materials

Wine, rice vinegar, salt, ginger, honey, cooking oil, Angelicae Sinensis Radix, Paeoniae Radix Alba, Salviae Miltiorrhizae Radix et Rhizoma, Scutellariae Radix, Dipsaci Radix, Chuanxiong Rhizoma, Cyperi Rhizoma, Corvallis Rhizoma, Olibanum, Bupleuri Radix, Eucommiae Cortex, Phellodendri Chinensis Cortex, Plantaginis Semen, Magnoliae Officinalis Cortex, Bambusae Caulis in Taenias, Glycyrrhizae Radix et Rhizoma, Lilii Bulbus, Stemonae Radix, Ephedrae Herba, Astragali Radix, Epimedii Folium, Gecko.

Methods

5.1 Stir-baking with wine

5.1.1 Angelicae Sinensis Radix

Mix the clean slices of Angelicae Sinensis Radix with wine, and stand for a while until the drugs are completely moistened. Put the drugs into a hot stir-baking pot, heat on a gentle fire, keep stir-baking until the surface of the drugs become dark yellow, take out and allow to cool. Use 10kg of wine for each 100kg of the slices of Angelicae Sinensis Radix.

5.1.2 Paeoniae Radix Alba

Mix the clean slices of Paeoniae Radix Alba with wine, stand for a while until the drugs are completely moistened. Put the drugs into a hot stir-baking pot, heat on a gentle fire, keep stir-baking until the surface of the drugs become yellowish, take them out and allow to cool. Use 10kg of wine for each 100kg of the slices of Paeoniae Radix Alba.

5.1.3 Scutellariae Radix

Mix the clean slices of Scutellariae Radix with wine, and stand for a while until the drugs are completely moistened. Put the drugs into a hot stir-baking pot, heat on a gentle fire, keep stir-baking until the surface of the drugs become dark yellow, take them out and allow to cool. Use 10kg of wine for each 100kg of the Scutellariae Radix.

5.1.4 Dipsaci Radix

Mix the clean slices of Dipsaci Radix with wine, and stand for a while until the drugs are completely moistened. Put the drugs into a hot stir-baking pot, heat on a gentle fire, keep stir-baking until the surface of the drugs become blackish, take them out and allow to cool. Use 10kg of wine for each 100kg of the Dipsaci Radix.

5.1.5 Salviae Miltiorrhizae Radix et Rhizoma

Mix the clean slices of Salviae Miltiorrhizae Radix et Rhizoma with wine, and allow to stand for a while until the drugs are completely moistened. Put the drugs into a hot stir- baking pot, heat on a gentle fire, keep stir-baking until the surface of the drugs become tawny, take them out and allow to cool. Use 10kg of wine for each 100kg of the Salviae Miltiorrhizae Radix et Rhizoma.

5.1.6 Chuanxiong Rhizoma

Mix the clean slices of Chuanxiong Rhizoma with wine, and stand for a while until the drugs are completely moistened. Put the drugs into a hot stir-baking pot, heat on a gentle fire, keep stir-baking until the surface of the drugs becomes heat colours, take them out and allow to cool. Use 10kg of wine for each 100kg of the Chuanxiong Rhizoma.

5.2 Stir-baking with vinegar

5.2.1 Cyperi Rhizoma

Mix the clean granules (or slices) of Cyperi Rhizoma with vinegar, and stand for a while until the drugs are completely moistened. Put the drugs into a hot stir-baking pot, heat on a gentle fire, keep stir-baking until the surface of the crude drugs becomes dark yellow, take them out and allow to cool. Use 20kg of vinegar for each 100kg of the Cyperi Rhizoma.

5.2.2 Corvallis Rhizoma

Mix the clean slices of Corvallis Rhizoma with vinegar, and stand for a while until the drugs are completely moistened. Put the drugs into a hot stir-baking pot, heat on a gentle fire, keep stir-baking until the surface of the crude drugs becomes dark yellow, take them out and allow to cool. Use 20kg of vinegar for each 100kg of the Corvallis Rhizoma.

5.2.3 Olibanum

Put the clean Olibanum into a hot stir-baking pot, heat on a gentle fire, keep stir-baking until the surface is smoking and slightly melted, spray vinegar and fry until the surface is lustrous, take them out and allow to cool. Use 10kg of vinegar for each 100kg of the Olibanum.

5.2.4 Bupleuri Radix

Mix the clean slices of Bupleuri Radix with vinegar, and stand for a while until the drugs are completely moistened. Put the drugs into a hot stir-baking pot, heat on a gentle fire, keep stir-baking until the surface of the crude drugs deeper in color, take them out and allow to cool. Use 20kg of vinegar for each 100kg of the Bupleuri Radix.

5.3 Stir-baking with salt-water

5.3.1 Eucommiae Cortex

Mix the pieces or slivers of Eucommiae Cortex with salt-water, and stand for a while until the drugs are completely moistened. Put the drugs into a hot stir-baking pot, heat on a gentle fire, keep stir-baking until the rubber threads broken off and the surface charred, take them out and allow to cool. Use 2kg of salt for each 100kg of the Eucommiae Cortex.

5.3.2 Phellodendri Chinensis Cortex

Mix the slivers or pieces of Phellodendri Chinensis Cortex with salt-water, and stand for a while until the drugs are completely moistened. Put the drugs into a hot stir-baking pot, heat on a gentle fire, keep stir-baking until the surface charred, take them out and allow to cool. Use 2kg of salt for each 100kg of the Phellodendri Chinensis Cortex.

5.3.3 Plantaginis Semen

Put the clean Plantaginis Semen into a hot stir-baking pot, heat on a gentle fire, keep stir-baking until it cracks, spray with salt-water and stir-bake to dryness. Take them out and allow to cool. Use 2kg of salt for each 100kg of the Plantaginis Semen.

5.4 Stir-baking with ginger juice

5.4.1 Magnoliae Officinalis Cortex

Put the slivers of Magnoliae Officinalis Cortex mixed well with ginger juice into a hot pot, heat on a gentle fire until the ginger juice is completely absorbed, take the drugs out and allow to cool. Use 10kg of fresh ginger for each 100kg of the Magnoliae Officinalis Cortex. Ginger juice can be prepared by frying (frying twice) or by ramming.

5.4.2 Bambusae Caulis in Taenias

Mix the Bambusae Caulis with ginger juice in a hot pot, heat on a gentle fire until drugs become yellow, take the drugs out and allow to cool. Use 10kg of fresh ginger for each 100kg of the Bambusae Caulis in Taenias. Ginger juice can be prepared by frying (frying twice) or by ramming.

5.5 Stir-baking with honey

5.5.1 Glycyrrhizae Radix et Rhizoma

Dilute refined honey with an appropriate quantity of lukewarm boiled water, add the decoction pieces of Glycyrrhizae Radix et Rhizoma, mix well, and allow to stand until the drugs are completely moistened. Put the drugs in a hot pot, heat on a gentle fire until it becomes yellow to deep yellow and not sticky to the fingers, take out and cool in the air. Use 25kg of refined honey for each 100kg of the Glycyrrhizae Radix et Rhizoma.

5.5.2 Astragali Radix

Dilute refined honey with an appropriate quantity of lukewarm boiled water, add the slicesof Astragali Radix, mix well, and allow to stand until the drugs are completely moistened. Put the drugs in a hot pot, heat on a gentle fire until it becomes yellow to deep yellow and not sticky to the fingers, take out and cool in the air. Use 25kg of refined honey for each 100kg of the Astragali Radix.

5.5.3 Stemonae Radix

Dilute refined honey with an appropriate quantity of lukewarm boiled water, add the slices of Stemonae Radix, mix well, and allow to stand until the drugs are completely moistened. Put the drugs in a hot pot, heat on a gentle fire until it not sticky to the fingers, take out and cool in the air. Use 12.5kg of refined honey for each 100kg of the Stemonae Radix.

5.5.4 Ephedrae Herba

Dilute refined honey with an appropriate quantity of lukewarm boiled water, add the sections of Ephedrae Herba, mix well, and allow to stand until the drugs are completely moistened. Put the drugs in a hot pot, heat on a gentle fire until it not sticky to the fingers, take out and cool in the air. Use 20kg of refined honey for each 100kg of the Ephedrae Herba.

5.5.5 Lilii Bulbus

Put the clean Lilii Bulbus into a hot stir-baking pot, heat on a gentle fire, keep stir-baking until the surface color deepens, add the dilute refined honey with an appropriate quantity of lukewarm boiled water stir-baking quickly until it becomes yellow and not sticky to the fingers, take out and cool in the air. Use 5kg of refined honey for each 100kg of the Lilii Bulbus.

5.6 Stir-baking with fat

5.6.1 Epimedii Folium

Stir-bake the slivers of Epimedii Folium with refined suet by gentle heating until an evenly lustre is produced, remove and cool. Using 20kg of refined suet per 100kg of Epimedii Folium.

5.6.2 Gecko Bake

Gecko on fire with sesame oil until it shows a yellow color and a crisp texture, remove its head, paws and squamae, and cut it into small pieces.

Results

6.1 Stir-baking with wine

6.1.1 Angelicae Sinensis Radix

The cut surface is dark yellow or pale brownish-yellow, somewhat with burnt specks. Odour is strongly aromatic, and slightly with wine aromatic odour.

6.1.2 Paeoniae Radix Alba

The finished products are externally pale yellow or pale brownish-yellow, sometimes burned spots visible, and slightly with wine aromatic odour.

6.1.3 Scutellariae Radix

Same shapes as the processing slices of Scutellariae Radix, show less burnt patches, slightly with wine aromatic odour.

6.1.4 Dipsaci Radix

The finished products are externally pale black or greyish-brown, slightly with wine aromatic odour.

6.1.5 Salviae Miltiorrhizae Radix et Rhizoma

The finished products are externally yellowish-brown, slightly with wine aromatic odour.

6.1.6 Chuanxiong Rhizoma

The finished products are externally color deepening, sometimes burned spots visible.

6.2 Stir-baking with vinegar

6.2.1 Cyperi Rhizoma

The finished products are externally blackish-brown, show less burnt patches, slightly with vinegar odour.

6.2.2 Corvallis Rhizoma

The cut surface is yellowish-brown, somewhat with burnt specks, slightly with vinegar odour.

6.2.3 Olibanum

The cut surface is yellowish-brown, lustrous, slightly with vinegar odour.

6.2.4 Bupleuri Radix

The surface color of the finished products is deeper than that of the raw products, slightly with vinegar aromatic odour.

6.3 Stir-baking with salt-water

6.3.1 Eucommiae Cortex

The surface color of the finished products is deeper than the raw products, externally charred, elasticity of the rubber threads weak when broken, and slightly salty.

6.3.2 Phellodendri Chinensis Cortex

The surface is deep yellow, occasionally showing charred stains, slightly salty.

6.3.3 Plantaginis Semen

The finished products are externally blackish-brown, slightly bulged, slightly salty.

6.4 Stir-baking with ginger juice

6.4.1 Magnoliae Officinalis Cortex

The finished products are externally blackish-brown, occasionally charred stains visible, slightly gingery odour.

6.4.2 Bambusae Caulis in Taenias

Yellow burned spots are occasionally visible on the surface, slightly gingery.

6.5 Stir-baking with honey

6.5.1 Glycyrrhizae Radix et Rhizoma

The finished products are externally reddish-brown or greyish-brown, slightly lustrous, cut surface yellow to deep yellow, texture sticky, with agreeable burnt smelling, taste sweet.

6.5.2 Astragali Radix

The finished products are externally pale brownish-yellow or pale brown, slightly lustrous; honeyed-fragrant, taste sweet.

6.5.3 Stemonae Radix

The finished products are externally brownish-yellow or brown, with less burnt specks, slightly sticky, taste sweet.

6.5.4 Ephedrae Herba

The finished products are externally dark yellow, somewhat lustrous, slightly viscous, honey aromatic, taste sweet.

6.5.5 Lilii Bulbus

Externally yellow, occasionally charred stains visible, slightly viscous.

6.6 Stir-baking with fat

6.6.1 Epimedii Folium

The finished products are externally pale yellow, fatty lustrous, slightly sebum in odour.

6.6.2 Gecko

The finished products are externally slightly yellow, texture crispy.

Notes

7.1 When using the method of mixing excipients first and then stir-frying medicine, the adjuvants should be mixed with medicine evenly and moistened until they are absorbed or permeated into the inner part of the medicine organization before stir-baking.

7.2 When stir-baking with wine, the container should be covered airtight to prevent the rapid evaporation of wine.

7.3 When the salt is dissolved, the amount of water used should be 4~5 times the amount of salt.

7.4 When ginger juice is prepared, the amount of water used is generally 1 ∶ 1 for the final ginger juice and ginger.

7.5 The time of stir-baking with honey can be slightly longer, as far as possible to remove water to avoid mildew, and pay attention to cool after airtight storage.

7.6 If the amount of liquid adjuvants is less and not easy to mix with drugs, it can be first added a proper amount of boiled water dilution to mix well run drugs.

7.7 Most of the drugs should be heated on a gentle fire and stirred frequently, so that the drugs are evenly heated, then stir-baked to a specified extent.

Questions

8.1 Briefly describe the similarities and differences of stir-baking with different liquid adjuvants.

8.2 Briefly describe the roles of the processing on each drug in the experiment.

8.3 Why use the method of frying the drug first and then add the auxiliary materials to stir-bake the Olibanum and other drugs?

8.4 How to prepare the adjuvants of stir-baking with honey, ginger juice, salt-water and fat, respectively?

实验五 煅法

PPT

实验目的

1. **掌握** 明煅法、煅淬法、闷煅法的操作方法、注意事项及成品质量。

2. **了解** 明煅法、煅淬法、闷煅法的目的和意义。

实验原理

1. **明煅法的作用** ①使药物质地酥脆，易于粉碎和煎出有效成分：如牡蛎、石决明等。②除去结晶水，增强收敛作用：如白矾、石膏、硼砂等。③缓和药性：如寒水石、石决明等。

2. **煅淬法的作用** ①使药物质地酥脆，易于粉碎，利于有效成分煎出：如代赭石、磁石等。②改变药性，增强疗效：如炉甘石等。③清除杂质，洁净药物。

3. **闷煅法的作用** ①改变药物性能，产生新的疗效，如血余炭和棕榈炭等。②增强或产生止血作用，如荷叶、丝瓜络等。③降低毒性和刺激性，如干漆等。

实验内容

1. **明煅** 明矾、石膏、龙骨。

2. **煅淬** 炉甘石、自然铜、磁石。

3. **闷煅** 棕榈、血余、灯心草。

实验器具和材料

1. **实验器具** 马弗炉、煅药炉、煅药锅、坩埚、坩埚钳、烧杯、量筒、电炉、乳钵、蒸发皿、搪瓷盘、台秤等。

2. **实验材料** 米醋、水；明矾、石膏、龙骨、炉甘石、自然铜、磁石、棕榈、血余、灯心草。

实验方法

（一）明煅法

煅白矾

煅炉甘石

1. **明矾** 取净明矾，敲成小块，称重，置耐火容器内，用武火加热至熔化，继续煅至无气体放出，呈白色蜂窝状时，取出，放凉，即得。

2. **石膏** 去净石膏块，称重，置耐火容器内火直接置火源上，用武火加热，煅至红透，取出，放凉，碾细，即得。

3. **龙骨** 取净龙骨，敲成小块，称重，置耐火容器内，用武火加热，煅至红透，取出，放凉，即得。

（二）煅淬法

1. **炉甘石** 取净炉甘石，置耐火容器内，用武火加热，煅至红透，取出，立即倒入水中浸淬，搅拌，倾取混悬液，残渣反复煅淬2~3次。合并混悬液，静置，倾去上层清水，下层沉淀干燥，研细。

2. 自然铜 取净自然铜，置耐火容器内，用武火加热，煅至红透，取出，立即倒入醋内浸淬，如此反复煅淬数次，至黑褐色，表面光泽消失并酥松，取出，放凉。每100kg自然铜，用米醋30kg。

3. 磁石 取净磁石，砸成小块，置耐火容器内，用武火加热，煅至红透，取出，立即倒入醋液内淬制，反复煅淬至酥脆，取出，干燥，碾碎。每100kg磁石，用米醋30kg。

（三）闷煅法

1. 棕榈炭 取净棕榈段或棕榈块，置适宜容器内，上扣一较小容器，两容器结合处用盐泥封固，上压重物，并贴一块白纸条或放大米数粒，先用文火后用武火煅至白纸或大米呈深黄色时，停火，待凉后，开锅取出中药。

2. 血余炭 取头发除去杂质，反复用稀碱水洗去油垢，清水漂净，晒干，置适宜容器内，上扣一较小容器，两容器结合处用盐泥封固，上压重物，并贴一块白纸条或放大米数粒，用武火加热至白纸或大米呈深黄色时，离火，待凉后，开锅取出中药。

3. 灯心草炭 取净灯心草，扎成小把，置适宜容器内，上扣一较小容器，两容器结合处用盐泥封固，上压重物，并贴一块白纸条或大米数粒，用武火煅至白纸条或大米呈深黄色时，停火，待凉后，开锅取出中药。

实验结果

（一）明煅法

1. 枯矾 成品呈蜂窝状的碎块或疏松的细粉，白色，质轻松，气微，味酸，极涩。

2. 煅石膏 成品为粉末状。白色，不透明。体较轻，质软。气微，味淡。

3. 煅龙骨 成品呈灰白色或灰褐色，质轻，酥脆易碎，表面显粉性，吸舌力强。

（二）煅淬法

1. 煅炉甘石 成品呈粉末状，白色或灰白色，质轻松细腻，无臭，味微苦。

2. 煅自然铜 成品呈粉末状，黑褐色，光泽消失，质酥脆，略有醋气

3. 煅磁石 成品呈粉末状，表面黑色，质硬而酥，无磁气，有醋气。

（三）闷煅法

1. 棕榈炭 成品形如棕榈，中间较厚，两侧较薄，表面呈灰褐色或黑褐色，微显光亮，内部呈棕褐色或黑褐色，质轻脆，易折断，味微苦涩。

2. 血余炭 成品呈不规则的小块，乌黑光亮，呈蜂窝状，研之清脆有声。体轻，质脆。用火烧之有焦发气，味苦。

3. 灯心草炭 成品表面呈黑色，质轻松，易碎，气微，味微涩。

注意事项

1. 煅明矾要用武火；一次煅透，中途不得停止加热；不得搅拌。

2. 自然铜煅制过程中，会产生硫的升华物或有毒的二氧化硫气体，故应在通风处操作。

3. 闷煅时，药料不宜放得过多，过紧，以容器的2/3为宜；应随时用湿泥封堵两容器结合处的盐泥裂缝；煅透后应放冷才能打开。

思考题

1. 简述明煅、煅淬、暗煅法的特点，分别适宜哪类药物。
2. 简述实验中各药的炮制目的。
3. 简述煅明矾为何不宜搅拌、中途不得停火的原因。

Experiment 5 Calcining

Aims

1.1 To master the method of operation, notes of operations and quality of calcining openly, calcining and quenching, carbonizing by calcining.

1.2 To understand the purpose and significance of calcining openly, calcining and quenching, carbonizing by calcining.

Principles

2.1 The effects of calcining openly

A. To make the drugs crisp, easy to be crushed and fried out the active composition, such as Ostreae Concha and Haliotidis Concha. B. To remove the crystal water and enhance convergence, such as Alumen, Gypsum Fibrosum and Borax. C. To mitigate drug effect , such as Gypsum rubrum and Haliotidis Concha.

2.2 The effects of calcining and quenching

A. To make the drugs crisp, easy to be crushed and fried out the active composition, such as Haematitum and Magnetitum. B. To change the property of drugs and enhance the effect, such as Calamina. C. To remove non-essential parts and cleaning the drugs.

2.3 The effects of carbonizing by calcining

A. To change the drug properties and produce the new curative effects, such as Crinis Carbonisatus and Trachycarpi Petiolus. B. To enhance or produce hemostatic effects, such as Nelumbinis Folium and Luffae Fructus Retinervus. C. To reduce toxicity and irritation, such as Toxicodendri Resina.

Contents

3.1 Calcining openly

Alumen, Gypsum Fibrosum and Fossil fragments.

3.2 Calcining and quenching

Calamina, Pyritum and Magnetitum

3.3 Carbonizing by calcining

Trachycarpi Petiolus, Crinis Carbonisatus and Junci Medulla.

Materials

4.1 Experimental apparatuses

Muffle furnace, drugs calcined furnace, calcined pan, crucible, crucible tongs, beaker, measuring cylinder, electric heater, mortar, evaporating dish, enamel tray, platform scale, etc.

4.2 Experimental materials

Vinegar, water, Alumen, Gypsum Fibrosum, Fossil fragments, Calamina, Pyritum, Magnetitum,

Trachycarpi Petiolus, Crinis Carbonisatus and Junci Medulla.

Methods

5.1 Calcining openly

5.1.1 Alumen

Take the Alumen, break it into small pieces and weigh it, then put it in a refractory container, heat it on a strong fire until it has melted, continue to burn it until no gas is released. When the Alum turns into white honeycomb, take the drugs out and allow to cool.

5.1.2 Gypsum Fibrosum

Take the clean Gypsum Fibrosum block and weigh it, put it in the refractory container directly on the fire source and heat it on a strong fire, calcine until the drugs become red. Take the drugs out, allow to cool and grind to a powder.

5.1.3 Fossil fragments

Take the clean Fossil fragments, break into small pieces and weigh it, put it in a refractory container and heat it on a strong fire, calcine until the drugs become red, take the drugs out and allow to cool.

5.2 Calcining and quenching

5.2.1 Calamina

Take the clean drugs, put them in a refractory container and heat on a strong fire, calcine crude drugs to red and immediately dip into water quenching system, stirring and pouring suspension, repeat this process 2~3 times. Combine the suspension, stewing, pour the upper water and take the precipitate out, dry and grind into a powder.

5.2.2 Pyritum

Take the clean drugs, put then in a refractory container and heat it on a strong fire, calcine crude drugs to red and immediately dip into vinegar quenching system, repeat this process 2~3 times until they are crisp enough, take the drugs out and allow to cool. Use 30kg of vinegar per 100kg of Pyritum.

5.2.3 Magnetitum

Take the Magnetitum, break it into small pieces, put it in a refractory container and heat on a strong fire, calcine crude drugs to red and immediately dip into vinegar quenching system, repeat this process 2~3 times until they are crisp enough, take the drugs out and allow to cool. Use 30kg of vinegar per 100kg of Magnetitum.

5.3 Carbonizing by calcining

5.3.1 Trachycarpi Petiolus carbon

Take the Trachycarpi Petiolus segments or Trachycarpi Petiolus and put it in a suitable container, attach a small container, seal the joint of the two containers with salt and mud, put heavy weights on the smaller container, paste a piece of white paper or put a few grains of rice, use a gentle heat and then burn on a strong fire until white paper or rice has been dark yellow, turn off the fire, allow to cool and take the Chinese medicines out.

5.3.2 Crinis Carbonisatus carbon

Take hair to remove non-essential parts, wash away the grease repeatedly with dilute alkali water, and rinse with clear water, dried, put it in a suitable container, attach a small container, seal the joint of the two containers with salt and mud, put heavy weights on the smaller container, paste a piece of white paper or put a few grains of rice, use a gentle heat and then burn on a strong fire until white paper or rice has been dark yellow, turn off the fire, allow to cool and take the Chinese medicines out.

5.3.3 Junci Medulla carbon

Take the clean Junci Medulla, bundle into small handfuls, put it in a suitable container, attach a small container, seal the joint of the two containers with salt and mud, put heavy weights on the smaller container, paste a piece of white paper or put a few grains of rice, use a strong fire until white paper or rice has been dark yellow, turn off the fire, allow to cool and take the Chinese medicines out.

Results

6.1 Calcining openly

6.1.1 Dried Alumen

The finished products are honeycombed fragments or loose powder, white, easy quality, weak smell, sour taste, very astringent.

6.1.2 Gypsum Ustum

The finished products are powder. White opaque. The quality is light and soft. The smell is weak and the taste is plain.

6.1.3 Calcined Fossil fragments

The finished products are grayish white or grayish brown, light, crisp and fragile, the surface shows powder, strong tongue force.

6.2 Calcining and quenching

6.2.1 Calcined Calamina

The finished products are powdery, white or grayish white, easy and delicate quality, no odor and taste slightly bitter.

6.2.2 Calcined Pyritum

The finished products are powdery, dark brown, glossy, crisp, slightly vinegar gas.

6.2.3 Calcined Magnetitum

The products are powder, black surface, hard and crisp, no magnetic gas, has vinegar gas.

6.3 Carbonizing by calcining

6.3.1 Trachycarpi Petiolus carbon

The finished products are like Trachycarpi Petiolus, thicker in the middle and thinner on both sides. The surfaces become brownish-black, and the inner parts become dark brown with light brightness. The interior is tan or dark brown, and it's light and fragile, easy to break and taste slightly bitter.

6.3.2 Crinis Carbonisatus carbon

The finished products are irregular small pieces, black and light, honeycomb, has clear sound when grinded. It has light weight, crisp quality, scorched gas when burned and bitter taste.

6.3.3 Junci Medulla carbon

The finished products are black, easy to fragile. The smell is weak and taste slightly bitter.

Notes

7.1 Calcined Alumen should be made on a strong fire. Once calcined thoroughly, do not stop heating halfway and do not stir.

7.2 The work should be done in a ventilated place as the calcining process of Pyritum will produce sulfur sublimates or toxic sulfur dioxide gases.

7.3 The work should be done in a suitable container, attach a small container, seal the joint of the two containers with salt and mud, allow to cool, and take the drugs out. But should be not put too more and too tight, 2/3 of the container is suitable.

Questions

8.1 Briefly describe the characteristics of calcining openly, calcining and quenching, carbonizing by calcining. Which kind of drug is suitable respectively?

8.2 Briefly describe the purposes of each drug in the experiment.

8.3 Why is calcined Alumen not suitable for being stirred and removed from heat in the middle of the work?

PPT

实验六　蒸煮燀法

实验目的

1. 掌握　蒸、煮、燀的基本操作、注意事项及成品质量。

2. 了解　蒸、煮、燀的炮制目的和意义及辅料对药物作用的影响。

实验原理

1. 蒸法的作用　①改变药物性能，扩大用药范围：如地黄等。②减少副作用：如大黄、黄精等。③保存药效，利于贮存：如桑螵蛸、黄芩等。④便于软化切片，如木瓜、天麻等。

2. 煮法的作用　①使药物软化，便于切片：如水煮黄芩。②消除或降低药物的毒副作用：如豆腐煮藤黄、甘草水煮远志等。③缓和药性：如甘草水煮远志。④增强疗效：如醋煮延胡索等。

实验内容

1. 蒸制　地黄、女贞子。

2. 煮制　草乌、远志。

3. 燀制　苦杏仁、白扁豆。

实验器具和材料

1. 实验器具　炒锅、锅铲、蒸锅、蒸笼、电子秤、烧杯、搪瓷盘等。

2. 实验材料　黄酒，甘草汁；地黄、女贞子、草乌、远志、苦杏仁、白扁豆。

实验方法

（一）蒸制

1. 地黄　取净生地黄，加入黄酒拌匀，隔水蒸至酒被吸尽（或加压蒸制），显乌黑色光泽，味转甜，取出，晒至外皮黏液稍干，切厚片，干燥。每 100kg 生地黄，用黄酒 30~50kg。

2. 女贞子　取净女贞子，用适量黄酒拌匀，稍闷后置适宜密闭蒸制容器内隔水炖，或直接通入蒸汽，蒸至酒被完全吸尽，色泽黑润时，取出，干燥。

（二）煮制

煮制草乌

1. 草乌　取净草乌，大小分档，用水浸泡至内无干心后，加水煮沸，保持微沸一定时间，选取个大的，切开无白心，口尝微有麻舌感，取出晾至六成干，切薄片，干燥。

2. 甘草汁煮远志　先将甘草片置锅内加适量水煎煮两次，过滤，合并滤液，弃去残渣，再将甘草汁浓缩至相当于甘草 10 倍量时，将净远志投入锅内，加热煮沸，保持微沸，并勤翻动，至甘草汁被吸尽，略干，取出干燥。每 100kg 远志，用甘草 6kg。

（三）燀制

1. 苦杏仁　取净苦杏仁投入沸水中燀约 10 分钟，燀至表皮微胀，易于挤脱时，取出置冷水中浸泡，取出搓开种皮和种仁，干燥后筛去种皮。

2. 白扁豆 取净白扁豆投入沸水中焯约 5 分钟，焯至表皮微胀，易于挤脱，取出置冷水中浸泡，取出搓开种皮和种仁，干燥后分别入药。

焯制苦杏仁

实验结果

（一）蒸法

1. 熟地黄 成品呈不规则团块状，表面乌黑色，有光泽，黏性大。质柔软而带韧性，不易折断，断面乌黑色，有光泽，气微或微有酒香气，味甜。

2. 女贞子 成品表面黑褐色，附有白色粉霜，微有酒气。

（二）煮法

1. 草乌 本品呈不规则类圆形或近三角形片，表面黑褐色，质脆，气微，味微辛辣，稍有麻舌感。

2. 甘草汁煮远志 成品呈黄色，味略甜，嚼之无刺喉感。

（三）焯法

1. 焯苦杏仁 成品表面白色，无种皮或分离成单瓣，表面乳白色，有特殊的香气，味苦。

2. 焯白扁豆 成品呈不规则的卷曲状种皮，乳白色，质脆易碎。

注意事项

1. 酒炖所用容器应密闭，以防黄酒挥发。
2. 煮时文火保持微沸，并勤翻动。辅料具挥发性的，宜加盖煮制。
3. 焯时水量宜大，待水沸后投入净药，时间不宜过长，制后及时干燥。
4. 在乌头煮制过程中应注意随时补充水以保证水量充足。

思考题

1. 简述实验中各药炮制的目的及注意事项。
2. 简述煮法炮制药物时，煮沸后为何需改用微火。
3. 简述焯苦杏仁时为何加水量需药物的 10 倍量。

Experiment 6 Steaming, boiling and blanching methods

Aims

1.1 To master the method of operation, notes of operations and quality of finished products of steaming, boiling and blanching.

1.2 To understand the purpose and significance of steaming, boiling and blanching and the effects of adjuvants on the action of the drugs.

Principles

2.1 The effects of steaming

A. To change the drugs properties, expand the scope of use, such as Rehmanniae Radix. B. To reduce side effects, such as Rhei Radix Et Rhizoma, Polygonati Rhizoma, etc. C. To preserve the drugs, conducive to storage, such as Mantidis Ootheca, Scutellariae Radix, etc. D. To make the drugs soften and cut easily , such as Chaenomelis Fructus, Gastrodiae Rhizoma, etc.

2.2 The effects of boiling

A. To make the drugs soften and cut sections easily, such as boiled Scutellariae Radix; B. To eliminate or reduce toxicity and side effects, such as boiled Garcinia morella with doufu, boiled Polygalae Radix with Glycyrrhizae Radix Et Rhizoma. C. To mitigate drug effect, such as boiled Polygalae Radix with Glycyrrhizae Radix Et Rhizoma. D. To enhance efficacy, such as boiled Corydalis Rhizoma with vinegar.

Contents

3.1 Steaming

Rehmanniae Radix, Ligustri Lucidi Fructus

3.2 Boiling

Aconiti kusnezoffii Radix, Polygalae Radix.

3.3 Blanching

Armeniacae Semen Amarum, Lablab Semen Album.

Materials

4.1 Experimental apparatuses

Frying pan, spatula, steamer, steam box, electronic scale, beaker, enamel tray, etc.

4.2 Experimental materials

Rice wine, Glycyrrhizae Radix Et Rhizoma juice; Rehmanniae Radix, Ligustri Lucidi Fructus, Aconiti kusnezoffii Radix, Polygalae Radix, Armeniacae Semen Amarum, Lablab Semen Album.

Methods

5.1 Steaming

5.1.1 Rehmanniae Radix

Take the crude Rehmanniae Radix, add rice wine and mix well, allow to stand until Rehmanniae Radix are moistened, keep steaming until the rice wine is completely absorbed. The color turns black and the taste becomes sweet. Take the drugs out, bask to dry, cut into thick slices and allow to dry. Use 30~50kg of rice wine per 100kg of Rehmanniae Radix.

5.1.2 Ligustri Lucidi Fructus

Take the Ligustri Lucidi Fructus, add rice wine and mix well, allow to stand until Fructus ligustri Lucidi are moistened, and put the drugs in a suitable steaming container until steam to the rice wine absorbed. The color turns black, take the drugs out and allow to dry.

5.2 Boiling

5.2.1 Aconiti kusnezoffii Radix

Take Aconiti kusnezoffii Radix and classify crude drugs by size, soaking in water until dry, add water to boil and keep boiling until no white colour is observed in the center of drugs and the taste is a little numb. Take the drugs out, put in air until 60% dry, cut into thin slices and allow to dry.

5.2.2 Boiled Polygalae Radix with Glycyrrhizae Radix Et Rhizoma juice

Firstly, put the Glycyrrhizae Radix Et Rhizoma slices in a wok and add appropriate amount water to boil twice, filter, combine filtrate and discard residue, and then condensed Glycyrrhizae Radix Et Rhizoma juice to amount of Glycyrrhizae Radix Et Rhizoma 10 times, put Polygalae Radix in a wok and keep boiling, stirring frequently until Glycyrrhizae Radix Et Rhizoma juice is completely absorbed, Take the drugs out and allow to dry. Use 6kg of Glycyrrhizae Radix Et Rhizoma per 100kg of Polygalae Radix.

5.3 Blanching

5.3.1 Armeniacae Semen Amarum

Put Armeniacae Semen Amarum in boiling water blanching about 10 minutes, blanch until the wrinkled testa become smooth and easily removable, take them out, put in cool water, remove the testa, and dry in the sun.

5.3.2 Lablab Semen Album

Put Lablab Semen Album in boiling water blanching about 5 minutes, blanch until the wrinkled testa become smooth and easily removable, take them out, put in cool water, remove the testa, and dry in the sun.

Results

6.1 Steaming

6.1.1 Rehmanniae Radix Praeparata

The finished product is irregular mass, the surface is black, shiny and viscous. The texture is soft and not easy to break, the fracture surface is black and shiny, the smell is faint or has slightly wine aroma, sweet taste.

6.1.2 Ligustri Lucidi Fructus

The finished product is black brown with white powder cream, and have the smell of wine.

6.2 Boiling

6.2.1 Aconiti kusnezoffii Radix

The finished product is irregular round or nearly triangular, the surface is dark brown, crisp, slightly gas, slightly spicy taste, a little numb.

6.2.2 Boiled Polygalae Radix with Glycyrrhizae Radix Et Rhizoma juice

The finished product is yellow with a slightly sweet smell and no prickly throat sensation.

6.3 Blanching

6.3.1 Blanched Armeniacae Semen Amarum

The finished product is white, no testa or separated into single petals, the surface is milky white with a special aroma, bitter taste.

6.3.2 Blanched Lablab Semen Album

The finished product is irregular and curly testa with milky white and fragile.

Notes

7.1 The containers used for stewing with rice wine should be closed to prevent rice wine from evaporating.

7.2 When boiling, keep a gentle fire boiling and stirring frequently. If the adjuvants are evaporate, it is advisable to cover and boil.

7.3 Put crude drugs in a large amount blanching water, stir for a short time, and take them out quickly and allow to dry.

7.4 We should pay attention to add water at any time to ensure adequate water in the process of boiling Aconiti kusnezoffii Radix.

Questions

8.1 Briefly describe the purposes and notes of operations of each drug processing in the experiments.

8.2 When boiling the drugs, why do you need to use a gentle fire after boiling?

8.3 Why blanching Armeniacae Semen Amarum must add 10 times the amount of water of the drug?

实验七 复制法

PPT

实验目的

1. **掌握** 复制法的操作方法、注意事项及成品质量。
2. **了解** 复制法的目的和意义。

实验原理

1. **降低或消除药物毒性** 如半夏用白矾、生姜制等。
2. **改变药性** 如天南星胆汁制，其性味由辛温转苦凉，功能也发生变化。
3. **增强疗效** 如白附子生姜、白矾制，增强了祛风逐痰的功效。
4. **矫臭矫味** 如紫河车酒制可除去腥臭味，便于服用。

实验内容

姜半夏、法半夏、制天南星、制白附子的炮制。

实验器具和材料

1. **实验器具** 不锈钢锅、锅铲、煤气灶、搪瓷盘、台秤、烧杯、石棉网、切药刀、砧板、烘箱等。
2. **实验材料** 半夏、天南星、白附子、生姜、白矾、甘草、生石灰。

实验方法

1. **姜半夏** 取净半夏，大小分开，用水浸泡至内无干心，另取生姜切片煎汤，加白矾与半夏共煮至透心，取出；晾至半干，切薄片，干燥。每 100kg 半夏，用生姜 25kg、白矾 12.5kg。

2. **法半夏** 取净半夏，大小分开，用水浸透至内无干心，取出，另取甘草适量，加水煎煮二次，合并煎液，倒入用适量生石灰配制的石灰液（生石灰饱和水溶液的上清液）中，搅匀，加入上述已浸透的半夏，浸泡，每日搅拌 1~2 次，并保持浸液 pH 12 以上，至剖面黄色均匀，口尝微有麻舌感时，取出，洗净，干燥。每 100kg 生半夏，用甘草 15kg，生石灰 10kg。

3. **制天南星** 取生天南星，加清水浸泡，每日换上 2~3 次，如水面起白沫，换水后加白矾（每 100kg 生天南星，加白矾 2kg），泡一日后，再换水浸泡至口尝微有麻舌感时取出，另取白矾、生姜片置锅内加适量水煮沸后，与天南星共煮至无干心时取出，除去姜片，晾至 4~6 成干，切薄片，干燥。每 100kg 生天南星，用生姜、白矾各 12.5kg。

4. **制白附子** 取生白附子，用水浸泡，每日换上 2~3 次，数日后如起泡沫，换水后加白矾（每 100kg 生白附子，加白矾 2kg），泡一日后再换水，至口尝微有麻舌感为度，取出。另取白矾及生姜片加适量水，煮沸后，与白附子煮至内无干心为度，捞出，除去生姜片，晾至 6~7 成干，切厚片，干燥。每 100kg 白附子，用生姜、白矾各 12.5kg。

实验结果

1. 姜半夏 为淡黄棕色片状，质硬脆，具角质样光泽。气微香，味辛辣，微有麻舌感，嚼之有粘牙感。

2. 法半夏 为黄色或淡黄色类球形或较为均匀的颗粒，质较松脆。气微，味淡略甘，微有麻舌感。

3. 制天南星 为黄白色或淡棕色薄片，半透明，质脆易碎。气微，味涩，微麻。

4. 制白附子 为黄白色至淡棕色片，呈半透明状，周边淡棕色，气微味微涩，无麻舌感或微有麻舌感。

注意事项

1. 药物浸泡时如起泡沫，加白矾防腐。
2. 药物应大小分档处理，以免炮制程度难以控制，影响炮制效果。
3. 本实验炮制的中药均有毒，在炮制时应避免与皮肤直接接触。

思考题

1. 简述半夏饮片规格及其炮制作用。
2. 简述半夏、天南星、白附子为何均采用白矾和生姜进行炮制。

Experiment 7 Complex processing method

Aims

1.1 To master operations and procautions of complex processing method, as well as the quality of finished products.

1.2 To understand the purpose and significance of complex processing method.

Principles

2.1 To recuce or eliminate drug toxicity

Such as processing Pinelliae Rhizoma with Alumen, Zingiberis Rhizona Recens and so on.

2.2 To Change drug effect

Such as processing Aeisaematis rhizome with bile, its property and flavor from pungent and warm to bitter and cold, along with function changes.

2.3 To enhance curative efficacy

Such as Typhonii Rhizoma is processed with Zingiberis Rhizona Recens and Alumen, which enhances the effect of dispelling wind and phlegm.

2.4 To neutralize the bad odor

Such as processing Hominis placenta with liquor, it can remove fishy smell and make it easy to take.

Contents

Pinelliae Rhizoma Praeparatumcum Zingibere Et Alumine, Fabanxia Pinelliae Rhizoma Praeparatum, Arisaematis Rhizoma Preparatum and Processed Rhizoma Typhonii.

Materials

4.1 Experimental apparatuses

Stainless steel pot, turner, gas stove, enamel tray, bench scale, beaker, asbestos mesh, herb cutting knife, cutting board, oven, etc.

4.2 Experimental materials Pinelliae Rhizoma, Arisaematis Rhizoma, Typhonii Rhizoma, Zingiberis Rhizona Recens, Alumen, Glycyrrhizae Radix Et Rhizoma, quicklime.

Methods

5.1 Pinelliae Rhizoma

Praeparatumcum Zingibere Et Alumine Pinelliae Rhizoma is taken cleanly, classify crude drugs by size and soak in water to prevent dryness. Take Zingiberis Rhizona Recens slices and decoct soup, boil with Alumen and Pinelliae Rhizoma until the centre of the drug is devoid of a dry core, then take Pinelliae Rhizoma out. Air-dried to semi dry, thin sliced, and drying. Use 25kg of Zingiberis Rhizona Recens and 12.5kg of Alumen per 100kg of Pinelliae Rhizoma.

5.2 Pinelliae Rhizoma Praeparatum

Pinelliae Rhizoma is taken cleanly and classifing crude drugs by size, soaking in water to prevent dryness. Take out and then take appropriate amount of Glycyrrhizae Radix Et Rhizoma, add water and boiling twice, combine the decoction, and pour into a lime solution prepared with an appropriate amount of quicklime. Serum, stir well, and add the soaked Pinelliae Rhizoma, soaking and then stir once or twice a day. And keep the pH of the leachate above 12 until the profile is evenly yellow and tastes slightly numbing, take out, wash and dry. For every 100kg raw Pinelliae Rhizoma, 15kg of Glycyrrhizae Radix Et Rhizoma and 10kg of quicklime are needed.

5.3 Arisaematis Rhizoma Preparatum (RhizomaArisaematis)

Take the crude Arisaematis Rhizoma,soaking it in clear water and changing water to 2~3 times a day. If the surface of the water froths, add Alumen (using 2kg of Alumen per 100kg of raw Arisaematis Rhizoma) after changing the water. Soaking it in water for a day, and then take it out when the taste is slightly numbing. Take another Alumenand Zingiberis Rhizona Recens slices, put them in a pot and boil with an appropriate amount of water, and boiling with Arisaematis Rhizoma until there is no dryness inside of it. Take them out and remove the Zingiberis Rhizona Recens slices, dry to 40% ~ 60%, cut into thin slices, and drying. Each 100kg of raw Arisaematis Rhizoma requires 12.5kg of Zingiberis Rhizona Recens and Alumen.

5.4 Processed Typhonii Rhizoma

Take crude Typhonii Rhizoma, then soaking it in water and change 2~3 times a day. If the surface of the water foams, add Alumen (using 2kg of Alumen per 100kg of crude Rhizoma Typhonii) after changing the water. Soak it in water for a day, and then take it out when the taste is slightly numbing. In addition, take the Alumen and Zingiberis Rhizona Recensslices, put them in the pot and add appropriate amount of water to boil them. Take them out when no dry heart, remove the Zingiberis Rhizona Recens slices, dry to 60%~70% , cut into thick slices and dry. Each 100kg of raw Typhonii Rhizoma requires 12.5kg of Zingiberis Rhizona Recens and Alumen.

Results

6.1 Pinelliae Rhizoma Praeparatumcum Zingibere Et Alumine

It is yellowish brown flake, hard and crisp, with keratinous luster. The smell is slightly fragrant and spicy with a slight tingling and slightly numbing and sticky to the chew.

6.2 Pinelliae Rhizoma Praeparatum

Yellow or light yellow globular or more relatively uniform particles, and its hardness is more crispy, tiny odor, the flavor is light and slightly sweetish, slightly numbing.

6.3 Arisaematis Rhizoma Preparatum

It is yellow white or light brown thin slices, translucent, brittle and fragile. It has tiny odor, astringent in flavor and slight tingling in tongue.

6.4 Processed Typhonii Rhizoma

Yellow-white to pale brown slices, translucent, peripheral light brown, tiny odor, slightly astringent in flavor, no or slightly numbing.

Notes

7.1 If the soaking medicine foams, add Alumen for antisepticise.

7.2 Crude drugs should be classfied by size in case of controlling the processing degree and then affect the processing effect.

7.3 All of the Chinese medicine processed in this experiment are toxic, so direct contact with skin should be avoided.

Questions

8.1 Briefly describe the specifications and processing functions of Pinellia ternate yinpian.

8.2 Why do all of Pinelliae Rhizoma, Aeisaematis rhizoma and Typhonii Rhizoma use Alumen and Zingiberis Rhizona Recens for processing?

PPT

实验八　发酵法、发芽法

实验目的

1. **掌握**　发酵法和发芽法的操作方法。
2. **了解**　发酵法和发芽法的目的、意义、影响因素及成品质量。

实验原理

1. **发酵的原理**　发酵过程主要是利用微生物自身产生的酶系对药物的营养成分进行利用和代谢形成各种代谢产物，从而使药物可以产生新的功效。

2. **发酵的作用**　①改变原有的性能，产生新的治疗作用，扩大药用品种，如淡豆豉、六神曲等。②增强疗效。药物在发酵过程中，大分子物质经微生物代谢后产生大量的小分子成分，更易被人体吸收利用，达到增强疗效和扩大用药范围的目的。

3. **发芽的意义**　通过发芽，淀粉被分解为糊精、葡萄糖和单糖，蛋白质被降解成为氨基酸，脂肪被分解成为甘油和脂肪酸，并产生各种消化酶类、维生素等，使药效物质基础发生改变，改变药物的原有性能，使其具有新的功效，扩大用药品种。

实验内容

1. **发酵法**　六神曲、淡豆豉。
2. **发芽法**　麦芽、大豆黄卷。

实验器具和材料

1. **实验器具**　蒸锅、漏水容器、发酵模具、烘箱等。

2. **实验材料**　苦杏仁、赤小豆、鲜青蒿、鲜苍耳草、鲜辣蓼、面粉或麦麸、黑大豆、新鲜大麦、鲜苘麻叶或粗纸、桑叶。

实验方法

（一）发酵法

1. **六神曲**　取苦杏仁、赤小豆粉碎，与面粉混合匀，加入鲜青蒿、鲜苍耳草、鲜辣蓼药汁(煎汁)，揉搓成“捏之成团，掷之即散”的粗颗粒软材，置模具中压制成扁平块(33cm × 20cm × 6.6cm)，用鲜苘麻叶或粗纸包严，按品字形堆放，上面覆盖鲜青蒿或湿麻袋等物。置温度为30~37℃，湿度为70%~80%的条件下，经4~6天即能发酵。待药面生出黄白色霉衣时取出，除去包裹物，切成2.5cm见方的小块，干燥。每100kg面粉(或面粉40kg加麦麸60kg)，用苦杏仁、赤小豆各4kg，鲜青蒿、鲜苍耳草、鲜辣蓼各7kg（干者用1/3），鲜青蒿、鲜苍耳草、鲜辣蓼药汁为鲜草榨汁合并其药渣煎煮液制备而成。

2. **淡豆豉**　取黑大豆洗净。另取桑叶、青蒿加水煎汤，将煎汁拌入净黑大豆中，待汤液被吸净后，置蒸制容器内蒸透，取出，稍凉，置容器内，用煎过汁的桑叶、青蒿渣覆盖，闷至发酵、长满黄衣时取出，去除桑叶、青蒿渣，加适量水搅拌，洗净捞出，置容器内，再闷15~20天，至充分发酵，有香气逸出时，取出，略蒸，干燥即得。每100kg黑大豆，用桑叶、青蒿各7~10kg。

（二）发芽法

1. 麦芽 取新鲜饱满的净大麦，用清水浸泡6~7成透，捞出，置能排水的容器内，用湿布覆盖，每天淋水2~3次，待芽长0.5cm时，取出，干燥。发芽率不得少于85%。

2. 大豆黄卷 取新鲜净大麦，用清水浸泡至表面起皱，捞出，置能排水的容器内，用湿布覆盖，每天淋水2~3次，待芽长0.5cm时，取出，干燥。

实验结果

（一）发酵法

1. 六神曲 为立方形小块，表面灰黄色，粗糙，内有斑点，质地较硬。有发酵香气，无霉气。

2. 淡豆豉 为椭圆形，表面黑色，皱缩不平，质柔软，断面棕黑色。气香，味微甘。

（二）发芽法

1. 麦芽 呈梭形，表面淡黄色，一端有幼芽，皱缩或脱落，下端有须根数条，纤细而弯曲。质硬，断面白色，粉性，气微，味微甘。

2. 大豆黄卷 呈肾形，表面黄色或黄棕色，微皱缩，芽黄色而卷曲，外皮质脆易裂开。气微，味淡，嚼之有豆腥味。

注意事项

1. 发酵法、发芽法均须控制温度和湿度。一般发酵时空气的相对湿度应控制在70%~80%；发酵的最佳温度为30~37℃。发芽法一般以18~25℃为宜。

2. 原料在发酵前应进行杀菌、杀虫的处理，以免杂菌影响发酵质量。

3. 发酵过程必须一次完成，不能中断或中途停顿。

4. 发酵品要芳香无霉味、酸败味。曲块表面霉衣黄白色，内部有斑点为佳；黑色质差。

5. 发芽前应测定发芽率，不得少于85%。

6. 发芽时应该避光，勤加检查、淋水，保持相应的湿度，防止发热霉烂。

思考题

1. 简述发酵法、发芽法的原理。
2. 简述发酵法、发芽法的适宜温湿度条件。
3. 简述发酵法、发芽法制备药物的目的。

Experiment 8 Fermenting and Sprouting methods

Aims

1.1 To master operations of both fermentation and germination methods.

1.2 To understand the purpose, significance and influence of influencing factors as well as quality of finished products.

Principles

2.1 The principles of fermentation

The fermentation process mainly uses the enzymes produced by microorganisms to utilize and metabolize the nutritional components of drugs to form various metabolites, so that drugs can produce new effects.

2.2 The functions of fermentation

A. Changing the original performance, produce new the rapeutic effects, and expand the medicinal varieties, such as Sojae Semen Praeparatum, Liushenqu(Medicated leaven), etc. B. Enhancing the efficacy. During the fermentation process of the drugs, macromolecular substances are metabolized by microorganisms to produce a large amount of small molecular components, which are more easily absorbed and utilized by the human body to achieve the purpose of enhancing the curative effect and expanding the scope of medication

2.3 The significance of germination

Through germination, starch is decomposed into dextrin, glucose and monosaccharides, protein is degraded into amino acids, fat is decomposed into glycerol and fatty acids, and various digestive enzymes, vitamins and so on are produced, which can change the basis of pharmacodynamic substances and the original properties of drugs, make them have new effects, and expand the variety of drugs.

Contents

3.1 Fermentating method

Medicated Leaven, Sojae Semen Praeparatu

3.2 Sprouting method

Hordei Fructus Germinatus Sojae Semen Germinatum（Da Dou Huang Juan）

Materials

4.1 Experimental apparatuses

Steamer, leaky container, fermentation mold, oven, etc.

4.2 Experimental materials

Armeniacae Semen Amarum, Vignae Semen, Fresh Artemisiae Annuae Herba, Fresh Xanthium Sibiricum, Fresh Polygonum or Wheat Bran, Black Soybean, Fresh Barley, Fresh Jute Leaf or Rough

Paper, Mori Folium.

Methods

5.1 Fermenting

5.1.1 Medicated Leaven

Take Armeniacae Semen Amarum and Vignae Semen, mix well with flour, add the juice (decoction) of Fresh Artemisiae Annuae Herba, Fresh Xanthium Sibiricum and fresh Polygonum, knead them into coarse particles that are "Pinch into a ball, disintegrates if throw it away" . The soft material is placed into a flat piece in (33cm × 20cm × 6.6cm) a medium pressure mold, wrapped with fresh jute leaf or rough paper, stacked according to the type of product, and covered with Fresh Artemisiae Annuae Herbaor wet sacks, etc. Under the condition of temperature of 30~37℃ and humidity of 70%~80%, it can fermente after 4~6 days. When the surface produces a yellow-white mold, removed the package and cut it into 2.5cm square pieces and dried. Each 100kg of flour (or 40kg of flour plus 60kg of wheat bran) was prepared with 4kg of Armeniacae Semen Amarum and Vignae Semeneach, Fresh Artemisiae Annuae Herba, Fresh Xanthium Sibiricum, fresh Polygonum 7kg each (1/3 of dry). The medical juice of Fresh Artemisiae Annuae Herba, fresh Xanthium Sibiricum and fresh Polygonum are prepared by extracting fresh grass juice and decoction of medicinal residue.

5.1.2 Sojae Semen Praeparatum

Wash black soybeans. In addition, take Mori Folium and Artemisia annual, add water to decoct the soup and mix the decoction into the black soybean. After the soup liquid is sucked off, put them into a steaming container for steaming throughly, take them out and cool them a little, then put them into a container by covering with the decocted Mori Folium and Artemisia annual dregs. They are taken out when black soybeans are fermented and full of yellow clothes. After removing Mori Folium and Artemisia annual dregs, stir with an appropriate amount of water, wash and take them out, then put them into a container. Stuffy for 15~20 days, fully fermented, when the aroma escapes, take them out and steam them slightly, then dry. Each 100kg of black soybean requires 7~10kg of Mori Folium and Artemisia annual.

5.2 Sprouting

5.2.1 Hordei Fructus Germinatus

Take fresh and full barley, soaking it in clean water for 60%~70% thoroughly, then take it out and put into a drainable container. cover it with a damp cloth, and flushing 2~3 times a day. When the bud length is 0.5cm it should be taken out and drying for later use. Germination rate shall not be less than 85%.

5.2.2 Sojae Semen Germinatum

Take fresh barley, soak it in clean water until the surface is wrinkled, then take it out and place it in a drainable container. Cover it with a wet cloth, and flushing 2~3 times a day, it should be taken out and drying for later use when the bud is 0.5cm long.

Results

6.1 Fermenting

6.1.1 Medicated Leaven

It is a small cubic block with gray yellow surface, rough surface, speckled inside, and hard texture.

It has fermented aroma and no mildew.

6.1.2 Sojae Semen Praeparatum

It is oval with black surface, uneven, soft hardness and a brown-black section. The flavor is sweet.

6.2 Sprouting

6.2.1 Malt Hordei Fructus Germinatus

The fractures is light yellow, with young shoots at one end, which are shrunk or shed, and a number of whiskers at the lower end, which are slender and curved. Hard, white cross-section, powdery, tiny odor, slightly sweet flavor.

6.2.2 Sojae Semen Germinatum

It is kidney-shaped with yellow or yellow-brown on the surface, slightly shrunk. The buds are yellow and curly, and the outer cortex is brittle and easy to crack. Tiny odor, mild flavor and has beany flavor when chewed.

Notes

7.1 Temperature and humidity should be both controlled for fermentation and germination. Generally, the relative humidity of air during fermentation should usually be controlled at 70%~80%, and the optimum temperature of fermentation at 30~37℃. While 18~25℃ is generally suitable for germination.

7.2 The raw materials should be sterilized and insecticidally treated before fermentation to avoid the influence of miscellaneous bacteria on fermentation quality.

7.3 The fermentation process must be completed at one time without interruption or pause.

7.4 The fermented products should be aromatic, and free from mildew and rancidity. The surface of the curved block is yellow-white, with spots inside. The black products' quality is poor.

7.5 The germination rate shall be determined before germination and shall not be less than 85%.

7.6 During germination, it should be protected from light, and inspected and flushing frequently to maintain the corresponding humidity to prevent fever and mildew.

Questions

8.1 Briefly describe the principles of fermentation and germination.

8.2 Briefly describe the suitable temperature and humidity conditions for fermentation and germination.

8.3 Briefly describe the purpose of preparing drugs by fermentation and germination.

实验九 其他制法

PPT

实验目的

1. **掌握** 煨、提净、水飞、制霜、干馏法的操作方法、注意事项及成品质量。
2. **了解** 煨、提净、水飞、制霜、干馏法的目的和意义。

实验原理

1. **煨法** 是将净制或切制后的药物用湿面或湿纸包裹，置于加热的滑石粉或热砂中，或将药物直接置于加热的麦麸中，或将药物铺摊吸油纸上，层层隔纸加热，以除去部分油质的方法。

2. **提净法** 主要针对某些矿物药，特别是一些可溶性无机盐类药物，经过溶解，过滤，除净杂质后，再进行重结晶，以进一步纯净药物的方法。

3. **水飞法** 主要针对某些不溶于水的矿物药，利用粗细粉末在水中悬浮性不同，将不溶于水的矿物、贝壳类药物经反复研磨，而分离制备极细腻粉末的方法。

4. **制霜法** 是药物经过加工处理，成为松散粉末或细小结晶，或煎熬成粉渣的方法。制霜法根据操作方法不同，可分为去油制霜、渗析制霜、升华制霜、煎煮制霜等。

5. **干馏法** 是将药物置于容器内，以火烤灼，使产生汁液的方法。制备有别于原药材的干馏物，以适合临床需要。

实验内容

1. **煨法** 肉豆蔻、木香。
2. **提净法** 芒硝。
3. **水飞法** 朱砂、滑石粉。
4. **制霜法** 巴豆霜、西瓜霜。
5. **干馏法** 蛋黄油。

实验器具和材料

1. **实验器具** 烘箱、炒锅、锅铲、煤气灶、搪瓷盘、台秤、铁丝匾、烧杯、石棉网、量筒、漏斗、滤纸、乳钵、筛子、草纸、压榨器、瓦罐、毛刷、砧板等。

2. **实验材料** 肉豆蔻、木香、朴硝、朱砂、滑石粉、巴豆、西瓜、鸡蛋、麦麸、面粉、滑石粉、萝卜、皮硝。

实验方法

（一）煨法

1. 肉豆蔻

（1）麦麸煨 将麦麸和净肉豆蔻同置预热的炒制容器内，用文火加热并适当翻动，至麦麸呈焦黄色，药物颜色加深时取出，筛去麦麸，放凉，即得。每 100kg 药物，用麦麸 40kg。

（2）面裹煨　取面粉，加适量水拌匀，制成均匀适宜的团块，再压成薄片，将净肉豆蔻逐个包裹或用清水将肉豆蔻表面湿润后，如水泛丸法裹面粉 3~4 层，倒入已炒热的滑石粉中，适当翻动，至面皮呈焦黄色时取出，筛去滑石粉，剥去面皮，放凉。每 100kg 肉豆蔻，用滑石粉 50kg。

2. 木香　取未干燥的木香片，在铁丝匾中，用一层草纸，一层木香片，间隔平铺数层，置炉火旁或烘干室内，烘煨至木香所含挥发油渗透到纸上，取出木香，放凉，备用。

（二）提净法

芒硝　取适量鲜萝卜，洗净，切成片，置煮制容器内，加适量水煮透，捞出萝卜，再投入适量天然芒硝(朴硝)共煮，至全部溶化，取出过滤或澄清以后取上清液，放冷。待结晶大部析出，取出置避风处适当干燥即得。其结晶母液经浓缩后可继续析出结晶，直至不再析出结晶为止，每 100kg 朴硝，用萝卜 20kg。

（三）水飞法

1. 朱砂粉　取原药材，用磁铁吸尽铁屑，置乳钵内，加适量清水研磨成糊状，然后加多量清水搅拌，倾取混悬液，下沉的粗粉再如上法，反复操作多次，直至手捻细腻，无亮星为止，弃去杂质，合并混悬液，静置后倾去上面的清水，取沉淀晾干或 40℃以下干燥，再研细即可。或取朱砂用磁铁吸除铁屑，球磨水飞成细粉，40℃以下干燥。

2. 滑石粉　取净滑石，砸碎，碾成细粉。或取滑石粗粉，加水少量，碾磨至细，再加适量清水搅拌，倾出上层混悬液，下沉部分再按上法反复操作数次，合并混悬液，静置沉淀，倾去上清液，将沉淀物干燥后再研细粉。

（四）制霜法

1. 巴豆霜　取净巴豆仁，碾如泥状，里层用纸，外层用布包严，蒸热，压榨去油，如此反复数次，至药物松散成粉，不再粘结成饼为度。或取净巴豆仁碾细，测定脂肪油含量，加适量的淀粉稀释，使脂肪油含量符合规定，混匀，即得。

2. 西瓜霜　取新鲜西瓜，沿蒂头切一厚片作顶盖，挖出部分瓜瓤，将皮硝填入瓜内，盖上顶盖，用竹签扦牢，用碗或碟托住，盖好，悬挂于阴凉通风处，待西瓜表面析出白霜时，随时刮下，直至无白霜析出，晾干。或取新鲜西瓜切碎，放入不带釉的瓦罐内，一层西瓜一层皮硝，将口封严，悬挂于阴凉通风处，数日后即自瓦罐外面析出白色结晶物，随析随收集，至无结晶析出为止。每 100kg 西瓜，用皮硝 15kg。

（五）干馏法

蛋黄油　鸡蛋煮熟后，剥取蛋黄置适当容器内，以文火加热，除尽水分后用武火炒熬，至蛋黄油出尽为止，滤尽蛋黄油装瓶备用。

实验结果

（一）煨法

1. 煨肉豆蔻　成品表面棕黄色或淡棕色，稍显油性，香气更浓烈，味辛辣。

2. 煨木香　形如木香片，棕黄色，气微香。

（二）提净法

芒硝　为棱柱状、长方形或不规则块状及粒状。无色透明或类白色半透明。质脆，易碎，断面显玻璃样光泽。气微，味咸。

（三）水飞法

1. 朱砂粉　为朱红色极细粉末，体轻，以手指撮之无粒状物，以磁铁吸之，无铁末。气微，无味。

2. 滑石粉 为白色或类白色、微细、无砂性的粉末，质细腻，手捻有滑润感。气微，无味。

（四）制霜法

1. 巴豆霜 为疏松的淡黄色粉末，微显油性，味辛辣。

2. 西瓜霜 为类白色至黄白色的结晶性粉末，气微，味咸，有清凉感。

（五）干馏法

蛋黄油 为棕褐色或深黄棕色油状液体，具青黄色荧光。

注意事项

1. 煨制时火力不宜过强，一般以文火缓缓加热，并适当翻动。
2. 提净法制备芒硝时加水量要适宜，以免影响结晶。
3. 水飞研磨过程中，水量宜少，搅拌混悬时加水量宜大，以除去有毒物质或杂质。
4. 朱砂干燥时，温度不宜过高，以晾干为宜。
5. 生巴豆有剧毒，在制霜过程中需要做好防护，戴手套及口罩，用过的布或纸立即烧毁，以免误用。
6. 西瓜霜的制作宜在秋凉季节进行，容易析出结晶。
7. 干馏蛋黄油时，先文火使水分蒸发，后武火加热出油。

思考题

1. 简述煨法与固体辅料炒的异同点。
2. 简述芒硝提净过程中所用萝卜的作用。
3. 简述朱砂、滑石粉水飞的主要目的。
4. 简述巴豆制霜时应注意的问题。
5. 简述传统制备西瓜霜的方法的优缺点。
6. 简述干馏法的炮制目的。

Experiment 9 Other methods

Aims

1.1 To master the operation methods, precautions and product quality of simmering, purification, powder-refining with water, making frost-like powder and retorting.

1.2 To understand the purpose and significance of simmering, purification, powder-refining with water, making frost-like powder and retorting.

Principles

2.1 The simmering method

It is a method that is used to wrap the medicine after being cleaned or cut with wet surface or paper, put it in the heated Talc or hot sand, or place the medicine directly in the heated wheat bran, or spread the medicine on the oil-absorbing paper and heat it layer by layer to remove part of the oiliness.

2.2 The purification method

It is a method that is mainly aimed at certain mineral drugs, especially some soluble inorganic salt drugs, After dissolving, filtering, removing non-essential parts, and then recrystallizing to further purify the drug.

2.3 Levigating method

It is a method that is mainly aimed at certain water-insoluble mineral medicines. The method uses coarse and fine powders with different suspension properties in water, and repeatedly grinds water-insoluble minerals and shellfishes to separate and prepare extremely fine powders.

2.4 The method of making frost-like powder

It is a method of processing the medicine into a loose powder or fine crystals, or cooking into a powder residue. According to different operation methods, the defrost method can be divided into making frost-like powder with degreasing , making frost-like powder with dialysis, making frost-like powder with stewing, making frost-like powder with decoction, etc.

2.5 Carbonizating

It is a method of producing juice by putting medicine in a container and bake it with fire. The dry distillate is different from that of the original medicine so as to meet the clinical needs.

Contents

3.1 The simmering method

Myristicae Semen and Radix Aucklandiae.

3.2 The purification method

Mirabilite.

3.3 Levigating method

Cinnabaris and Talc.

3.4 The frosty method

Crotonis Semen Pulveratum and Mirabilitum Praeparatum.

3.5 Carbonizating method

Yolk oil.

Materials

4.1 Experimental apparatuses

Oven, wok, spatula, gas stove, enamel tray, platform scale, iron wire plaque, beaker, asbestos mesh, measuring cylinder, funnel, filter paper, mortar, sieve, straw paper, presser, crock, brush, anvil, etc.

4.2 Experimental materials

Myristicae Semen, Aucklandiae Radix, Mirabilite, Cinnabaris Talc, Crotonis Fructus, watermelon, egg, wheat bran, flour, Talc, radish and Mirabilite.

Methods

5.1 The simmering method

5.1.1 Myristicae Semen

5.1.1.1 Simmered by the wheat bran

Put the wheat bran and the pure Myristicae Semen in the preheated frying container, heat them on a gentle fire and turn properly until the wheat bran is burnt yellow, take them out when the medicine color is deepens, sifting the wheat bran and cool them. Using 40kg of wheat bran per 100kg of drug.

5.1.1.2 Simmered with flour

Take flour, add an appropriate amount of water and mix them well to make a uniform and suitable mass, then press it into thin slices, wrap the cleaning Myristicae Semen one by one or wet the surface of Myristicae Semen with water, wrap the flour in 3~4 layers with water like flooding method, pour it into the heated talcum powder, turn it properly, take it out when the skin is burnt yellow, sifting the talcum powder, peel the dough and let it cool. For 100kg of Myristicae Semen, use 50kg of talcum powder.

5.1.2 Aucklandiae Radix

Take non-drying Aucklandiae Radix slices. In the iron wire plaques, use a layer of straw paper, a layer of Aucklandiae Radix slices, and tile several layers at intervals. Place it by the fire or in a drying room, bake and simmer until the volatile oil contained in the Aucklandiae Radix permeates into the paper, take out the radix auckladiae, let it cool and set aside.

5.2 The purification method

Mirabilite

Take an appropriate amount of fresh radish, clean it, cut it into pieces, put it into a boiling container, add an appropriate amount of water to boil it thoroughly, remove radish. Then put them in a proper amount of natural mirabilite and cook it together until it dissolves completely, take it out to filtrate then cool it. When most of the crystallization precipitates out, take it out and put it in the shelter to dry properly. After concentrating the crystallization mother liquor, crystals can continue to be precipitated until crystals are no longer precipitated. For each 100kg of pumice, 20kg of radish is used.

5.3 Levigating method

5.3.1 Cinnabar powder

Take the original medicinal materials, use iron magnets to remove iron filings, place them in a mortar, grind them into a paste with an appropriate amount of water, and then add a large amount of water to stir. Sink the coarse powder, and repeat the operation as above until there is no bright stars. Remove non-essential parts, combine the suspensions, and then pour off the clear water after standing, take the sediment to dry below 40℃, and then finely grind. Or use cinnabar to remove iron filings with a magnet, refine it with ball and water into fine powder, and dry below 40℃.

5.3.2 Talc

Take cleaning talc, smash it and grind it into a fine powder. Or take coarse talcum powder and grind it to a fine level with a small amount of water. stir with an appropriate amount of water, pour out the upper suspension, and repeat the operation for the sinking part several times according to the above method, Combine the suspensions, settle them in a static state, pour out the supernatant, dry the precipitate, and then grind the fine powder.

5.4 The method of making frost-like powder

5.4.1 Crotonis Semen Pulveratum

Grind the cleaning Crotonis Fructus kernel into muddy stuff. The inner layer is covered with paper and the outer layer is wrapped tightly with cloth. steaming it and press to remove oil. This is repeated several times until the medicine is loose and powdered. Or take the cleaning Crotonis Fructus kernel and grind it, determine the content of fatty oil, add some starch to dilute, make the content of fat oil in accordance with the provisions, mix it evenly.

5.4.2 Mirabilitum Praeparatum

Take fresh watermelon, cut a thick slice along the tip of the stalk as the top cover, dig out some of the pulp, fill the inside of the melon with the mirabilite, cover the top cover, fasten it with bamboo sticks, hold it with a bowl or dish, cover it, hang it in a cool and ventilated place, when the white frost comes out on the surface of the watermelon, scrape it off at any time until no white frost comes out and dry it. Or take fresh watermelon and chop it, put them into an unglazed crock, one layer of watermelon and one layer of nitrate, seal the mouth tightly, hang them in a cool and ventilated place, and white crystals will be precipitate from the outside of the crock after a few days, collect them until no crystals precipitate. Use 15kg of mirabilite per 100kg of watermelon.

5.5 Carbonizating method

The yolk oil

After eggs are boiled, peel the yolk and put it into a proper container, heat it over gentle fire, fry the yolk with strong fire after removing the water, until the yolk oil goes out, filter it and bottle it for later use.

Results

6.1 The simmering method

6.1.1 Stewed Myristicae Semen

The surface of stewed Myristicae Semen is brownish yellow or light brown, slightly oily, with stronger fragrance and a pungent flavor.

6.1.2 Stewed Aucklandiae Radix

The shape of Aucklandiae Radix is like sliced radix aucklandiae, which is brown yellow and slightly fragrant.

6.2 The purification method

Mirabilite

It is prismatic, rectangular or irregular block and granular. It is colorless transparent or white-like translucent. It is brittle and fragile, with a glass-like gloss on the cross section. The odor is slight and the flavor is salty.

6.3 Water flying method

6.3.1 Cinnabaris

Cinnabaris is vermilion extremely fine powder, light in weight, free of particles by fingers, attracted by magnets, free of iron dust. The air is slight and no flavor.

6.3.2 Talc

Talc is white or quasi-white, fine and non-sandy powder, with fine quality and smooth feeling in hand twisting. The air is slight and no flavor.

6.4 Levigating

6.4.1 Crotonis Semen Pulveratum

It is very fine vermilion powder, light, no granular matter with fingers, no iron powder with magnets. The odor is tiny and the flavor is pungent.

6.4.2 Mirabilitum Praeparatum

It is white or off-white powder without sand. It feels smooth and its odor is tiny and the flavor is salty.

6.5 Carbonizating

The yolk oil

It is a brown or dark yellow brown oily liquid with a greenish yellow fluorescence.

Notes

7.1 When simmering, the fire power should not be too strong. Generally, drugs are heated slowly with gentle fire and turned over properly.

7.2 When preparing mirabilite by the purification method, the amount of water should be appropriate to avoid affecting the crystallization.

7.3 In the process of powder-refining with water, the amount of water should be less, and the amount of water during mixing and suspension should be more to remove toxic components or non-essential parts.

7.4 When the Cinnabaris is dry, the temperature should not be too high. It is better to dry it in the air.

7.5 Crude Crotonis Fructus is highly toxic. In the process of making frost-like powder, it is necessary for people to protect themselves by wearing gloves and masks, and burn the used cloth or paper immediately to avoid misuse.

7.6 Mirabilitum Praeparatum should be made in autumn or cool season so that it is easy to crystallize.

7.7 When the yolk oil is retorted, the water is evaporated by gentle fire first, and then the oil comes out by heating with strong fire.

Questions

8.1 Briefly describe the similarities and differences between simmering method and solid adjuvant.

8.2 Briefly describe the role of radish which is used in the process of mirabilite extraction.

8.3 Briefly describe the main purpose of Cinnabaris and Talc.

8.4 What should be paid attention to when making Crotonis Semen Pulveratum?

8.5 Briefly describe the advantages and disadvantages of the traditional method of preparing Mirabilitum Praeparatum.

8.6 Briefly describe the purposes of retorting.

第三章 中药炮制综合性实验

实验一 净制对牡丹皮有效成分含量的影响实验

PPT

实验目的

1. **掌握** 中药材净制方法及操作要点。

2. 通过对牡丹皮不同部位成分含量测定结果，说明净制对中药成分的影响。

实验原理

1. 中药材源于天然动、植物不同部位，同时中药材在采集、贮存和运输过程中，常混有杂质。去除杂质和非药用部位，可以提高有效成分相对含量，保证用药卫生及剂量的准确。

2. 按照《中国药典》（2020年版）“牡丹皮”项下含量测定方法，采用高效液相色谱法（HPLC）对牡丹皮主要有效成分丹皮酚进行含量测定。

实验内容

1. 牡丹皮原药材的净制。

2. 牡丹皮不同样品中丹皮酚的含量测定。

实验器具和材料

1. 实验器具 高效液相色谱仪、超声波提取仪、粉碎机、切药刀、搪瓷盘等。

2. 实验材料 牡丹皮、丹皮酚对照品；甲醇等。

实验方法

1. 牡丹皮原药材的净制 取牡丹皮原药材，除去细根和泥沙，刮去粗皮，除去木心，干燥。

2. 牡丹皮不同样品中丹皮酚的含量测定

（1）色谱条件与系统适用性试验 以十八烷基硅烷键合硅胶为填充剂，以甲醇－水（45∶55）为流动相，检测波长为274nm理论塔板数按丹皮酚峰计算不应低于5000。

（2）对照品溶液的制备 取丹皮酚对照品适量，精密称定，加甲醇制成每1ml含20μg的溶液，即得。

（3）供试品溶液的制备 取牡丹皮原药材与净制牡丹皮粗粉各0.5g，精密称定，置具塞锥形瓶中，精密加入甲醇 50ml，密塞，称定重量。超声 30 分钟，放冷。再次称定重量，用甲醇补足减失的重量，摇匀，过滤，精密量取续滤液 1ml，置 10ml 容量瓶中，加甲醇稀释至刻度，摇匀，即得。

（4）测定法　分别精密吸取对照品溶液与供试品溶液各 10μl，注入液相色谱仪，测定，即得。按干燥品计分别计算出牡丹皮原药材与净制牡丹皮中丹皮酚的百分含量。

实验结果

表 3-1　净制对牡丹皮中丹皮酚含量的影响

样品组	样品取样量 / g	丹皮酚含量 / %
牡丹皮原药材		
净制牡丹皮		

注意事项

1. 牡丹皮药材刮去粗皮时，不宜用铁质器具加工。
2. 测定丹皮酚含量时，要保持不同样品的操作条件一致。

思考题

1. 简述中药材净选加工的目的。
2. 简述牡丹皮净制后丹皮酚含量变化的原因。

Chapter 3 Comprehensiveness Experiment of Chinese Medicine Processing

Experiment 1 Effects of Cleaning on the Content of Active Ingredients in Moutan Cortex

Aims

1.1 To understand and master the cleaning methods and key operation points of Chinese medicinal materials.

1.2 To measure the content of ingredients in different parts of the skin of Paeonia suffruticosa Andr (Moutan Cortex, MC), the effect of the Cleaning on the ingredients of Chinese medicine can be explained.

Principles

2.1 Chinese medicinal materials are derived from different parts of natural animals and plants, and they are frequently mixed with impurities during the processes of collection, storage and transportation. Removal of non-essential and non-medicinal parts can increase the relative contents of active ingredients and ensure the hygiene of medicines and the accuracy of dosage.

2.2 The content of paeonol, the main active ingredients in MC, is determined by using high performance liquid chromatography (HPLC) in accordance with the content determination method under "MC" in the Chinese Pharmacopoeia (2020 Edition).

Contents

3.1 Cleaning of the original MC.

3.2 Determination of the contents of paeonol in MC of different samples.

Materials

4.1 Experimental apparatuses

HPLC, ultrasonic extraction instrument, pulverizer, medicine cutter, and enamel tray, etc.

4.2 Experimental materials

MC, paeonol standard references sample; methanol, etc.

Methods

5.1 Cleaning of MC original medicinal materials

The original MC medicinal materials are taken, fine roots and sediment are removed, the rough skin is scraped, the duramen is removed and the samples are dried.

5.2 Determination of paeonol content in MC of different samples

5.2.1 Chromatographic conditions and systematic adaptation tests

Octadecylsilane-bonded silica gel is used as the filler. Methanol water (45 ∶ 55) is used as the mobile phase. The detection wavelength is 274nm. The number of theoretical plates is calculated based on the paeonol peak and it should not less than 5000.

5.2.2 Preparation of standard reference sample solution

An appropriate amount of paeonol reference sample is taken and weighted accurately. Methanol is added to make a solution containing 20μg/ml of standard reference sample.

5.2.3 Preparation of the test solution

The crude powder of MC original medicinal materials and cleansed MC are 0.5g respectively, and are accurately weighed and placed in a conical flask with plug. Methanol (50ml) is added precisely. The samples are ultrasound for 30 minutes and let cool and weighed again, the lost weight is make up with methanol, shake well, filter, and 1ml of the filtrate is measured accurately and placed in a 10ml volumetric flask, methanol is added to the mark and shake well.

5.2.4 Assay Method

Each of the reference sample solution (10μl) is accurately pipette and the test solution is added into the HPLC for measurement. The percentages of paeonol in the original MC and the pure MC are calculated based on the dried product.

Results

Table 3–1 Effect of Cleaning on paeonol content in MC

Sample set	Amount of sample/g	Relative contents of paeonol/%
MC original medicinal materials		
Cleaned MC		

Notes

7.1 It is not advisable to use iron utensils to remove rough skin from MC.

7.2 When measuring paeonol content, the operating conditions of different samples should be kept consistent.

Questions

8.1 Briefly describe the purpose of the cleaning of Chinese medicinal materials.

8.2 Briefly describe the reasons for the change in paeonol content after the MC is cleaned.

PPT

实验二　切制对甘草中成分含量的影响实验

实验目的

1. **掌握**　中药材软化切制方法及操作要点。

2. 通过对甘草不同软化方法切制品中甘草酸和甘草苷含量比较，说明甘草洗润软化的意义。

实验原理

1. 中药材干燥状态细胞皱缩，需软化后才能切制成各种规格的饮片。药材用水清洗浸润，表面先湿润，从而在药材表面与中心之间形成湿度差，水分逐渐向中心部位渗透直至药材被软化。药材软化的过程除了与其体形大小有关外，还与药材的组织结构、水温等有关。

2. 甘草酸和甘草苷为甘草的主要有效成分。切制过程中不同的软化方法对甘草中甘草酸和甘草苷含量有较大的影响，软化时加水量过多会导致有效成分流失。本实验分别采用洗润法（《中国药典》2020 年版）和泡法软化甘草，再经切片、干燥，制得供试品。用 70% 乙醇超声提取供试品中甘草酸和甘草苷，用 HPLC 同时测定甘草酸和甘草苷的含量。

实验内容

1. 甘草的软化切制。

2. 甘草不同饮片中甘草酸和甘草苷的含量测定。

实验器具和材料

1. **实验器具**　高效液相色谱仪、超声波清洗器、电子天平、切药机、烘箱、盆、竹匾、砂布、切药刀、搪瓷盘、容量瓶、移液管、锥形瓶、漏斗、微孔滤膜（0.45μm）等。

2. **实验材料**　甘草、甘草苷对照品、甘草酸铵对照品；乙醇、磷酸、色谱乙腈、纯净水等。

实验方法

1. 甘草的软化切制

（1）洗润法软化　取甘草药材，除去杂质，用水快速洗净，及时取出，置适宜容器内，以湿物覆盖，保持湿润状态，至药材内外湿度一致时，取出，切厚片（厚度为 2~4mm），干燥。

（2）泡法软化　取甘草药材，除去杂质，洗净，置适宜容器内，加入清水至淹没药材，上压重物，浸泡至内外湿度一致时，取出，切厚片（厚度为 2~4mm），干燥。

2. 甘草不同饮片中甘草酸和甘草苷的含量测定

（1）色谱条件与系统适用性试验　以十八烷基硅烷键合硅胶为填充剂；以乙腈为流动相 A，以含 0.05% 磷酸溶液为流动相 B，梯度洗脱，洗脱程序见表 3-2；检测波长为 237nm。理论板数按甘草苷峰计算应不低于 5000。

表 3-2 梯度洗脱程序

时间（分钟）	流动相 A（%）	流动相 B（%）
0~8	19	81
8~35	19→50	81→50
35~36	50→100	50→0
36~40	100→19	0→81

（2）对照品溶液的制备　取甘草苷对照品、甘草酸铵对照品适量，精密称定，加 70% 乙醇分别制成每 1ml 含甘草苷 20μg、甘草酸铵 0.2mg 的溶液，即得（甘草酸重量 = 甘草酸铵重量 /1.0207）。

（3）供试品溶液的制备　取不同软化方法制备的甘草片粉末（过三号筛）各约 0.2g，精密称定，置具塞锥形瓶中，精密加入 70% 乙醇 100ml，密塞，称定重量，超声处理 30 分钟，放冷，再称定重量，用 70% 乙醇补足减失的重量，摇匀，滤过，取续滤液，即得。

（4）测定法　分别精密吸取对照品溶液与供试品溶液各 10μl，注入液相色谱仪，测定，即得。按干燥品计，分别计算不同软化法制备的甘草中甘草酸和甘草苷的百分含量。

实验结果

表 3-3 不同软化法对甘草饮片中甘草酸和甘草苷含量的影响

样品组	样品取样量 / g	甘草酸含量 / %	甘草苷含量 / %
洗润法			
泡法			

注意事项

1. 甘草切制时，除软化方法不同外，切片厚度、干燥温度和时间应一致。
2. 测定甘草酸和甘草苷含量时，要保持不同软化品的操作条件一致。

思考题

1. 简述软化切制过程影响饮片质量的主要因素。
2. 简述不同软化方法制备的甘草片中甘草酸和甘草苷含量差异的原因。

Experiment 2　Effect of cutting on the content of components in Glycyrrhizae Radix Et Rhizoma

Aims

1.1　To master the methods and key points of operation of raw Chinese Medicine softening and cutting.

1.2　To explained the significance of Glycyrrhizae Radix Et Rhizoma softening by washing and moistening by comparing the content of glycyrrhizic acid and liquiritin in different softening methods.

Principles

2.1　Raw Chinese medicine have some shrinkage cells in dried state, which needs to be softened before it can be cut into Yinpian (decoction pieces/processed Chinese medicine). Clean and infiltrate the raw Chinese medicine with water, wet the surface first, thus form a humidity difference between the surface and the center of the raw Chinese medicine, the water gradually permeates into the center until the raw Chinese medicine is penetrated. The softening process of raw Chinese medicine is not only related to their body size, but also their tissue structure and water temperature and so on.

2.2　Main active components of Glycyrrhizae Radix Et Rhizoma are glycyrrhizic acid and liquiritin. The content of glycyrrhizic acid and liquiritin in Glycyrrhizae Radix Et Rhizoma is greatly affected by different softening methods in the cutting process, too much water in softening process will lead to the loss of main active components. In this experiment, the methods of soaking and moistening refer to soften Glycyrrhizae Radix Et Rhizoma (《Chinese Pharmacopoeia》2020), then after slicing and drying, the test sample being examined is prepared. Glycyrrhizic acid and liquiritin are ultrasonic extracted by 70% ethanol, and the content of glycyrrhizic acid and liquiritin is determined by HPLC at the same time.

Contents

3.1　Softening and cutting of Glycyrrhizae Radix Et Rhizoma.

3.2　Determination of the content of glycyrrhizic acid and liquiritin in different Yinpian (decoction pieces/processed Chinese medicine) of Glycyrrhizae Radix Et Rhizoma.

Materials

4.1　Experimental apparatuses

High performance liquid chromatography, ultrasonic cleaner, electronic scale, medicine cutting machine, oven, basin, bamboo plaque, gauze, herb cutting knife, enamel tray, volumetric flask, transfer pipette, conical flask, funnel, millipore filter (0.45μm) and so on.

4.2 Experimental materials

Glycyrrhizae Radix Et Rhizoma, glycyrrhizic acid (reference sample), ammonium gycyrrhizate (reference sample), ethyl alcohol, phosphoric acid, chromatography acetonitrile, distilled water and so on.

Methods

5.1 Softening and cutting of Glycyrrhizae Radix Et Rhizoma.

5.1.1 Softening by washing and moistening

Take Glycyrrhizae Radix Et Rhizoma raw Chinese medicine, remove impurities, wash with water quickly and take out in time, place it in a suitable container, cover it with wet material and keep it wet. When the internal and external humidity of the raw Chinese medicine are the same, take it out, cut into thick slices (the thickness is 2~4mm), and dry.

5.1.2 Softening by soaking method

Take Glycyrrhizae Radix Et Rhizoma raw Chinese medicine, remove impurities, wash with water, place it in a suitable container, add clear water to submerge the medicinal materials, press a heavy object on it, soak until the internal and external humidity are the same, take out and cut into thick slices (the thickness is 2~4mm), and dry.

5.2 Determination of glycyrrhizic acid and liquiritin in different Yinpian (decoction pieces/processed Chinese medicine) of Glycyrrhizae Radix Et Rhizoma.

5.2.1 Chromatographic conditions and systematic adaptation test

Use octadecane bonded silica gel as filler, acetonitrile as mobile phase A, gradient elution 0.05% phosphoric acid solution as mobile phase B, gradient elution and elution program is shown in table 3-2, and the detection wavelength is 237nm. theoretical plates should be no less than 5000, according to the calculation of glycyrrhizin peak.

Table 3-2 Gradient elution procedure

Time (minutes)	Mobile Phase A (%)	Mobile Phase B (%)
0~8	19	81
8~35	19→50	81→50
35~36	50→100	50→0
36~40	100→19	0→81

5.2.2 Preparation of reference sample

Take proper liquiritin (reference sample) and ammonium glycyrrhizate (reference sample), accurately weigh and add 70% ethanol to make a solution containing 20μg liquiritin (reference substance) and 0.2mg ammonium glycyrrhizinate per 1ml, then reference solution is prepared (weight of glycyrrhizic acid = weight of ammonium glycyrrhizinate / 1.0207).

5.2.3 Preparation of test sample solution

Take 0.2g licorice powder (passing No.3 sieve) prepared by different softening methods, weigh accurately, conical flask with plug, precisely add 100ml of 70% ethanol, sealed with plug , weigh and ultrasonic treatment for 30 minutes, then cool down, weigh again, add 70% ethanol to make up the lost weight, shake well, filter and take the continuous to obtain the test solution.

5.2.4 Determination method

Accurately pipette 10μg of the reference solution and the test samples respectively into the liquid chromatograph for determination, the operation is completed. Calculate the percentage of glycyrrhizic acid and liquiritin in different softening methods according to the dried product.

Results

Table 3-3 Effect of different softening methods on the content of glycyrrhizic acid and liquiritin in Glycyrrhizae Radix Et Rhizoma Yinpian (decoction pieces/processed Chinese medicine)

Sample group	Sample quantity/g	Glycyrrhizic acid content/%	Liquiritin content/%
Washing and moistening method			
Soaking method			

Notes

7.1 Except different softening methods, the slice thickness, drying temperature and time should be the same.

7.2 When determining the content of glycyrrhizic acid and liquiritin, the operating conditions of different softened products should be the same.

Questions

8.1 Briefly describe the main factors influencing the quality of Yinpian (decoction pieces/processed Chinese medicine) in softening and cutting process.

8.2 Briefly describe the reason for the difference of glycyrrhizic acid and liquiritin content in Glycyrrhizae Radix Et Rhizoma decotion pieces prepared by different softening methods.

PPT

实验三　炒黄对王不留行浸出物的影响实验

实验目的

1. **掌握**　炒黄的炮制方法和药物炮制的作用。
2. 通过王不留行炒制前后浸出物的含量变化，说明炮制对药物浸出物产生的影响。

实验原理

1. 王不留行属于种子类药物，含有大量油脂，并有坚硬致密的种皮，不利于水分的浸润和渗透。采用加热炒制，表层组织失水收缩，内部组织的水分受热气化产生膨胀压，达到一定程度可使表皮组织明显破裂，利于水分进入和成分溶出；同时内聚力降低，质地疏松有利于粉碎。炒王不留行爆花率与含水量和种子成熟度有关，爆花率越高，成分溶出率越高。

2. 王不留行具有活血通经，下乳消肿，利尿通淋的功能，含有三萜皂苷、黄酮、氨基酸、微量元素、类脂、糖类等成分，临床应用多入汤剂。按照《中国药典》（2020 年版）四部 2201“浸出物测定法”，以水为溶媒加热提取，比较王不留行炒黄前后水溶性浸出物的含量变化，验证炒黄有利于成分煎出炮制原理的科学性。

实验内容

1. 王不留行的炮制。
2. 王不留行不同炮制品中浸出物的测定。

实验器具和材料

1. 实验器具　电子天平、炒锅、锅铲、煤气灶（控温电炉或电磁炉等）、搪瓷盘、电热套、烘箱、冷凝器、蒸发皿、布氏漏斗、干燥器、水浴锅、250ml 锥形瓶、25ml 刻度吸管、100ml 刻度吸管、300ml 抽滤瓶、滤纸等。

2. 实验材料　王不留行、蒸馏水等。

实验方法

1. 王不留行的炮制　取净王不留行 100g，置热锅内，用中火加热，炒至大多数爆开百花，取出，晾凉。

2. 王不留行不同炮制品浸出物的测定　分别取王不留行生品和炒制品约 5g，精密称定，置 250ml 锥形瓶中，加水 100ml，密塞，称定重量，静置 1 小时，加热回流 1 小时，放冷后，取下锥形瓶，称定重量，用水补足减失的重量，摇匀，用干燥滤器滤过，精密量取续滤液 25ml，置已干燥至恒重的蒸发皿中，在水浴上蒸干后，于 105℃干燥 3 小时，移至干燥器中，冷却 30 分钟，迅速精密称定重量，计算供试品中水溶性浸出物的含量。

实验结果

表 3-4 王不留行不同炮制品中浸出物含量比较

样品组	样品取样量 / g	浸出物重量 / g	浸出物含量 / %
王不留行			
炒王不留行			

注意事项

1. 炒王不留行时，锅预热，火力宜大，用中火，防止火力过小产生僵子。
2. 浸出物测定宜选择爆花率 80% 以上的样品。
3. 样品提取过程中应控制温度，防止温度过高导致爆沸。
4. 不同炮制品浸出物制备过程中应条件一致，防止产生误差影响实验结果的准确性。

思考题

1. 简述影响炒王不留行爆花率的主要因素。
2. 简述王不留行炮制品比较研究的评价指标除水浸出物外，还可选择哪些指标。

Experiment 3 The influence of stir-frying to yellow on extractives of Vaccariae Semen

Aims

1.1 To master operation and principle of the stir-frying to yellow of Vaccariae Semen.

1.2 To understand the significance of processing on extractives of medicinal materials through comparison of the extracts amount of Vaccariae Semen before and after processing.

Principles

2.1 Vaccariae Semen, a seed medicinal material containing lots of oils & fats, has hard and dense testa; therefore, it's hard to be moistened and penetrated by moisture content. The stir-frying processing could result in water loss and drying shrinkage of surface tissue, and subsequently lead to the formation of moisture content swelling pressure in internal tissues of the seeds, which could be beneficial for the moisture content infiltration and extractive of the active composition in seeds. Besides, the cohesion decline of the seed tissue could also beneficial for powdering of the medicinal materials. Importantly, for stir-frying of the Vaccariae Semen, the puffed rice ratio has a positive correlation relationship with the extractive rate.

2.2 Vaccariae Semen possesses the functions of "activating blood to promote menstruation, promoting lactation to detumescence, and disinhibit urine and free strangury" , and the main phytochemical compositions are triterpene saponins, flavonoids, lipoids, saccharides, and amino acids, etc. Furthermore, decoction is the most common used medication form in clinic. According to Chinese Pharmacopoeia (2020 Edition), volume Ⅳ, 2201 "Extracts determination", heating extraction is carried out with the water as the solvent, and subsequently the extracts amount of Vaccariae Semen before and after processing are compared to verify the processing mechanisms and significance of stir-frying to yellow on Vaccariae Semen.

Contents

3.1 Processing method of the Vaccariae Semen.

3.2 Determination of extracts from Vaccariae Semen and its processed products.

Materials

4.1 Experimental apparatuses

Electronic scale/balance, experimental apparatus wok, turner, electric stove, enamel tray, electric jacket, oven, condensing apparatus, evaporating dish, Buchner funnel, desiccator, water bath, conical flask (250ml), graduated pipette (25ml, 100ml), suction flask (300ml), filter paper, etc.

4.2 Experimental materials

Vaccariae Semen, distilled water, etc.

Methods

5.1 Processing of the Vaccariae Semen

A total of 100g Vaccariae Semen are weighed accurately to place in the hot fry pan, and medium fire is used to process the Vaccariae Semen. After most of the Vaccariae Semen become puffed rice, the processed Vaccariae Semen are took out and then cooled.

5.2 Determination of the extractives' contents from Vaccariae Semen and its processed products

A total of 5g Vaccariae Semen crude Chinese medicine and its processed product are exactly weighed respectively, and then the samples are placed in a 250ml conical flask, and 100ml distilled water is added. The conical flasks are sealed with plug and weighed exactly, and then reacted under stationary condition for 1 hour. After that, the samples are heated reflux with water for 1 hour, and then allowed to cool and replenished the lost with water. Subsequently, the extracts are filtrated, and 25ml subsequent filtrate are measured accurately in a invariable weight evaporating dish. The sample in the evaporating dish is evaporated to dry for 3 hours after water bath (105℃) successively. Then, the samples are placed in the desiccator to cool for 30 minutes, and subsequently the test samples are weighed accurately and the extractives' contents are calculated according to the experimental data.

Results

Table 3-4 Comparison of extractives' contents from Vaccariae Semen and its processed products

Samples	Sampling amount/g	Weight of extracts/g	Extracts contents/%
Vaccariae Semen			
Stir-fried Vaccariae Semen			

Notes

7.1 Big fire should be used to preheat the fry pan, and medium fire should be used to process the Vaccariae Semen in order to avoid to produce the "Jiangzi" .

7.2 For determining the extracts contents, stir-fried Vaccariae Semen with the 80% puffed rice ratio should be selected.

7.3 Avoiding bumping in the extracting process.

7.4 The same extracting conditions should be carried out for each sample to avoid error influences.

Questions

8.1 Briefly describe the main influence actors for the puffed rice ratio of Vaccariae Semen.

8.2 What are other indexes that we can selected to study the influence of stir-frying to yellow processing on Vaccariae Semen besides extractives' contents?

PPT

实验四　炒炭对槐米成分及止血作用的影响实验

实验目的

1. **掌握**　炒炭的炮制方法及对药物的影响。

2. 通过对槐米和槐米炭中鞣质含量及止血作用影响，说明“炒炭存性”的意义。

实验原理

药物高温条件下加热炒炭，其组织与成分均产生不同程度的物理与化学变化，炒炭的药物可产生或增强止血作用，炮制上有“血见黑则止”的学说。槐米炒炭后具有止血作用的鞣质含量增加，鞣质具有还原性，在常温或酸性溶液中可被高锰酸钾氧化，据此测定鞣质的含量。观察槐米炒炭前后对小鼠出血时间和凝血时间的影响，验证槐米炒炭后鞣质增加与止血作用的相关性。

实验内容

1. 槐米炭的炮制。
2. 槐米不同炮制品中鞣质含量测定。
3. 槐米不同炮制品止血实验。

实验器具和材料

1. 实验器具　温度计、10ml 吸量管、500ml 烧瓶、乳钵、漏斗、玻璃漏斗、500ml 容量瓶、500ml 量筒、10ml 量筒、棕色瓶、25ml 酸式滴定管、10ml 刻度吸管、抽滤瓶、小砂轮、电子天平、电炉、5ml 注射器、毛细管（φ1mm）、剪刀、秒表、小鼠灌胃器、兔开口器等。

2. 实验材料　槐米；高锰酸钾、靛胭脂、浓硫酸、氯化钠、碳酸钡、碳酸钡、明胶、滤纸条等。

实验方法

1. 槐米炭的炮制　取净槐米，置预热后的炒制容器内，用中火加热，炒至焦褐色，喷洒少量清水、灭尽火星，文火炒干，取出，放凉，备用。

2. 槐米不同炮制品中鞣质含量测定　分别取槐米生品和炒炭品，置于研钵内研成粗粉，精密称定约 10g，加蒸馏水 300ml，小火煮沸 30 分钟，过滤。药渣再加水 100ml 提取 2 次，合并滤液，定容于 500ml 容量瓶中，静置过夜，次日滤去析出的沉淀物。精密吸取滤液 100ml 于 1000ml 锥形瓶中，加蒸馏水 500ml，0.6% 靛胭脂 5ml，硫酸 20ml，0.02mol/L 高锰酸钾溶液滴定至出现黄绿色，消耗高锰酸钾的毫升数为“A”。

（1）空白溶液测定　精密吸取上述提取液 100ml，加入新鲜配制的 2.5% 明胶液 30ml，用氯化钠饱和，加入 10% 稀硫酸 10ml 及硫酸钡 10g，振摇数分钟，于干滤纸过滤。吸取滤液 10ml，同上法用 0.02ml/L 高锰酸钾溶液滴定，消耗高锰酸钾的毫升数为“B”。

（2）鞣质的含量测定　以鞣酸为标准，每毫升 0.1mol/L 高锰酸钾溶液，相当于 0.004157g 鞣酸。

$$X=\frac{(A-B)\times 0.004157\times T\times 100}{W}\times\frac{M_1}{M_2}$$

式中，X：样品中鞣质含量（%）；A：高锰酸钾的用量（毫升数）；B：空白中高锰酸钾的用量（毫升数）；T：稀释度；W：取样量；M_1：滴定用高锰酸钾的毫摩尔数；M_2：0.1mol/L 用高锰酸钾的毫摩尔数。

3. 槐米不同炮制品止血实验

（1）药液的准备　称取生药和炭药各 100g，分别置于 1000ml 烧杯中，加水 400ml 煎煮 1 小时，用纱布过滤，残渣加水 200ml，再煎煮 30 分钟，纱布过滤，合并滤液浓缩至 100ml。

（2）出血时间测定　取体重 18~22g 小鼠 30 只，随机分成 3 组，称重，标号。按 0.8ml/20g 的剂量，分别将生药水煎液和炭药水煎液给两组小鼠灌胃。30 分钟后，剪去小鼠尾部 3mm，每隔 30 秒，用滤纸轻轻吸取血滴，但不能挤压尾部，直至血流自然停止，用秒表记录出血时间。另以生理盐水组对照，对所得结果进行统计学分析。

（3）凝血时间测定　取体重 18~22g 小鼠 30 只，随机分成 3 组，称重，标号。按 0.8ml/20g 剂量，分别将生药水煎液和炭药水煎液给两组小鼠灌胃。30 分钟后，用毛细管（φ1mm）于小鼠眼球静脉取血，至管内血柱达 5cm 后取出，当血液进入毛细管时开始计时，每 30 秒轻轻折断毛细管约 0.5cm，若有血丝出现即为凝血，测得凝血时间。另以生理盐水为对照组，对所测得结果进行统计学分析。

实验结果

表 3–5　槐米不同炮制品中鞣质含量测定

样品组	样品取样量 / g	鞣质含量 / %
槐米		
槐米炭		

表 3–6　槐米不同炮制品出血时间与凝血时间实验（$\bar{x}\pm s$）

样品组	给药剂量	数量 / n	出血时间	凝血时间
对照组				
槐米				
槐米炭				

注意事项

1. 槐米炒炭时，铁锅温度不能超过 250℃，槐米温度不能超过 210℃，出炭率不得低于 82%。
2. 加明胶和酸性氯化钠溶液后，必须振摇。
3. 测定出血时间时，应将小鼠固定，并尽量使之保持安静。
4. 测定凝血时间时，应轻折毛细管，并缓缓向左右拉开。

思考题

1. 简述鞣质含量测定的原理，如何除去测定中的干扰物。
2. 简述槐米生品和炒炭品止血作用有何不同。

Experiment 4 The influence of carbonizing by stir-frying on chemical compositions and hemostatic effects of the Flos Sophorae Immaturus

Aims

1.1 To master operation of the carbonizing by stir-frying processing and its influences on medicinal materials.

1.2 To understand the significance of the "stir-frying the crude drugs into black on outside and brown in inside" through studying the influence of carbonizing by stir-frying processing on chemical constituents and hemostatic effects of the Flos Sophorae Immaturus.

Principles

Under high temperature condition, various physical and chemical reactions would be occurred in the tissues and chemical compositions of medicinal materials. In addition, carbonizing by stir-frying processing is recognized to produce or enhance the hemostatic effects in medicinal materials due to the theory of "Blood can be coagulated by Black " in traditional Chinese medicine. It's reported that tannins possesses good hemostatic effects, and interestingly the contents of tannins in carbonized Flos Sophorae Immaturus are significant higher than that of in crude Flos Sophorae Immaturus. The contents of tannins could be determined based on the principle that tannins has good reducibility and can be oxidized by the potassium manganite in acid solution. Furthermore, by determine the hemostatic indexes (bleeding time & blood clotting time), the relationship between the tannins contents in medicinal materials and its hemostatic effect will be explored.

Contents

3.1 Preparation of the carbonized Flos Sophorae Immaturus.

3.2 Determination of tannins' contents in Flos Sophorae Immaturus and its processed product.

3.3 Determination of hemostatic effects of Flos Sophorae Immaturus and its processed product.

Materials

4.1 Experimental apparatuses

Electronic scales, thermometer, 10ml pipet, 500ml flask, mortar, funnel, glass funnel, 500ml volumetric flask, measuring cylinder (500ml and 10ml), brown bottle, 25ml acid burette, graduated pipette (10ml), suction flask, grinding wheel, electronic scale/balance, electric heater, injection syringe (5ml), capillary (φ1mm), scissor, second chronograph, intragastric device for mouse, mouth gag for rabbit, etc.

4.2 Experimental materials

Flos Sophorae Immaturus, potassium manganite, indicarminum, concentrated sulphuric acid, sodium chloride, barium carbonate, gelatin, filter paper, etc.

Methods

5.1 Preparation of the carbonized Flos Sophorae Immaturus

Flos Sophorae Immaturus are stir-fried using medium fire to be black-brown-colored superficially in a pre-heated fry pan. Then, a small amount of clear water is sprayed to extinguish the spark of medicinal materials, and the processed Flos Sophorae Immaturus are subsequently stir-fried using gentel fire to be dried. Finally, the processed Flos Sophorae Immaturus are took out and allowed to cool for later use .

5.2 Determination of the tannins' contents in Flos Sophorae Immaturus and its processed product

A total of 10g powder of the Flos Sophorae Immaturus crude Chinese medicine and its processed product are weighed accurately respectively, and then the samples are boiled with 300ml distilled water for 30 minutes using small fire, and filtrated, subsequently the dregs of decoction are decocted another twice with 100ml distilled water for 30 minutes using small fire. All the filtrates are combined and metered fixed volume in a 500ml volumetric flask, and then the solution are static stayed overnight, and filtrated in the next day. The filtrates (100ml) are accurately pipetted in a 1000ml conical flask, and 500ml distilled water, 5ml 0.6% indicarminum, 20ml sulfuric acid are added. Subsequently, 0.02mol/L potassium permanganate solution is titrated with the solution until the solution color change into green yellow, and the used volume (milliliter amount) of the 0.02mol/L potassium permanganate solution is recorded as "A" .

5.2.1 Blank solution determination

100ml solution mentioned above is accurately pipetted in a conical flask, and 30ml fresh 2.5% gelatin solution is added, then the mixed solution is saturated with sodium chloride, and subsequently 10ml 10% dilute sulphuric acid and 10g barium sulfate are added. After shaking several minutes, the mixed solution is filtrated with dry filter paper. Then, 10ml filtrates are pipetted in a conical flask, and subsequently 0.02mol/L potassium permanganate solution is titrated with the solution until the solution color change into green yellow, and the used volume (milliliter amount) of the 0.02mol/L potassium permanganate solution is recorded as "B" .

5.2.2 Determination of the tannins' contents

Taking the tannin as standard reference, one milliliter of the 0.1mol/L potassium permanganate solution is equivalent to 0.004157g tannins.

$$X=\frac{(A-B)\times 0.004157\times T\times 100}{W}\times\frac{M_1}{M_2}$$

X: Tannin contents (%); A: milliliter amount of the 0.02mol/L potassium permanganate solution in sample solution; B: milliliter amount of the 0.02mol/L potassium permanganate solution in blank solution; T: dilution; W: sampling weight; M_1: millimole number of the titrated with potassium permanganate solution; M_2: millimole number of the 0.1mol/L potassium permanganate solution.

5.2.3 Determination of the hemostatic effects of Flos Sophorae Immaturus and its processed product

5.2.3.1 Sample preparation

A total of 100g powder of the Flos Sophorae Immaturus and its processed product are exactly weighed respectively, and then the samples are boiled with 400ml distilled water for 1hour in a 1000ml beaker, and then filtrated with gauze, subsequently the dregs of decoction are boiled with 200ml distilled water for 30 minutes again. The filtrates are combined and concentrated to 100ml.

5.2.3.2 Determination of the bleeding time

Total 30 mice (18~22g) were divided into 3 groups randomly and weighed, including control group, Flos Sophorae Immaturus group and carbonized Flos Sophorae Immaturus group. The testing drugs including extracts of Flos Sophorae Immaturus group and carbonized Flos Sophorae Immaturus group are administrated orally at the doses of 0.8ml/20g. Then, 30 minutes after the drug administration, the 3mm tail from the tip of the mouse is cut, and a filter paper is used to examine the bleeding every 30 seconds since the tail cutting until blood clotting, but it can't squeeze the tail. The bleeding time is recorded as the evaluating index, and the normal saline is used as the blank control.

5.2.3.3 Determination of the blood clotting time

Total 30 mice (18~22g) were divided into 3 groups randomly and weighed, including control group, Flos Sophorae Immaturus group and carbonized Flos Sophorae Immaturus group. The testing drugs including extracts of Flos Sophorae Immaturus group and carbonized Flos Sophorae Immaturus group are administrated orally at the doses of 0.8ml/20g. Then, 30 minutes after the drug administration, a capillary tube (φ1mm) is used to collect blood from the eyeball vein with 5cm blood column. Time recording start from the initial of the blood collecting, and 0.5cm capillary tube is broke off to observe the blood clotting every 30 seconds, and the blood clotting time is recorded when the blood clotting occurred, and the normal saline is used as the blank control.

Results

Table 3–5 Determining tannins' contents in Flos Sophorae Immaturus and its processed product

Group	Sampling weight/g	Tannins' contents/%
Flos Sophorae Immaturus		
Carbonized Flos Sophorae Immaturus		

Table 3–6 Determining hemostatic effects in Flos Sophorae Immaturus and its processed product（$\bar{x}\pm s$）

Group	Dose	Number/n	Bleeding time	Blood clotting time
Control				
Flos Sophorae Immaturus				
Carbonized Flos Sophorae Immaturus				

Notes

7.1 For preparation of the carbonized Flos Sophorae Immaturus, the temperature of the fry pan and medicinal materials are no more than 250℃ and 210℃, respectively, and the carbonized products yield was no less than 82%.

7.2 After the adding of gelatin and acid sodium chloride solution, the mixed solution must be shook several minutes.

7.3 For determination of the bleeding time, the mouse should be fixed and kept quiet.

7.4 For determination of the blood clotting time, the capillary tube should be broke off gently with careful observation on the blood clotting.

Questions

8.1 What is the principle for determination of the tannin in medicinal materials and how to remove the chaff interference in the determination?

8.2 Briefly describe the differences in the hemostatic effects between Flos Sophorae Immaturus crude Chinese medicine and carbonized Flos Sophorae Immaturus.

PPT

实验五　砂炒对马钱子质量及毒性的影响实验

实验目的

1. **掌握**　砂炒的炮制方法及对药物的影响。
2. 通过对砂烫马钱子质量及毒性的影响实验，说明砂烫马钱子的炮制原理及目的意义。

实验原理

1. 河砂由于质地坚硬，传热较快，与药物接触面积较大，可使其受热均匀。故适用于炒制质地坚硬或韧性较大的动物类药物，同时砂炒可使某些药物的毒性成分结构改变或破坏，从而降低其毒性。马钱子砂烫时，高温使马钱子中的毒性成分破坏，毒性降低，可供内服；同时，使马钱子质地酥脆，易于粉碎。马钱子主要成分为士的宁和马钱子碱，其既是镇痛有效成分也是有毒成分。马钱子生品砂烫炮制时，使其中所含士的宁、马钱子碱等毒性较大的生物碱的醚键断裂、开环，转化成为异士的宁、异马钱子碱、士的宁氮氧化物、马钱子碱氮氧化物、异士的宁氮氧化物、异马钱子碱氮氧化物等毒性较小的生物碱。此外，马钱子碱相对比士的宁易于分解破坏（这与其结构上的 C_2—OCH_3、C_3—OCH_3 取代有关），致使马钱子碱的含量大幅下降，士的宁的含量则下降较少，而马钱子碱的药理强度仅为士的宁的 1/40，通过炮制可除去疗效较差而毒性较大的马钱子碱，从而降低了马钱子的毒性。

2. 在碱性条件下，士的宁以游离形式存在，且易溶于三氯甲烷。因此，选取三氯甲烷和氢氧化钠试液作为提取马钱子中目标成分的溶剂。以 C_{18} 为固定相，亲水性溶液为流动相，采用 HPLC 测定供试品溶液中的士的宁和马钱子碱含量；采用薄层色谱法，以硅胶 G 为吸附剂，碱性弱极性溶液为展开剂，以士的宁和马钱子碱为对照进行马钱子生品与砂烫品的鉴别；通过对马钱子生品和砂烫品的 LD_{50} 测定，比较马钱子生品和砂烫品的毒性。

实验内容

1. 砂烫马钱子的炮制。
2. HPLC 测定马钱子不同炮制品中士的宁和马钱子碱的含量。
3. 马钱子不同炮制品的 TLC 鉴别。
4. 马钱子不同炮制品的小鼠 LD_{50} 测定。

实验器具和材料

1. **实验器具**　高效液相色谱仪、烘箱、水浴锅、超声波清洗器、粉碎机、电子天平、炒锅、电炉、锅铲、搪瓷盘、三号筛、10ml 容量瓶、刻度吸管、分液漏斗、50ml 具塞锥形瓶等。

2. **实验材料**　马钱子、士的宁、马钱子碱对照品、河砂；硅胶 G、CMC-Na、C_{18} 色谱柱、氢氧化钠、碘化铋钾、甲苯、丙酮、三氯甲烷、浓氨水、庚烷磺酸钠、磷酸二氢钾、甲醇、无水乙醇、浓硫酸、浓盐酸、磷酸、乙腈、水，中速定量滤纸、pH 试纸等。

3. **实验动物**　健康小鼠（18~22g），雌雄各半。

实验方法

1. 砂烫马钱子的炮制 取净马钱子，称重。取洁净的河砂放入锅内，用武火加热至灵活状态时，投入大小一致的净马钱子，不断翻动，烫至鼓起并显棕褐色或深棕色，取出，筛去河砂，摊开放凉，称重，计算得率。砂烫后的马钱子两面均膨胀鼓起。表面棕褐色或深棕色，质坚脆，平行剖面可见棕褐色或深棕色的胚乳。微有香气，味极苦。河砂用量以能掩盖药物为度。

2. HPLC 测定马钱子不同炮制品中士的宁和马钱子碱的含量

（1）色谱条件及系统适应性试验 以十八烷基硅烷键合硅胶为填充剂；以乙腈 -0.01mol/L 庚烷磺酸钠与 0.02mol/L 磷酸二氢钾等量混合溶液（用 10% 磷酸调节 pH 至 2.8）（21：79）为流动相；检测波长为 260nm。理论板数按士的宁峰计算应不低于 5000。

（2）对照品溶液的制备 取士的宁对照品 6mg、马钱子碱对照品 5mg，精密称定，分别置 10ml 量瓶中，加三氯甲烷适量使溶解并稀释至刻度，摇匀。分别精密量取 2ml，置同一 10ml 量瓶中，用甲醇稀释至刻度，摇匀，即得（每 1ml 含士的宁 0.12mg、马钱子碱 0.1mg）。

（3）供试品溶液的制备 取马钱子不同炮制品粉末（过三号筛）约 0.6g，精密称定，置具塞锥形瓶中，加氢氧化钠试液 3ml，混匀，放置 30 分钟，精密加入三氯甲烷 20ml，密塞，称定重量，置水浴中回流提取 2 小时，放冷，再称定重量，用三氯甲烷补足减失的重量，摇匀，分取三氯甲烷液，用铺有少量无水硫酸钠的滤纸滤过，弃去初滤液，精密量取续滤液 3ml，置 10ml 量瓶中，加甲醇至刻度，摇匀，即得。

（4）测定法 精密吸取各供试品溶液 10μl，注入液相色谱仪，测定，即得。分别以干燥品计算马钱子不同炮制品中士的宁和马钱子碱的百分含量。

3. 马钱子不同炮制品的 TLC 鉴别

（1）对照品溶液的制备 分别精密称取士的宁、马钱子碱对照品适量，加三氯甲烷制成每 1ml 各含 2mg 对照品混合溶液，作为对照品溶液。

（2）供试品溶液的制备 取马钱子生品和砂烫品粉末各 0.5g，分别置具塞锥形瓶中，加入三氯甲烷 – 乙醇（10：1）混合溶液 5ml 与浓氨试液 0.5ml，密塞，振摇 5 分钟，放置 2 小时，滤过，滤液作为供试品溶液。

（3）鉴别 精密吸取供试品溶液和对照品溶液各 10μl，分别点于同一硅胶 G 薄层板上，以甲苯 – 丙酮 – 乙醇 – 浓氨试液（4：5：0.6：0.4）为展开剂，展开，取出，晾干，喷以稀碘化铋钾试液。供试品色谱中，在与对照品色谱相应的位置上，显相同颜色的斑点。

4. 马钱子不同炮制品的小鼠 LD_{50} 测定 分别称取马钱子生品和砂烫品粉末约 5g，精密称定，加入三氯甲烷 100ml 与浓氨试液 5ml，密塞，轻轻振摇，超声提取 1 小时，滤过，滤液置分液漏斗中，用硫酸溶液（3→100）提取 5 次，每次 50ml，合并硫酸液，加浓氨试液调节 pH 值至 9~10，加入三氯甲烷萃取 5 次，每次 100ml，合并三氯甲烷液，回收三氯甲烷至干，制成马钱子生品和制品总生物碱。取马钱子生品和砂烫品总生物碱各 10mg，精密称定，分别用 1mol/L 盐酸 0.5ml 溶解，再用 1mol/L 氢氧化钠调 pH 至 6~6.5，并稀释至适当浓度。选取健康小鼠，随机分为 4 组，每组 4 只，参照药理实验方法学中急性毒性预试的试验方法，进行预试，确定 100% 致死剂量（$D_{最大}$）和 0% 致死剂量（$D_{最小}$），再按适当的等比级数确定给药剂量。生品和砂烫品各选用小鼠 50 只，分为 5 个剂量组，腹腔注射各样品 0.2ml/kg，记录给药后 2 小时内小鼠的死亡情况，统计死亡率，并用 Bliss 法计算 LD_{50} 及 95% 可信限。

实验结果

表 3-7 马钱子不同炮制品中士的宁和马钱子碱的含量测定

样品组	样品取样量 /g	士的宁含量 /%	马钱子碱含量 /%
生马钱子			
砂炒马钱子			

表 3-8 马钱子生品、砂烫品急性毒性实验

样品组	剂量 mg/kg	动物数 /*n*	死亡数 /*n*	LD_{50}
生马钱子				
砂炒马钱子				

注意事项

1. 马钱子的毒性较强，在炮制和提取时要戴橡胶手套操作，注意做好安全防护。
2. 用过的河砂应妥善处理。

思考题

1. 简述马钱子炮制过程中主要生物碱成分发生变化。
2. 简述选用马钱子总生物碱进行急性毒性实验，而非煎煮液的原因。
3. 简述砂炒马钱子减毒的基本原理。

Experiment 5 The effect of Sand-fried on quality and toxicity of Strychni Semen

Aims

1.1 To master the processing method of sand sand-fried and its effect on drugs.

1.2 To clarify the processing principle and purpose of sand-fried Strychni through the experiments of quality and toxicity on sand-fried Strychni Semen.

Principles

2.1 Because of its hard texture and rapid heat transfer, river sand has a large contact area with the drug, which makes it evenly heated. Therefore, river sand is suitable to sand-fry hard or tough animal drugs. The method of sand fried can change or destroy the structure of toxic composition of some drugs, and reduce their toxicity. When sand-fried Strychni Semen, high temperature can destroy toxic composition, reduce toxicity, which can be used internally. Meanwhile, the texture of the Strychni Semen becomes crispy and easy to crush. The main ingredients of Strychni Semen are strychnine and brucine, which are both analgesic and toxic composition. During the processing, ether bonds and ring of toxic alkaloids such as strychnine and brucine are broken and opened, therefore converting to less toxic alkaloids, such as nitrogen oxide compounds of isostrychnine, isobrucine, strychnine, brucine, isostrychnine and isobrucine, etc. In addition, brucine is easy to decompose and break down compared with strychnine (this is related to the substitution of C_2—OCH_3 and C_3—OCH_3 on the structure), resulting in a significant decrease in brucine content and a slight decrease in strychnine. However, the pharmacological strength of brucine is only 1/40 of strychnine. By processing, the less effective and more toxic brucine can be removed, so the toxicity of Strychni Semen are reduced.

2.2 In alkaline conditions, strychnine is in dissociate state and easily dissolved in chloroform. Therefore, chloroform and sodium hydroxide solutions are selected as the solvents for the target composition in Strychni Semen. C_{18} is used as the stationary phase, and the hydrophilic solution is used as the mobile phase. HPLC is used to determine the content of strychnine and brucine in the test sample solution. Thin layer chromatography is used to identify Strychni Semen crude Chinese medicine and sand-fried Strychni Semen. Silica gel G, weak alkaline solution and strychnine and brucine are used as the adsorbent, developing agent, and reference. The LD_{50} of Strychni Semen crude Chinese medicine and sand-fried Strychni Semen is measured to compare the toxicity of Strychni Semen crude Chinese medicine and sand-fried Strychni Semen.

Content

3.1 Processing of Strychni Semen.

3.2 Determine the content of strychnine and brucine in different processed products by HPLC.

3.3 TLC identification of different processed products of Strychni Semen.

3.4 Determine LD_{50} of different processed products of Strychni Semen in mice.

Materials

4.1 Experimental apparatuses

High performance liquid chromatography, oven, water bath, ultrasonic cleaner, shredder, electronic scale/balance, experimental apparatus wok, truner, electric heater, enamel tray, No. 3 sieve, 10ml volumetric flask, calibration suction pipet, separatory funnel, 50ml conical flask with plug, etc.

4.2 Experimental materials

Strychni Semen, strychnine and brucine reference sample, river sand, silica gel G, CMC—Na, C_{18} columns, sodium hydroxide, bismuth potassium iodide, toluene, acetone, chloroform, concentrated ammonia, heptanesulfonate sodium, potassium dihydrogen thophosphate, methanol, absolute ethanol, concentrated sulfuric acid, concentrated hydrochloric acid, phosphoric acid, acetonitrile, water; medium-speed quantitative filter paper, pH test paper, etc.

4.3 Experimental animals

Healthy mice (18~22g), half male and half female.

Method

5.1 Processing of Strychni Semen.

Take the cleaning Strychni Semen and weigh it. Take the clean river sand and put it into the pot. When heating with strong fire to smooth, cleaning Strychni Semen with same size is put into the pot, then keep stirring, scald until it turns brown and dark brown, take out, sieve the river sand, spread and cool, weigh and calculate yield. After sand-fried, Strychni Semen swell on both sides, with surface brown or dark brown, and the quality is crisp. The endosperm with brown or dark brown can be seen in parallel sections. Sand-fried Strychni Semen is slightly fragrant and extremely bitter. The amount of river sand is to cover the drug.

5.2 Strychnine and brucine content in different processed products of Strychni Semen by HPLC.

5.2.1 Chromatographic conditions and systemetic adaptation tests

Octadecylsilane-bonded silica gel is used as a filler. A mixed solution of acetonitrile–0.01mol/L sodium heptanesulfonate and 0.02mol/L potassium dihydrogen phosphate in an equal amount is used (adjust the pH to 2.8 with 10% phosphoric acid) (21 ∶ 79) as mobile phase. The detection wavelength is 260nm. The number of theoretical plates should not be less than 5000 according to strychnine peak.

5.2.2 Preparation of reference sample solution

Take Strychnine reference sample 6mg and brucine reference sample 5mg, weigh accurately, and place them in 10ml volumetric flask, respectively. Add an appropriate amount of chloroform to dissolve, dilute to the mark, and shake well. Measure accurately 2ml reference solution, place them in the same 10ml volumetric flask, dilute to the mark with methanol, and shake (each 1ml contains 0.12mg of strychnine and 0.1mg of brucine).

5.2.3 Preparation of test sample solution

Take about 0.6g powder of different processed products of Strychni Semen (passed through No. 3 sieve), weigh accurately, place in conical flask with plug, add 3ml of sodium hydroxide solution, mix well, and place for 30 minutes. Add 20ml of chloroform accurately, sealed with plug, weigh, and place in water bath for 2 hours with reflux extraction. Allow to cool, then weigh again. To replenish the weight loss with chloroform. Shake well to distribute chloroform. Filter with a small amount of anhydrous sodium sulfate filter paper, discard the initial filtrate, measure accurately the remaining 3ml of the subsequent filtrate, place it in a 10ml volumetric flask, add methanol to the mark, and shake to obtain.

5.2.4 Measure method

10μl of each test sample solution is accurately pipetted, injected into a liquid chromatograph, and measured. The dried products are used to calculate the percentage of strychnine and brucine content in different processed products of Strychni Semen.

5.3 TLC identification of different processed products of Strychni Semen.

5.3.1 Preparation of reference sample solution

Precisely weigh appropriate reference sample strychnine and brucine, add chloroform to make a mixed solution containing 2mg of reference sample per 1ml, and use as the reference sample solution.

5.3.2 Preparation of test sample solution

Take Strychni Semen crude Chinese medicine and sand-fried Strychni Semen powder 0.5g each, put them into conical flask with plug, add 5ml chloroform–ethanol (10 : 1) mixed solution and ammonia test solution 0.5ml, sealed with plug, shake 5 minutes, leave for 2 hours, filter, and the filtrate is used as the test sample solution.

5.3.3 Thin-layer identification

Accurately pipette 10μl each of the test sample solution and the reference sample solution, spotted then on the same silica gel G thin-layer plate, and the toluene–acetone–ethanol–ammonia test solution (4 : 5 : 0.6 : 0.4) is used as developing solvent. Fold, remove, dry, spray with diluted iodized bismuth potassium solution. In the chromatogram of the test sample, the spots of the same color are displayed at the positions corresponding to the chromatogram of the reference sample.

5.4 Determine LD_{50} in mice with different processed products.

Weigh around 5g of Strychni Semen crude Chinese medicine and sand-fried Strychni Semen powder, weigh accurately, add 100ml chloroform and 5ml ammonia test solution, be airtight, shake slightly, ultrasonic extraction for 1 hour, and filter. The filtrate was placed in a separatory funnel, and extracted with sulfuric acid solution (3 to 100) for 5 times, 50ml each time. Combine sulfuric acid solution, add ammonia test solution to adjust the pH to 9~10, and add chloroform extraction 5 times,100ml each time. Chloroform solution is combined, and recovered to dryness, and the total alkaloids of Strychni Semen crude Chinese medicine and processed Strychni Semen are made. Take 10mg of total alkaloids from Strychni Semen crude Chinese medicine and sand-fried Strychni Semen powder respectively, weigh accurately, and dissolve them in 0.5ml of 1mol/L hydrochloric acid, then adjust the pH to 6~6.5 with 1mol/L sodium hydroxide, and dilute to the proper concentration. Healthy mice were selected and randomly divided into 4 groups, 4 in each group. According to the test method of acute toxicity pretest in pharmacological experiment methodology, pretest was performed to determine the 100% lethal dose (D_{max}) and 0% lethal dose (D_{min}). Then determine the dose according to the geometrical progression. Fifty mice are selected for each group, and divided into 5 dose groups. Each sample is injected intraperitoneally with 0.2ml/kg. The mouse deaths are recorded within 2 hours after administration, and the mortality is calculated and Bliss method is used to calculate LD_{50} and 95% confidence limit.

Results

Table 3–7 Determination of strychnine and brucine in different processed production of Strychni Semen

Sample	Sample weight/g	Strychnine content/%	brucine content/%
Raw Strychni Semen			
sand-fried Strychni Semen			

Table 3–8 Acute toxicity test of Strychni Semen crude Chinese medicine and sand-scorched Strychni Semen

Sample	dose(mg/kg)	Number of animals/*n*	Number of deaths/*n*	LD_{50}
Raw Strychni Semen				
sand-fried Strychni Semen				

Notes

7.1 Strychni Semen is highly toxic. When processing and extracting, we should wear rubber gloves and pay attention to safety protection.

7.2 The used river sand should be disposed of properly.

Questions

8.1 What happened to the main alkaloids during the processing of Strychni Semen?

8.2 Why use the total alkaloids of Strychni Semen for acute toxicity test instead of decoction?

8.3 Briefly describe the attenuation principles of sand-fried Strychni Semen.

PPT

实验六　酒炙对大黄成分及泻下作用的影响实验

实验目的

1. **掌握**　酒炙的炮制方法及其对药物的影响。
2. 通过大黄酒炙前后蒽醌含量测定及泻下实验，说明大黄炮制的意义。

实验原理

1. 液体辅料与药物一起炮制，在炮制过程中，辅料渗入药物中，使得药物在性味、功效、作用趋向、归经和理化性质方面均能发生某些变化，从而起到降低毒性、抑制偏性、增强疗效、矫臭矫味、有效成分易于溶出等作用，有利于疗效的发挥。酒味甘辛，性大热。气味芳香，能升能散，行药势，具有活血通络、散寒、去腥的作用，酒炙能改变性，缓和寒性，免伤脾胃阳气，并可借酒升提之力引药上行。大黄生品泻下力强，酒炙后泻下力减弱，活血作用增强。

2. 大黄主要含有结合蒽醌和游离蒽醌，游离蒽醌类有大黄酸、大黄素、大黄酚、芦荟大黄素、大黄素甲醚，为大黄抗菌的有效成分；结合蒽醌有单蒽醌类的苷，如大黄素、大黄酚和芦荟大黄素的双葡萄苷，还有双蒽酮苷类，如番泻苷A、B、C、D、E、F，为大黄泻下的主要成分。大黄酒炙后番泻苷A、B含量下降，酒炙使一部分蒽醌苷类成分转化为游离型蒽醌，导致游离蒽醌含量有所上升，故而泻下作用减弱，抗菌消炎作用加强。酒炙后结合型蒽醌类成分含量下降与传统认为酒炙减弱大黄泻下作用相一致。采用HPLC测定大黄炮制前后番泻苷A、B的含量变化；采用小肠推进实验观察炮制前后泻下作用的变化，验证大黄炮制的意义。

实验内容

1. 酒大黄的炮制。
2. 大黄不同炮制品中番泻苷A、番泻苷B的含量测定。
3. 大黄不同炮制品小鼠小肠推进实验。

实验器具和材料

1. **实验器具**　炒锅、锅铲、煤气灶、搪瓷盘、高效液相色谱仪、超声波清洗器、电子天平、高速万能粉碎机、2ml注射器、灌胃针头、手术剪、眼科镊、直尺、烧杯、硅板等。

2. **实验材料**　大黄、番泻苷A对照品、番泻苷B对照品；黄酒、炭末、甲醇、纯净水等。

3. **实验动物**　健康雄性小鼠（18~22g）。

实验方法

1. **酒大黄的炮制**　取净大黄片或块50g，用黄酒5g喷淋拌匀，闷润30分钟，待酒被吸尽后，入热锅内，用文火微微翻炒至干，表面呈深棕色或棕褐色，取出晾凉，除净碎屑。

2. 大黄不同炮制品中番泻苷 A、番泻苷 B 的含量测定

（1）色谱条件与系统适用性试验 C_{18} 色谱柱（150mm×4.6mm，5μm），Agilent Zorbax Extend C_{18} 保护柱（10mm×4.6mm，5μm）；流动相为 0.1% 磷酸水（A）- 乙腈（B），梯度洗脱，洗脱程序见表 3-9；进样量 10μl；柱温 30 ℃；体积流量 1ml/min；检测波长为 340nm。

表 3–9 梯度洗脱程序

时间（分钟）	流动相 A 0.1% 磷酸水（%）	流动相 B 乙腈（%）
0~27	87	13
27~40	87→84	13→16
40~47	84	16
47~50	84→62	16→38
50~60	62→47	38→53
60~65	47→40	53→60
65~75	40	60

（2）对照品溶液的制备 精密称取番泻苷 A 和番泻苷 B 对照品适量，加入甲醇 - 水（3：2）溶解并定容，分别制成 110.0μg/ml 番泻苷 A、95.6μg/ml 番泻苷 B 对照品储备液，精密量取上述对照品溶液各 2ml，混匀，即得。

（3）供试品溶液的制备 分别取大黄、酒大黄药材粉末（过三号筛）各约 0.2g，精密称定，置具塞锥形瓶中，加入 80% 甲醇 30ml，称定重量，超声提取 1 小时，放冷，用 80% 甲醇补足损失的重量，混匀，滤过，取续滤液过 0.22μm 微孔滤膜，取续滤液，即得。

（4）测定法 精密吸取各供试品溶液 10μl，注入液相色谱仪，测定，即得。按干燥品计，分别计算各样品中番泻苷 A、番泻苷 B 的含量。

3. 大黄不同炮制品小鼠小肠推进实验

（1）样品液的制备。分别取大黄、酒大黄各 50g，加入水 250ml，煎煮 20 分钟，过滤，滤液浓缩至 50ml。配制炭末生理盐水混悬液 0.1g/ml（含炭末 0.1g/ml）、大黄水煎液 1g/ml（含炭末 0.1g/ml）、酒大黄水煎液 1g/ml（含炭末 0.1g/ml）。

（2）取禁食 12 小时、体重 18~22g 的小鼠 30 只，随机均分为 3 组，每组 10 只，用苦味酸做标记。分别用上述 3 种炭末液 0.3ml/10g 体重灌胃。给药 30 分钟后脱颈椎处死，切开腹腔分离肠系膜，剪取上端至幽门，下端至回盲肠的肠管，置于托盘上。轻轻将小肠拉成直线，测量肠管长度作为一小肠总长度，从幽门至炭末沿的距离作为一炭末在肠内推进距离，取各组小鼠平均值，用公式计算炭末推进百分率。

炭末推进率 = 炭末在肠内推进距离（cm）/ 小肠全长（cm）×100%

实验结果

表 3–10 大黄不同炮制品中番泻苷 A、番泻苷 B 的含量测定

样品组	样品取样量 /g	番泻苷 A 含量 /%	番泻苷 B 含量 /%
生大黄			
酒大黄			

表 3-11 大黄不同炮制品小鼠小肠推进实验（$\bar{x}\pm s$）

样品组	给药剂量	数量 /*n*	肠内推进距离 /cm	推进率 /%
对照组				
生大黄				
酒大黄				

注意事项

1. 药物加入一定量酒拌匀闷润过程中，容器上面应加盖，以免酒被迅速挥发。

2. 酒炙一般为药物每 100kg，用黄酒 10~20kg。若酒的用量较少，不易拌匀药物时，可加适量水稀释。

3. 酒炙药物一般文火。勤翻动，炒至近干，颜色加深时，即可取出，晾凉。

思考题

1. 根据实验结果，探讨大黄酒炙的意义。

2. 简述大黄入煎剂为何需后下。

Experiment 6 Effects of stir fried Rhei Radix et Rhizoma with rice wine on composition and purgative activity

Aims

1.1 To master the method of stir fried with rice wine and its effect on drug.

1.2 To understand the significance of stir fried Rhei Radix et Rhizoma with rice wine through determination the content of anthraquinone and purgative effect before and after processing.

Principles

2.1 The liquid adjuvant is processed together with the drug. During the processing, the adjuvant materials is inhaled into the drug, so that property and flavor, efficacy, trend of action, meridian tropism, and physicochemical properties of drug can be changed. Therefore, stir fried with rice wine could reduce toxicity, inhibit partiality, enhance curative effect, neutralize the bad odor and easily dissolve active composition, which is beneficial to extractive curative effect. The rice wine is sweet and pungent in flavor and hot in property. The taste is fragrant, which can rise, disperse, guide the drug's ascending tendency. It has the effects of promoting blood circulation, alleviate coldness, and remove fishy smell. Stir fried with rice wine can change drug's properties, moderate cold property, avoid hurting spleen and stomach yang, and use raising property of rice wine to guide the medicine to the upper. The Rhei Radix et Rhizoma crude Chinese medicine has a strong effect on purgation, however, the purgative effect decreases and the effect of promoting circulation strengthens after stir fried with rice wine.

2.2 Bound anthraquinone and dissociate anthraquinone are the main contains of Rhei Radix et Rhizoma. Dissociate anthraquinones include rhein, emodin, chrysophanol, aloe-emodin, and emodin methylether, which are active composition of Rhei Radix et Rhizoma. Combined anthraquinones include monoanthraquinone glycosides, such as bis-glucosides of emodin, chrysophanol, and aloe-emodin, and bis-anthrone glycosides, such as sennanosides A to F, which are the main composition of purgation. After stir fried with rice wine, the content of sennax A and B are decreased, and parts of anthraquinone glycosides are converted into dissociate anthraquinone by stir-frying with wine, resulting in an increase in the content of dissociate anthraquinone. Therefore, the purgative effect is weakened and the antibacterial and anti-inflammatory effect is strengthened. The decrease in the content of bound anthraquinones after stir fried with rice wine is consistent with the conventional wisdom that stir fried with rice wine can reduce the effect of purgation. HPLC is used to determine the content of sennanoside A and B before and after stir fried Rhei Radix et Rhizoma with rice wine. The small intestine propulsion experiment is used to observe the change of purgation effect before and after processing, and to verify the significance of Rhei Radix et Rhizoma processing.

Content

3.1 Stir fried Rhei Radix et Rhizoma with rice wine.

3.2 Determination the content of sennanoside A and B in different processed Rhei Radix et Rhizoma products.

3.3 Small intestine propulsion experiment of mice with different processed Rhei Radix et Rhizoma products.

Materials

4.1 Experimental apparatuses

Wok, truner, electric stove, enamel tray, high performance liquid chromatography, ultrasonic cleaner, electronic scale/balance, high-speed universal shredder, 2ml syringe, gavage needles, surgical scissors, ophthalmic tweezers, ruler, beaker, silicon plate, etc.

4.2 Experimental materials

Rhei Radix et Rhizoma, reference sample of sennanoside A and sennanoside B; rice wine, charcoal powder, methanol, distilled water, etc.

4.3 Experimental animals

Healthy male mice (18~22g).

Method

5.1 Stir fried Rhei Radix et Rhizoma with rice wine.

Take 50g of Rhei Radix et Rhizoma tablets or slices, flush with 5g of rice wine, mix well, and moisten for 30 minutes. After the wine is exhausted, put drug into the hot pot and stir fried with gentle fire until dry. The surface of Rhei Radix et Rhizoma is dark brown or tan. Take it out and remove debris.

5.2 Determination the content of sennanoside A and sennanoside B in different Rhizoma Rhei processed products.

5.2.1 Chromatographic conditions and systematic adaptation test

C_{18} column (150mm × 4.6mm, 5μm), Agilent Zorbax Extend C_{18} guard column (10mm × 4.6mm, 5μm), mobile phase is 0.1% phosphoric acid water (A)–acetonitrile (B), gradient elution, the elution procedure is shown in Table 3–9. The injection volume is 10μl, the column temperature is 30℃, the

Table 3–9 Gradient elution procedure

Time (minutes)	Mobile phase A 0.1% phosphoric acid water (%)	Mobile phase B Acetonitrile(%)
0~27	87	13
27~40	87→84	13→16
40~47	84	16
47~50	84→62	16→38
50~60	62→47	38→53
60~65	47→40	53→60
65~75	40	60

volume flow rate is 1ml/min, and the length of detection wavelength is 340nm.

5.2.2 Preparation of reference sample solution

Precisely weigh appropriate amount of sennanoside A and sennanoside B reference sample with methanol-water (3 : 2) and dissolve to volume. The concentration of sennanoside A and B reference sample stock solution is 110.0μg/ml and 95.6μg/ml, respectively. Measure accurately each of the above reference sample solution 2ml, and mix to obtain.

5.2.3 Preparation of the test sample solution

Weigh about 0.2g powder (passed through No. 3 sieve) of raw and stir fried Rhei Radix et Rhizoma with rice wine, respectively, weigh accurately, and put them into two conical flask with plug. Add 30ml 80% methanol, weigh them, ultrasonic extraction for 1 hour, allow to cool, replenish the weight loss with 80% methanol, mix well, filter, take the subsequent filtrate through a 0.22μm millipore filter, and use the subsequent filtrate.

5.2.4 Method

Accurately pipette 10μl each test sample solution, and inject them into the liquid chromatograph for determination, respectively. Calculate the contents of sennanoside A and sennanoside B in each sample by dried product.

5.3 Small intestine propulsion experiment in mice with different Rhei Radix et Rhizoma products.

5.3.1 Preparation of sample solution

Take 50g of raw and processed Rhei Radix et Rhizoma, add water 250ml, boiling for 20 minutes, filter, and concentrate the filtrate to 50ml. Preparation of charcoal saline 0.1g/ml (containing charcoal powder 0.1g/ml), Rhei Radix et Rhizoma decoction 1g/ml (containing charcoal powder 0.1g/ml), stir fried Rhei Radix et Rhizoma with rice wine decoction 1g/ml (containing charcoal powder 0.1g/ml).

5.3.2 Thirty mice that were fasted for 12 hours and weighed 18~22g are randomly divided into 3 groups, 10 in each group, marked with picric acid. Intragastric administration 0.3ml/10g of body weight of the three kinds of above-mentioned charcoal liquid. Thirty minutes after the administration, the mice are sacrificed and the mesentery is separated by incision of the abdominal cavity. Cut the bowel from the upper end to the pylorus and the lower end to the ileum and place on a tray. Gently pull the small intestine into a straight line and measure the length of the intestine as the total length of the small intestine, and the distance from the pylorus to the edge of the charcoal is the propulsive distance of charcoal in the intestine. Take the average of the length in each group, and calculate the percentage of carbon powder propulsion with the formula.

Charcoal powder propulsion rate=Charcoal propulsion distance in the intestine (cm)/full length of small intestine (cm) × 100%

Results

Table 3–10 Determination of sennanoside A and sennanoside B in different processed products of Rhei Radix et Rhizoma

Sample	Sample volume/g	Sennanoside A content/%	Sennanoside B content/%
Raw Rhet Radix et Rhizoma			
Stir fried Rhet Radix et Rhizoma with rice wine			

Table 3-11 Small intestine propulsion experiment of mice with different processed Rhei Radix et Rhizoma products ($\bar{x}\pm s$)

Sample	Dose	Amount/*n*	Charcoal propulsion distance in the intestine/cm	Charcoal powder propulsion rate/%
Control				
Raw				
Stir fried with rice wine				

Notes

7.1 During adding wine to the drug, mixing and moistening, the container should be covered with a lid to prevent the rice wine from being rapidly evaporated.

7.2 Use 10~20kg of rice wine per 100kg drug for stir fried with rice wine. If the amount of rice wine is less, it is not easy to mix. Appropriate amount water could be added to dilute.

7.3 Gentle Fire is used for stir fried with rice wine. Stir-fry as quickly as possible, take the drugs out until the drugs nearly dry and the color deepened, and let the drugs cool.

Questions

8.1 According to the results, explore the significance of stir fried Rhei Radix et Rhizoma with rice wine.

8.2 Why do Rhei Radix et Rhizoma need to be decocted later?

实验七 醋炙延胡索对延胡索乙素含量和镇痛作用的影响

PPT

实验目的

1. **掌握** 延胡索的炮制方法及炮制原理。

2. 通过延胡索炮制前后生物碱的含量测定及镇痛实验了解延胡索炮制的意义。

实验原理

1. 延胡索的炮制及其增效原理 按照2020年版《中国药典》延胡索项下的炮制方法，采用醋炙法炮制延胡索，可以增强其行气止痛作用，广泛用于身体各部位的多种疼痛。延胡索中具有止痛作用的有效成分延胡索乙素和丑素等，均属于难溶于水的游离生物碱，醋炙后可使游离生物碱与醋酸结合成易溶于水的醋酸盐，提高溶出率。由于延胡索生物碱的含量高低与止痛效力成正比，故醋炙后因延胡索乙素等生物碱溶出率增加而增强了止痛作用。

2. 小鼠镇痛实验原理 采用HPLC测定延胡索炮制前后延胡索乙素的含量变化，采用小鼠腹腔注射醋酸溶液，引起疼痛刺激，如腰部收缩、扭体以及蠕行等不同方式的痛觉反应。通过比较空白组、阳性对照组及给药组，以反映醋炙延胡索的镇痛作用。

实验内容

1. 延胡索的炮制。
2. 延胡索不同炮制品中延胡索乙素含量测定。
3. 延胡索不同炮制品镇痛作用实验。

实验器具和材料

1. 实验器具 炒锅、锅铲、煤气灶、搪瓷盘、切药刀、标准筛(50目,即三号筛)、研钵、高效液相色谱仪、万分之一电子天平、水浴锅、容量瓶(10ml、5ml)、圆底烧瓶(50ml)、平底烧瓶(100ml)、移液管(25ml、50ml)、回流及回收装置、玻璃漏斗、锥形瓶、量筒、微孔滤膜、微量进样器、流动相过滤装置、台式天平、烧杯(1000ml)、秒表、注射器、小鼠笼等。

2. 实验材料 延胡索、米醋、甲醇(分析纯和色谱纯)、浓氨水、0.1%磷酸、三乙胺、蒸馏水、生理盐水、0.6%醋酸溶液、苦味酸、延胡索乙素对照品等。

3. 实验动物 健康雌性和雄性小鼠(18~22g)。

实验方法

1. 醋延胡索的炮制

(1)醋炙法 取净延胡索饮片，称重，加入定量的米醋拌匀，闷润至醋被吸尽后，置炒制容器内，文火加热，炒干，取出晾凉。称重，计算得率。

（2）醋煮法　取净延胡索饮片，称重，加入定量的米醋和适量清水（以平药面为宜），浸润1小时，置煮制容器内，文火加热煮至透心、醋液被吸尽时，取出，晾至6成干，切厚片，晒干。称重，计算得率。

每100kg延胡索，用米醋20kg。

2. 延胡索不同炮制品中延胡索乙素含量测定　照高效液相色谱法（通则0512）测定。

（1）色谱条件与系统适用性试验　以十八烷基键合硅胶为填充剂，以甲醇-0.1%磷酸溶液（三乙胺调pH至6.0）（55：45）为流动相；检测波长为280nm。理论塔板数按延胡索乙素峰计算应不低于3000。

（2）对照品溶液的制备　取延胡索乙素对照品适量，精密称定，加甲醇制成每1ml含46μg的溶液，即得。

（3）供试品溶液的制备　分别取上述醋炙、醋煮炮制品粉末（过三号筛）约0.5g，精密称定，置平底烧瓶中，精密加入浓氨试液-甲醇（1：20）混合溶50ml，称定重量，冷浸1小时后加热回流1小时，放冷，再称定重量，用浓氨试液-甲醇（1：20）混合溶液补足减失的重量，摇匀，滤过。精密量取续滤液25ml，蒸干，残渣加甲醇溶解，转移至5ml量瓶中，并稀释至刻度，摇匀，滤过，取续滤液，即得。

（4）测定法　分别精密吸取对照品溶液与供试品溶液各10μl，注入液相色谱仪，测定，即得。本品按干燥品计算，分别计算延胡索不同炮制品中延胡索乙素的百分含量，含延胡索乙素（$C_{21}H_{25}NO_4$）不得少于0.050%。

3. 醋酸扭体法比较延胡索炮制前后的镇痛作用

（1）供试品溶液的制备　取延胡索生品及不同醋炮制品各25g分别煎煮，第一次加水400ml、第二次加水250ml，煎煮2次，每次25分钟，脱脂棉滤过，合并滤液，浓缩至100ml备用。

（2）实验方法　取小鼠随机分为5组，每组10只，雌雄各半，分别灌以生理盐水、2%阿司匹林、延胡索生品供试液、延胡索醋炙品供试液、延胡索醋煮品供试液，0.3ml/10g，40分钟后，各鼠腹腔注射0.6%醋酸0.1ml/10g，注射后立即启动秒表，记录扭体潜伏期及0~15分钟、15~30分钟的扭体次数。

实验结果

表3-12　延胡索乙素含量测定表

组号	药物	取样量/g	延胡索乙素含量/%
1	生延胡索		
2	醋炙延胡索		
3	醋煮延胡索		

表3-13　动物扭体潜伏期和单位时间内的扭体次数

组号	药物	给药量/ml	扭体潜伏期/秒	0~15分钟	15~30分钟
1	生理盐水				
2	2%阿司匹林				
3	生延胡索				
4	醋炙延胡索				
5	醋煮延胡索				

根据上述实验结果数据，进行统计学分析。

注意事项

1. 炮制延胡索时，注意火候，以醋液刚好被吸尽为宜。

2. 测定延胡索乙素含量时，要保证进样量准确，以免造成误差过大，另外注意高效液相色谱仪的正确操作。

3. 醋酸溶液应临用临配。

4. 镇痛实验需 30% 以上动物不产生扭体反应才能认为镇痛阳性。扭体反应表现为腹部内凹、伸展后肢、臀部抬高。

思考题

1. 简述延胡索生品、醋制品中的延胡索乙素含量有何不同。

2. 简述醋炙和醋煮两种炮制工艺区别与炮制作用差异。

Experiment 7 The influence of stir-frying Corydalis Rhizoma with rice vinegar on the content of tetrahydropalmatine and its analgesic effect

Aims

1.1 To master operation and principle of processing Corydalis Rhizoma.

1.2 To understand the significance of processing Corydalis Rhizoma through determination of alkaloids in Corydalis Rhizoma and measurement of its analgesic effect before and after processing.

Principles

2.1 Processing of Corydalis Rhizoma and its synergistic principle

According to Chinese Pharmacopoeia (2020 Edition), Corydalis Rhizoma should be processed by stir-frying with rice vinegar, which could enhance its activities of promoting *Qi* circulation and relieving pain, and could be widely used for various pains in various parts of the body. The effective components of Corydalis Rhizoma, such as tetrahydropalmatine B and Corydalis L are insoluble free alkaloids. After vinegar processing, the free alkaloids can combine with acetic acid to form water-soluble acetate and improve the dissolution rate. Because the content of Corydalis Rhizoma alkaloid is directly proportional to the analgesic effect, the analgesic effect can be enhanced by the increase of dissolution rate of tetrahydropalmatine and other alkaloids after vinegar processing.

2.2 Experimental principle of analgesia in mice

The content of tetrahydropalmatine B before and after processing of Corydalis Rhizoma is determined by HPLC. Mice are injected intraperitoneally with acetic acid solution to induce pain stimulation, such as waist contraction, writhing, peristalsis and so on. The analgesic effect of Corydalis Rhizoma with vinegar will be reflected by comparing the blank group, the control group and the administration group.

Contents

3.1 Processing of Corydalis Rhizoma.

3.2 Determination of tetrahydropalmatine B in different processed products of Corydalis Rhizoma.

3.3 Analgesic effect of different processed products of Corydalis Rhizoma.

Materials

4.1 Experimental apparatuses

Wok, truner, electric stove, enameled tray, herb cutting knife, standard sieve (50 mesh, i.e. No.3 sieve), mortar, HPLC, one thousandth electronic balance, water bath pot, volumetric flask (10ml,

5ml), round bottom flask (50ml), flat bottom flask (100ml), pipette (25ml, 50ml), reflux and recovery device, beaker, glass funnel, conical flask , measuring cylinder, syringe, microporous filter membrane, microinjector, mobile phase filter, table balance, beaker (1000ml), stopwatch, syringe, mouse cage, etc.

4.2 Experimental materials

Corydalis, rice vinegar, methanol (analytical pure and chromatographic pure), concentrated ammonia water, 0.1% phosphoric acid, triethylamine, distilled water, normal saline, 0.6% acetic acid solution, picric acid, corydalis, etc.

4.3 Experimental animals

Healthy female and male mice (18~22g).

Methods

5.1 Processing of Corydalis Rhizoma vinegar.

5.1.1 Vinegar roasting method

Take the pure Corydalis Rhizoma Yinpian (decoction pieces/processed Chinese medicine), weigh them, add in the quantitative rice vinegar and mix them well, dry them until the vinegar is moistened, put them in the frying container, heat them gently, fry them dry, take them out and cool them. Weigh and calculate the yield.

5.1.2 Vinegar boiling method

The method of vinegar boiling is to take pure Corydalis Rhizoma Yinpian (decoction pieces/ processed Chinese medicine), weigh them, add quantitative rice vinegar and proper amount of clear water (it is better to use plain noodles), moisten them for 1 hour, put them in a cooking container, heat them gently until they are completely absorbed, take them out, air them to 60% dry, cut thick pieces and dry them in the sun. Weigh and calculate the yield.

Every 100kg of Corydalis Rhizoma use 20kg of rice vinegar.

5.2 Determination of tetrahydropalmatine B in different processed products of Corydalis Rhizoma.

According to high performance liquid chromatography (general rule 0512).

5.2.1 Chromatographic conditions and system suitability test

Octadecyl bonded silica gel as filler, methanol–0.1% phosphoric acid solution (triethylamine adjusted pH to 6.0) (55 ∶ 45) as mobile phase, detection wavelength of 280nm. The number of theoretical plates shall not be less than 3000 calculated according to the peak of tetrahydropalmatine.

5.2.2 Preparation of reference solution

Take a proper amount of tetrahydropalmatine reference, weigh accurately, add methanol to make a solution containing 46μg/ml.

5.2.3 Preparation of test solution

Take about 0.5g of the both processed products powder (passing No.3 screen) respectively, weigh accurately, put it in a flat bottom flask, add precisely 50ml of concentrated ammonia test solution methanol (1 ∶ 20) mixed solution, weigh it, heat and return it for 1 hour after cold soak, cool it, weigh it again, use concentrated ammonia test solution methanol (1 ∶ 20) mixed solution to make up the lost weight, shake it well and filter it. Accurately measure 25ml of the continuous filtrate, evaporate it to dryness, dissolve the residue with methanol, transfer it to 5ml measuring bottle, dilute it to the scale, shake it well, filter it, and take the continuous filtrate.

5.2.4 Determination method

Take 10μl of the reference solution and the test solution respectively, inject them into the liquid chromatograph, and determine them. The content of tetrahydropalmatine ($C_{21}H_{25}NO_4$) in different processed products of Corydalis Rhizoma shall be calculated as per the dry product, and the content of tetrahydropalmatine ($C_{21}H_{25}NO_4$) shall not be less than 0.050%.

5.3 Analgesic effect of different processed products of Corydalis Rhizoma.

5.3.1 Preparation of test solution

Extract 25g of Corydalis Rhizoma crude Chinese medicine and different processed products of vinegar, decoct respectively, add 400ml of water for the first time, 250ml of water for the second time, decoct twice, each time for 25 minutes, filter the absorbent cotton, combine the filtrate, and concentrate to 100ml for standby.

5.3.2 Method

The mice are randomly divided into 5 groups, 10 mice in each group, half male and half female. They are respectively infused with saline, 2% aspirin, Corydalis Rhizoma crude Chinese medicine, Corydalis Rhizoma vinegar, Corydalis Rhizoma vinegar boiled, 0.3ml/10g. 40 minutes later, each rat is injected with 0.6% acetic acid 0.1ml/10g.After injection, the stopwatch is immediately started to record twisting body Incubation period and the number of writhing in 0~15 minutes and 15~30 minutes.

Results

Table 3–12 Determination table of tetrahydropalmatine content in Corydalis Rhizoma

Group	Sample	Sampling quantity/g	Content of tetrahydropalmatine/%
1	Raw Corydalis Rhizoma		
2	Stir-frying Corydalis Rhizoma with vinegar		
3	Boiled Corydalis Rhizoma with vinegar		

Table 3–13 Latency to the first contortion and the number of writhes in per unit time of mice

Group	Sample	Dosage /ml	Latency to the first contortion/second	0~15minutes	15~30minutes
1	Normal saline				
2	2% Aspirin				
3	Raw Corydalis Rhizoma				
4	Stir-frying Corydalis Rhizoma with vinegar				
5	Boiled Corydalis Rhizoma with vinegar				

According to the above data, statistical analysis is conducted.

Notes

7.1 When processing Corydalis Rhizoma, one should pay close attention to duration of heating and it is appropriate to stop heating only after rice vinegar is sucked up.

7.2 When determining the content of tetrahydropalmatine B, it is necessary to ensure that the injection quantity is accurate, so as to avoid excessive error, and pay attention to the correct operation of the high performance liquid chromatograph.

7.3 Acetic acid solution should be prepared for clinical use.

7.4 In the analgesic experiment, more than 30% of the animals do not produce writhing reaction in order to be considered to be positive for analgesia. The torsion reaction showed that the abdomen is concave, the hind limbs are extended, and the buttocks are raised.

Question

8.1 What's the difference in content of tetrahydropalmatine B between Corydalis Rhizoma crude Chinese medicine and rice vinegar stir-fried Corydalis Rhizoma.What does it indicate?

8.2 Briefly describe the difference of processing and effect between broiling with vinegar and stir-frying with vinegar.

PPT

实验八　煅制石膏质量评价实验

实验目的

1. **掌握**　明煅的炮制方法及对药物的影响。

2. 通过石膏煅制前后定性及定量评价实验，说明明煅法对石膏的影响。

实验原理

1. 石膏味辛、甘，性大寒，归肺、胃经，具有清热泻火，除烦止渴的功效。经过煅制成为煅石膏后，味甘、辛、涩，性寒，归肺、胃经，具有收湿、生肌、敛疮、止血的功效。石膏的主要化学成分是 $CaSO_4 \cdot 2H_2O$。煅制时，当温度达到一定程度就会失去结晶水变成煅石膏。煅石膏的主要化学成分是 $CaSO_4$。

2. 石膏中 Ca^{2+} 与氨羧络合剂乙二胺四醋酸二钠（EDTA）能定量地形成金属络合物，其稳定性较 Ca^{2+} 与指示剂形成的络合物为强。在适宜的 pH 范围内以 EDTA 滴定，当到达终点时，EDTA 夺取与指示剂结合的 Ca^{2+}，指示剂被游离而显色，显示终点到达。根据 EDTA 滴定液的消耗量即可计算样品中 Ca^{2+} 的含量。

实验内容

1. 石膏的煅制。
2. 石膏煅制前后的定性分析。
3. 石膏煅制前后主要化学成分的含量测定。

实验器具和材料

1. 实验器具　红外光谱仪、玛瑙研钵、压片机、电子天平、马福炉、坩埚、坩埚钳、铁架台、试管、软木塞、称量瓶、锥形瓶、酸式滴定管、碱式滴定管等。

2. 实验材料　石膏；KBr、EDTA、铬黑 T 、钙黄绿素、甲基红、醋酸、稀盐酸、氨试液、氢氧化钾试液、氧化锌试剂等。

实验方法

1. 石膏的煅制　取石膏药材 5g，打碎，除去杂石，置坩埚中，厚度 1~4cm，放入马福炉内，加热煅烧至红透，取出，置干燥器中冷却，备用。

2. 石膏煅制前后的定性分析

（1）水分　称取石膏和煅石膏约 2g，分别置具有小孔软木塞的试管内，灼烧。如管壁有水生成，药物变为不透明体，则为石膏；不出现上述现象，则为煅石膏。

（2）钙盐　称取石膏和煅石膏粉末约 0.2g，分别置试管内，加稀盐酸 10ml，加热使溶解。溶液加甲基红指示剂 1 滴，用氨试液中和，再滴加盐酸至恰显酸性即生成白色沉淀，分离，沉淀不溶于醋酸，可溶于稀盐酸。

（3）硫酸盐　称取石膏和煅石膏粉末约 0.2g，分别置试管内，加稀盐酸 10ml，加热使溶解。滴加氯化钡试液即生成白色沉淀，分离，沉淀在盐酸中不溶解。

（4）红外光谱　称取石膏、煅石膏样品约 1mg，分别与 KBr 200mg 于玛瑙研钵中研磨粉碎至 200 目，然后置压片机中压制成透明薄片，置红外光谱仪上于 4000~600cm^{-1} 扫描测定。所得图谱经计算机自动基线矫正和自动纵坐标标准化处理，比较分析石膏炮制前后红外光谱的异同。

3. 石膏煅制前后主要化学成分的含量测定

（1）石膏中 $CaSO_4 \cdot 2H_2O$ 的含量测定　取石膏细粉约 0.2g，精密称定，置锥形瓶中，加稀盐酸 10ml，加热使溶解，加水 100ml 和甲基红指示剂 1 滴，滴加氢氧化钾试液至溶液呈浅黄色，再继续多加 5ml，加钙黄绿素指示剂少量，用 EDTA 滴定液（0.05mol/L）滴定，至溶液的黄绿色荧光消失并呈橙色。每 1ml EDTA 滴定液（0.05mol/L）相当于 8.608mg 的含水硫酸钙（$CaSO_4 \cdot 2H_2O$）。

（2）煅石膏中 $CaSO_4$ 的含量测定　取煅石膏细粉约 0.15g，精密称定，照石膏中 $CaSO_4 \cdot 2H_2O$ 的含量测定方法，自“置锥形瓶中，加稀盐酸 10ml”起，依法测定。每 1ml EDTA 滴定液（0.05mol/L）相当于 6.807mg 的硫酸钙（$CaSO_4$）。

实验结果

表 3-14　石膏煅制前后主要化学成分的含量测定

样品组	样品取样量 /g	$CaSO_4 \cdot 2H_2O$ 含量 /%	$CaSO_4$ 含量 /%
石膏			
煅石膏			

注意事项

1. 煅制石膏时温度很高，应注意安全，避免烫伤。

2. 煅后石膏温度降至 100℃左右时，应及时放入干燥器中冷却，以免吸收空气中的水分而影响煅制效果。

思考题

1. 简述测定石膏中 $CaSO_4 \cdot 2H_2O$ 的含量，滴加氢氧化钾至呈浅黄色之后，为何需继续多加 5ml。

2. 简述哪些物理、化学指标可用于快速、灵敏、准确地评价石膏和煅石膏的质量。

Experiment 8 Experiment of calcined gypsum quality evaluation

Aims

1.1 To master the processing method of calcining of gypsum and its influence on drugs.

1.2 To reveal the influence of calcining on gypsum through qualitative and quantitative evaluation experiments before and after calcining of gypsum.

Principles

2.1 Gypsum flavor xin and gan, mssive cold, belong to the lung, stomach meridian, with the effect of heat-clearing, fire-draining, thirst-cooling , and restless-arresting. After calcining into calcined gypsum, sweet, spicy and astringent, cold, belong to the lung, stomach meridian, with the effect of hygroscopia, muscle, collect sores, hemostasis. The main chemical component of gypsum is $CaSO_4 \cdot 2H_2O$. During calcining, when the temperature reaches a certain level, the crystallized water is lost and becomes calcined gypsum. The main chemical component of calcined gypsum is $CaSO_4$.

2.2 Ca^{2+} and ammonia carboxylic complexer EDTA can quantitatively form metal complexes in gypsum, and its stability is stronger than that formed by Ca^{2+} and indicator. Titrates with EDTA within the appropriate pH range, and when the end point is reached, EDTA captures the Ca^{2+} bound to the indicator, which is dissociated and colored to indicate the end point arrival. The amount of Ca^{2+} in the sample can be calculated based on the consumption of EDTA volumetric solution.

Contents

3.1 Calcining of gypsum.

3.2 Qualitative analysis before and after calcining of gypsum.

3.3 Determination of main chemical components of gypsum before and after calcining.

Materials

4.1 Experimental apparatuses

Infrared spectrophotometer, agate mortar, tablet press, electronic scale, muffle furnace, crucible, crucible tongs, iron stand, test tube, bored cork, weighing bottle, conical bottle, acid burette, base burette, etc.

4.2 Experimental materials

Gypsum, KBr, EDTA, chrome black T, calcein, methyl red, acetic acid, dilute hydrochloric acid, ammonia test solution, potassium hydroxide test solution, zinc oxide reagent, etc.

Methods

5.1 Calcining of gypsum.

Take 5g of the gypsum materials, smash them and remove mixed stones, placed in a crucible with a thickness of 1~4cm, put into a maffle furnace, heat and calcine them until red through, then remove them, store in a desiccator and cool for later use.

5.2 Qualitative analysis of gypsum before and after calcining.

5.2.1 Moisture content

About 2g of gypsum and calcined gypsum are used, and put separately into tubes with corks with small holes, then ignited. If water is formed on the wall of the tube and the drug becomes opaque, it is gypsum. If the above phenomenon does not occur, it is calcined gypsum.

5.2.2 Calcium salt

About 0.2g of gypsum and calcined gypsum powder are used, respectively placed in a test tube, and 10ml of diluted hydrochloric acid is added, and heated to dissolve.Add 1 drop of methyl red indicator to the solution, neutralize it with ammonia test solution, and then add hydrochloric acid to the solution until it is just acidic, that is, white precipitate is formed. The precipitation is insoluble in acetic acid, but soluble in dilute hydrochloric acid.

5.2.3 Sulfate

About 0.2g of gypsum and calcined gypsum powder is weighed, respectively placed in a test tube, 10ml of dilute hydrochloric acid is added, and heated to dissolve.Add barium chloride test solution to produce white precipitation, separation, precipitation in hydrochloric acid is insoluble.

5.3.4 Infrared spectroscopy

About 1mg of gypsum and calcined gypsum samples were taken, respectively, and KBr 200mg were ground and pulverized in agate mortar to 200 mesh, and then transparent thin slices were made by pressing machine, which were scanned and determined by infrared spectrometer at 4000~600cm^{-1}.The obtained spectra were compared and analyzed by computer automatic baseline correction and automatic ordinate standardization.

5.3 Determination of main chemical components of gypsum before and after calcining.

5.3.1 $CaSO_4 \cdot 2H_2O$ content determination in gypsum

About 0.2g of gypsum powder was weighed precisely, placed in a conical flask, add 10ml dilute hydrochloric acid, heat to dissolve, add 100ml water and methyl red indicator 1 drop, titrate with potassium hydroxide test solution to solution until it is light yellow. Then continue to add 5ml, add a little calcein indicator, titrate with EDTA standard solution titration (0.05mol/L), until the yellow-green fluorescence of solution disappear and orange fluorescence occur. Each 1ml EDTA titrant (0.05mol /L) is equivalent to 8.608mg of hydrated calcium sulfate ($CaSO_4 \cdot 2H_2O$).

5.3.2 The content determination of $CaSO_4$ in calcined gypsum

About 0.15g fine powder of calcined gypsum is weighed precisely. According to the method of '$CaSO_4 \cdot 2H_2O$ content determination in gypsum'. Each 1ml EDTA titrant (0.05mol /L) is equivalent to 6.807mg of calcium sulfate ($CaSO_4$).

Results

Table 3-14 Determination of main chemical components of gypsum before and after calcining

Sample	Sampling quantity/g	$CaSO_4 \cdot 2H_2O$ content/%	$CaSO_4$ content/%
Gypsum			
Calcined gypsum			

Notes

7.1 The temperature of calcined gypsum is very high, be careful to avoid scald.

7.2 When the temperature of calcined gypsum drops to about 100℃, it should be cooled in a dryer in time to avoid absorbing moisture in the air and affecting the calcining effect.

Questions

8.1 After the determination of $CaSO_4 \cdot 2H_2O$ in gypsum and the dripping of potassium hydroxide test solution until it is pale yellow, why do we need to add 5ml more?

8.2 What physical and chemical indicators can be used to evaluate the quality of gypsum and calcined gypsum rapidly, sensitively and accurately?

PPT

实验九 煅淬对自然铜成分含量的影响实验

实验目的

1. **掌握** 煅淬的炮制方法。
2. 通过自然铜煅制前后成分含量比较实验，说明煅淬法对自然铜的影响。

实验原理

1. 自然铜主含二硫化亚铁（FeS_2），经煅制后，二硫化亚铁分解为硫化亚铁，经醋淬后表面部分产生醋酸亚铁，且能使药物质地疏松易碎，便于粉碎，并使药物中铁离子溶出增加，易于被人体吸收。且炮制后自然铜中 Pb 等有毒物质，由于高温煅烧氧化而减少或清除。

2. 自然铜中的 Fe^{2+} 可与重铬酸钾发生氧化还原反应，引起颜色变化，根据消耗的重铬酸钾滴定液的体积计算 Fe^{2+} 的含量。以下式计算 Fe^{2+} 的含量：

$$P（\%）= 6C_{K_2Cr_2O_7}Vm_{K_2Cr_2O_7}M_{Fe} / M$$

$C_{K_2Cr_2O_7}$: $K_2Cr_2O_7$ 的摩尔浓度。

$V_{K_2Cr_2O_7}$: 滴定时消耗 $K_2Cr_2O_7$ 的体积。

M_{Fe}: Fe 的原子质量。

M: 样品的重量。

3. 原子吸收法测定自然铜中铅。由铅灯发出的特征谱线通过供试品蒸气时，被蒸气中铅的基态原子所吸收，吸收遵循一般分光光度法的吸收定律，通过测定辐射光强度减弱的程度可求出供试品中铅的含量。通常借助比较标准品和供试品的吸光度，求得供试品中铅元素的含量。

4. DDC-Ag 法测定自然铜中砷。利用金属锌与酸作用产生新生态的氢，与药物中的微量亚砷酸盐反应生成具有挥发性的砷化氢，用二乙基二硫代氨基甲酸银溶液吸收，使之还原生成红色胶态银，在 510nm 处测定吸收度，同条件下与一定量标准砷溶液吸光度进行比较，以判定砷盐的限量或含量。

实验内容

1. 自然铜的炮制。
2. 自然铜不同炮制品中铁含量测定。
3. 自然铜不同炮制品中铅含量测定。
4. 自然铜不同炮制品中砷含量测定。

实验器具和材料

1. **实验器具** 原子吸收分光光度计、可见 - 紫外分光光度计、电子天平、电炉、研钵、研锤、坩锅、坩埚钳、石棉网、250ml 锥形瓶、50ml 容量瓶、移液管（1.0、2.0、5.0、10ml）、玻璃漏斗、50ml 烧杯、量杯、酸式滴定管、100 目筛等。

2. **实验材料** 自然铜；活性炭、15% 硫酸 - 磷酸混合液、0.5% 二苯胺磺酸钠、重铬酸钾标准液（0.05mol/L）、标准铅溶液（100μg/ml）、标准砷溶液（5μg/ml）、DDC-Ag 液等。

实验方法

1. 自然铜的炮制 取净自然铜，大小分档，置坩埚内，用电炉加热，煅至红透时取出立即投入醋液中淬制，待冷后取出，继续煅烧，醋淬，反复煅淬至自然铜呈暗红褐色，外表脆裂，光泽消失，质地酥脆，取出，摊开放凉，干燥后粉碎。每 100kg 自然铜，用醋 30kg。

2. 试剂配制

（1）15% 硫酸 - 磷酸混合液　在不断搅拌下把 150ml 浓硫酸加入到 700ml 水中，冷却后加入 150ml 磷酸。

（2）准铅溶液（100μg/ml）、标准砷溶液（5μg/ml）　参考《中国药典》(2020 年版)。

（3）DDC-Ag 液　称取 0.6g 二乙基二硫代氨基甲酸银溶于含 3% 的三乙醇胺三氯甲烷溶液中，放置过夜，滤过，于棕色瓶中避光保存。

3. 自然铜不同炮制品中铁含量测定 分别取生、煅自然铜粉末约 3.0g，精密称定，置 250ml 锥形瓶中，加水 100ml，煮沸 25 分钟，加入活性炭 0.1g，继续煮沸 10 分钟，过滤。滤渣加水 80ml，煮沸 20 分钟，过滤，合并滤液，加入硫酸 - 磷酸混合液 15ml、0.5% 二苯胺磺酸钠 3 滴，用重铬酸钾滴定液（0.05mol/L）滴定至稳定的蓝紫色，并将滴定结果用空白试验校正。每 1ml 重铬酸钾滴定液相当于 3.351mg 的铁。

4. 自然铜不同炮制品中铅含量测定

（1）标准曲线的绘制　分别精密吸取标准铅溶液（100μg/ml）0、0.5、1.0、1.5、2.0ml 于 50ml 容量瓶中，用水稀释至刻度，摇匀。用原子吸收分光光度计在波长 283nm、灯电流 1mA、狭缝宽度 0.1mm、燃烧器高度 12mm、燃气流量 1.5L/min、助燃气流量 6L/min 条件下测定吸收度。以浓度为横坐标 X，吸收度为纵坐标 Y，计算求得回归方程，计算相关系数。

（2）供试品溶液制备　分别取生、煅自然铜粉末约 1g，精密称定，置锥形瓶中，加重蒸馏水 100ml，煮沸 1 小时（随时补充重蒸馏水），滤过。滤渣继续加重蒸馏水 50ml，煮沸 20 分钟，过滤。合并滤液，浓缩至约 25ml，放冷后移入 50ml 容量瓶中，加浓盐酸 2.8ml，再加重蒸馏水至刻度，摇匀，作为供试品溶液。

（3）测定法　以 2% 盐酸作为空白测定供试品溶液吸收度，根据回归方程，求得相应铅的浓度。

5. 自然铜不同炮制品中砷含量测定

（1）最大吸收波长的选择　精密吸取标准砷溶液 2.0ml 于砷化氢发生器的锥形瓶中，加 1 ∶ 1 硫酸溶液 7ml，以去离子水补至 40ml，加入 30% 碘化钾 5ml、40% 氯化亚锡 1.5ml，放置 15 分钟，加入 50% 酒石酸 1ml，放置 5 分钟，加入无砷锌粒 5g，立即接上装有醋酸铅棉花导气管的瓶塞，导管通入盛有 5ml DDC-Ag 吸收液的吸收管中，反应 15 分钟后，用三氯甲烷补至 5ml，置 1cm 吸收池中，以去离子水加相同试剂为空白，用可见 - 紫外分光光度计于 400 ~700nm 波长范围扫描，在 525 ~530nm 波长处有最大吸收。

（2）酸度范围　在 1.5 ~1.8mol/L 硫酸酸度范围内吸收值稳定。

（3）呈色稳定性　经呈色稳定性试验，结果呈色后溶液吸收值在 3 小时内稳定。

（4）标准曲线制备　精密吸取标准砷溶液 0、1.0、2.0、3.0、4.0、5.0ml（相当于 0.0、5.0、10.0、15.0、20.0、25.0μg 砷），分别置于砷化氢发生器的锥形瓶中，加 1 ∶ 1 硫酸溶液 7ml，以去离子水补至 40ml，按上述“最大吸收波长的选择 ”方法自“加入 30% 碘化钾 5ml”起操作，以分光光度计在 527nm 处测定吸光度。计算回归方程，砷在 0 ~25μg 范围内与吸光度呈线性相关。

（5）供试品测定　分别取生、煅自然铜粉末 0.1g，精密称定，置于 50ml 烧杯中，加 10ml 王水溶解，小火蒸至近干后加入 1 ∶ 1 硫酸溶液 10ml，加热至冒白烟。冷却后加去离子水煮沸，冷却，转移到 50ml 容量瓶中，用去离子水稀释至刻度，滤过。精密吸取滤液 25ml 于砷化氢发生瓶中，加 1 ∶ 1 硫酸溶液 7ml，以下按“标准曲线制备项”下“以去离子水补至 40ml”起操作，同时作一空白，以标准曲线项下 0 管调“0”点，测定吸光度，按回归方程计算砷含量。

实验结果

表 3–15 自然铜不同炮制品中化学成分含量测定

样品组	样品取样量 /g	铁含量 /%	铅含量 /%	砷含量 /%
生自然铜				
煅自然铜				

注意事项

1. 自然铜煎煮时宜用小火，并需不断搅拌，防止瓶底结块与爆溅。加活性炭时应离火，以免引起爆沸。

2. 煅自然铜溶液颜色较深，影响终点观察，可再加混合酸 15ml。

思考题

1. 简述重铬酸钾法测定二价铁离子含量时，滴定前为何需加入硫酸 – 磷酸混合液。
2. 简述原子吸收法测定铅含量时，供试品水煎液定容前为何需加入盐酸。

Experiment 9 Experiment of effects of calcining and quenching on the composition of Pyritum

Aims

1.1 To master the processing method of calcining and quenching.

1.2 To demonstrate the effect of calcined quenching on Pyritum by comparing the composition of Pyritum before and after calcining and quenching.

Principles

2.1 Pyritum mainly contains ferrous disulfide (FeS_2). After calcination, ferrous disulfide is decomposed into ferrous sulfide. After quenching with vinegar, ferrous acetate is generated on the surface. After processing, Pyritum becomes crisp and easy to be powdered. The efficient ingredients content can increase in the water-soluble extractives. At the same time, Pb and other toxic substances in Pyritum are reduced or eliminated due to calcination and oxidation at high temperature.

2.2 Fe^{2+} in Pyritum can undergo oxidation-reduction with potassium dichromate to cause color change. The Fe^{2+} content is calculated according to the volume of potassium dichromate titrant consumed. The following formula is used to calculate the Fe^{2+} content:

$$P(\%) = 6C_{K_2Cr_2O_7}Vm_{K_2Cr_2O_7}M_{Fe}/ M$$

$C_{K_2Cr_2O_7}$: mol concentration of $K_2Cr_2O_7$.

$V_{K_2Cr_2O_7}$: the volume of $K_2Cr_2O_7$ consumed during titration.

M_{Fe}: atomic mass of Fe.

M: the weight of the sample.

2.3 Determination of lead in Pyritum by atomic absorption spectrophotometry. When the characteristic spectral line emitted by the lead lamp passes through the vapor of the test sample, it is absorbed by the ground state atoms of lead in the vapor. The absorption follows the absorption law of general spectrophotometry. Usually by comparing the absorbance of the standard product and the test sample, the content of lead in the test sample can be obtained.

2.4 The determination of arsenic in Pyritum by DDC-Ag method. Using Zinc and acid to generate new ecosystem of hydrogen, and drug trace arsenite reactions generated in the volatile arsine, with silver diethyldithio-car-bamate solution absorption, make the reduction of generated red colloidal silver, determination of absorbance at 510nm, and with a certain amount standard arsenic solution under the condition of absorbance comparison, to determine contents of arsenic salt.

Contents

3.1 Processing of Pyritum.

3.2 Determination of iron content in different processed products of Pyritum.

3.3 Determination of lead content in different processed products of Pyritum.

3.4 Determination of arsenic content in different processed products of Pyritum.

Materials

4.1 Experimental apparatuses

Atomic absorption spectrophotometer, visible-ultraviolet spectrophotometer, electronic scale/balance, electric heater, mortar, hammer, crucible, crucible tongs, asbestos mesh, 250ml conical flask, 50ml volumetric flask, pipette (1.0, 2.0, 5.0, 10ml), glass funnel, 50ml beaker, beaker, acid burette, 100-mesh sieve, etc.

4.2 Experimental materials

Pyritum, activated charcoal, 15% sulfuric acid-phosphoric acid mixture, 0.5% sodium diphenylamine sulfonate, potassium dichromate standard solution (0.05mol/L), standard lead solution (100 μg /ml), standard arsenic solution (5g/ml), DDC-ag solution, etc.

Methods

5.1 Processing of Pyritum.

Take Pyritum, classify crude drugs by size, put them into the crucible and use the electric heater to heat, when they are calcined to red, immediately dip into the vinegar liquid to quench. Repeatedly to calcine and quench, until the drug appear dark brown, gloss disappear, texture becomes crisp, spread and cool , crush after drying. Use 30kg of vinegar per 100kg of Pyritum.

5.2 Reagent preparation.

5.2.1 15% sulfuric acid-phosphoric acid mixture

150ml concentrated sulfuric acid is added to 700ml water under constant agitation, and 150ml phosphoric acid is added after cooling.

5.2.2 Standard lead solution (100g/ml) and standard arsenic solution (5g/ml)

Reference to Chinese Pharmacopoeia (2020 Edition).

5.2.3 DDC-Ag solution

0.6g silver diethyldithio-car-bamate is dissolved in triethanolamine trichloromethane solution containing 3%, allow it to stand overnight, filtered and protected from light.

5.3 Determination of iron content in different processed products of Pyritum.

Both raw and calcined Pyritum powder are about 3.0g, weigh accurately, placed in a 250ml conical bottle, add 100ml water, boil for 25 minutes, add 0.1g activated charcoal, continue to boil for 10minutes and filter. The filter residue is added with 80ml water, boiled for 20 minutes, filtered and combined with filtrate. The mixture of sulfuric acid and phosphoric acid is added with 15ml and 3 drops of 0.5% sodium diphenylamine sulfonate. The titrant of potassium dichromate (0.05mol/L) is titrated to a stable blue-purple color. Every 1ml of potassium dichromate titrant is equivalent to 3.351mg of iron.

5.4 Determination of lead content in different processed products of Pyritum.

5.4.1 Drawing of standard curve

Standard lead solution (100g/ml) 0, 0.5, 1.0, 1.5 and 2.0ml are accurately pipetted into a 50ml volumetric bottle, diluted with water to the scale and shaken well. Absorption is measured by atomic absorption spectrophotometer at wavelength 283nm, lamp current 1mA, gap width 0.1mm, burner height 12mm, gas flow 1.5L/min and auxiliary gas flow 6L/min. Taking the concentration as X and the absorption as Y, the regression equation is calculated and the correlation coefficient is calculated.

5.4.2 Preparing the test sample solution

Take raw and calcined Pyritum powder of about 1g, weigh accurately, place it in a conical bottle, add 100ml distilled water, boil it for 1 hour (adding double distilled water at any time) and filter it. The filter residue is further weighted with 50ml distilled water, boiled for 20 minutes, and filtered. The filtrate is combined and concentrated to about 25ml. Allow to cool, the filtrate is transferred to a 50ml volumetric bottle. 2.8ml of concentrated hydrochloric acid is added.

5.4.3 Determination method

2% hydrochloric acid is used as blank to determine the absorbance of the test sample solution, and the corresponding lead concentration is obtained according to the regression equation.

5.5 Determination of arsenic content in different processed products of Pyritum.

5.5.1 Choose the maximum absorption wavelength

Accurately pipette the standard arsenic solution 2.0ml in the conical flask of arsine generator, add 1 ∶ 1 sulfuric acid solution 7ml, with deionized water to 40ml, add 30% potassium iodide 5ml, 40% stannous chloride 1.5ml, placed for 15 minutes, add 1ml 50% tartaric acid and place for 5 minutes, join arsenic-free zinc grain of 5g, immediately connect to cork containing lead acetate cotton airway access catheter containing 5ml DDC-Ag absorbing liquid absorption tube, 15 minutes after the reaction, add chloroform to 5ml, put in the 1cm absorption cuvette, Deionized water is added with the same reagent as blank, and the scanning is performed with a visible-UV spectrophotometer in the wavelength range of 400~700nm, with the maximum absorption at the wavelength of 525 ~530nm.

5.5.2 The acidity range

The absorption value is stable within the acidity range of 1.5 ~1.8mol /L sulfuric acid.

5.5.3 Color rendering stability

After color rendering stability test, the solution absorption value is stable within 3hour after color rendering.

5.5.4 Preparation of standard curve

Accurately pipette the standard arsenic solution 0, 1.0, 2.0, 3.0, 4.0, 5.0 ml (0.0, 5.0, 10.0, 15.0, 20.0, 25.0 μg arsenic), respectively put in to the conical flask with arsine generator, add 1 ∶ 1 sulfuric acid solution 7ml, with deionized water to 40ml, according to the above method of 5.5.1 since "join 30% potassium iodide 5ml" operation, determine absorbance at 527nm with spectrophotometer. According to the regression equation, arsenic is linearly correlated with the absorbance in the range of 0~25g.

5.5.5 Determination of arsenic content in the test sample

0.1g of the raw and calcined Pyritum powder is weighed accurately. The powder is placed in a 50ml beaker, dissolved with 10ml of chloroazotic acid, steamed to dry nearly, then add 10ml of 1∶1 sulfuric acid solution, and heat to produce white smoke and cool it. Then boil it with deionized water and cool, transfer to a 50ml volumetric flask, dilute to volume with deionized water, and filter. Add 7ml of 1∶1 sulfuric acid solution to 25ml of filtrate in the arsine generator bottle, and start the operation according to "fill to 40 ml with deionized water" under 5.5.4. Meanwhile, make a blank, adjust the "0" point with 0 tube under the standard curve, measure the absorbance, and calculate the arsenic content according to the regression equation.

Results

Table 3–15 Determination of chemical composition in different processed products of Pyritum

Sample	Sample quantity/g	Iron content/%	Lead content/%	Arsenic content/%
Raw Pyritum				
Calcined pyritum				

Notes

7.1 Use low heat when decoct Pyritum, and keep stirring to prevent caking and spillage at the bottom of the bottle. We should be keep out of the fire to add activated charcoal, so as not to cause explosive boiling.

7.2 If the color of calcined pyritum solution is darker which affect the evaluation of end point observation, 15ml of mixed acid could be added.

Question

8.1 When potassium dichromate method is used to determine the content of ferrous ions, why should sulfuric acid-phosphoric acid mixture be added before titration?

8.2 When determining the content of lead by atomic absorption spectrometry, why should hydrochloric acid be added to the decoction before the volume is fixed?

PPT

实验十　蒸制对黄芩成分含量的影响实验

实验目的

1. **掌握**　蒸制法及其对药物的影响。
2. 通过黄芩蒸制前后成分含量实验，说明黄芩炮制的意义。

实验原理

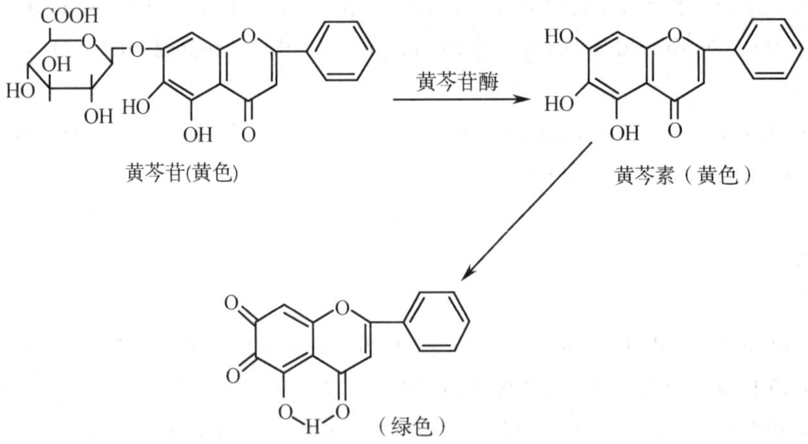

图 3-1　黄芩苷水解的分子结构图

1. 蒸制是利用水蒸气加热药物的方法，借助于水蒸气的穿透力和热量，可以使药物中的一些成分在加热过程中和水分子的作用下发生变化，如水解、结构破坏、含量下降或产生新成分等，从而达到改变药物性味、产生新的功能、扩大临床适用范围、便于切制或使药物便于保存等炮制目的。采用蒸制法炮制黄芩，以此起到杀酶保苷的作用。黄芩在软化过程中，如用冷水处理，易变绿色（图 3-1）。这是由于黄芩所含的酶在一定温度和湿度下，可酶解黄芩中的黄芩苷和汉黄芩苷，产生葡萄糖醛酸和两种苷元，即黄芩素和汉黄芩素。其中黄芩苷元为邻位三羟基黄酮，本身不稳定，容易被氧化成醌类物质而变绿，使疗效降低。黄芩苷的水解与酶的活性有关，以冷水浸，酶的活性最大。而采用蒸或燀等加热方法可破坏酶使其活性消失，有利于黄芩苷的保存。实验表明，黄芩经过蒸制或沸水煮，既可杀酶保苷，又可使药物软化，便于切片，也可保证饮片质量和原有的色泽。

2. 按照《中国药典》(2020 年版)“黄芩”项下含量测定方法，采用 HPLC 对黄芩主要有效成分黄芩苷进行含量测定，分析比较黄芩蒸制对其主要有效成分黄芩苷的影响。

实验内容

1. 黄芩的炮制。
2. 黄芩不同炮制品中黄芩苷的含量测定。

实验器具和材料

1. 实验器具 高效液相色谱仪、C_{18}色谱柱、电子天平、筛子、蒸锅、电炉、铁架台、冷凝管、橡皮膏、量筒、容量瓶、移液管等。

2. 实验材料 黄芩、黄芩苷对照品；甲醇、乙醇、磷酸、水等。

实验方法

1. 黄芩的炮制

（1）黄芩 取黄芩原药材除去杂质，洗净。大小分档，置蒸制容器内隔水加热，蒸至“圆汽”后半小时，质地软化，取出，趁热切薄片，干燥。

（2）冷浸黄芩 取黄芩原药材除去杂质，洗净，加水浸泡至质地软化，取出，切薄片，干燥。

2. 黄芩不同炮制品中黄芩苷的含量测定

（1）色谱条件与系统适用性试验 以十八烷基硅烷键合硅胶为填充剂；以甲醇 – 水 – 磷酸（47∶53∶0.2）为流动相；检测波长 280nm。理论塔板数按黄芩苷峰计算应不低于 2500。

（2）对照品溶液的制备 取在 60℃减压干燥 4 小时的黄芩苷对照品适量，精密称定，加甲醇制成每 1ml 含 60μg 的溶液，即得。

（3）供试品溶液的制备 取黄芩不同炮制品中粉约 0.3g，精密称定，加 70% 乙醇 40ml，加热回流 3 小时，放冷，滤过，滤液置 100ml 量瓶中，加甲醇至刻度，摇匀，即得。

（4）测定法 分别精密吸取对照品溶液与供试品溶液各 10μl，注入液相色谱仪，测定，即得。按干燥品计，分别计算黄芩不同炮制品中黄芩苷的百分含量。

实验结果

表 3–16 黄芩不同炮制品中黄芩苷的含量测定

样品组	样品取样量 /g	黄芩苷含量 /%
黄芩		
冷浸黄芩		

注意事项

1. 黄芩药材应大小分档炮制。
2. 实验操作时，样品及对照品应平行进行，否则影响实验结果。

思考题

1. 简述何种软化方法能够提高黄芩饮片质量。
2. 简述黄芩蒸制前后黄芩苷含量有何不同。

Experiment 10 The Influence of steaming on the Composition of Scutellariae Radix

Aims

1.1 To master steaming and its influence on medicinal herbs.

1.2 To indicate the significance of processing Scutellariae Radix through testing the composition of Scutellariae Radix before and after processing.

Principles

2.1 Serving as the method of heating herbs by water vapor, while taking the aid of penetrating power and heat of that, steaming can make some of the composition change in the heating process and under the action of water molecules, such as hydrolysis, the content decline, structural failure and the generation of new composition, so as to achieve the processing purposes like property and flavor upgrading, generating new functions, expanding the clinical application scope, convenient for cutting or preserving, etc. The Scutellariae Radix is processed by steaming method, which can kill enzyme and protect glycosides. Scutellariae Radix, in the process of softening, if treated with cold water, is easy to turn green. This is because the Scutellariae Radix contains enzymes, at a certain temperature and humidity, it is capable of enzymatic hydrolysis of baicalin and wogonosiden, producing glucuronic acid and two aglycons, namely baicalein and wogonin. Baicalein is an ortho-trihydroxy brass, which is unstable and easy to be oxidized into quinones and turn green, then reduce the curative effect. The hydrolysis of baicalin is related to the activity of the enzyme which is maximized when immersed in cold water. However, steaming or blanching can destroy the enzyme and make its activity disappear, which is beneficial to the preservation of baicalin. The results show that taking the means of steaming or boiling could not only kill the enzyme and protect the anhydride in Scutellariae Radix, but also soften the herb,

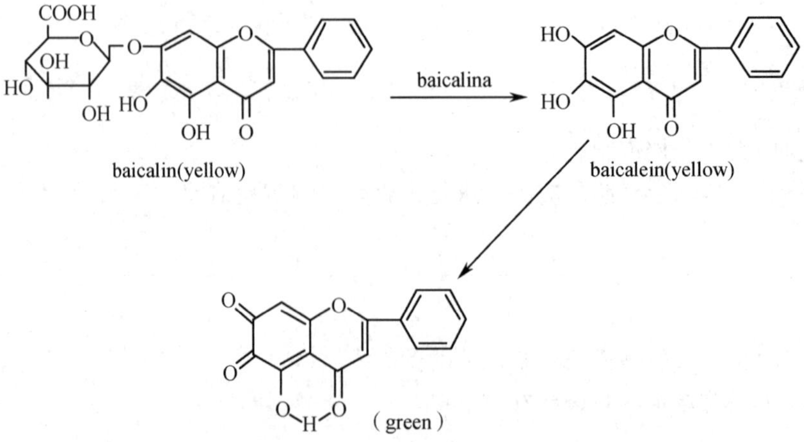

Graph 3-1 Molecular structure diagram of baicalin hydrolysis

making it easier to be cut into slices, meanwhile, guarantee the quality and original color of Yinpian (decoction pieces/processed Chinese medicine).

2.2 According to the content determination method of "baicalin" in Chinese pharmacopoeia (2020 edition), the main effective composition of baicalin is determined by HPLC, and the effect of steaming of baicalin on its main effective composition is analyzed and compared.

Contents

3.1 Processing of Scutellariae Radix.

3.2 Determination of baicalin in different processed products of Scutellariae Radix.

Materials

4.1 Laboratory apparatuses

High performance liquid chromatograph, C_{18} chromatographic column, electronic scale/balance, sieve, steamer, electric heater, iron stand, condensing tube, rubber tube, measuring cylinder, volumetric flask, pipette, etc.

4.2 Laboratory materials

Scutellariae Radix, Baicalin reference sample, methanol, ethanol, phosphoric acid, water, etc.

Methods

5.1 Processing of Scutellariae Radix.

5.1.1 Scutellariae Radix

Remove non-essential parts from Scutellariae Radix raw Chinese medicine and wash the latter. Classify crude drugs by size and heat them with water in the steam vessel, until the steam has filled in it for half an hour, by then, the Scutellariae Radix getting soft in the texture, take them out, cut into thin slices hot, and dry them.

5.1.2 Soak Scutellariae Radix into cold water

Remove non-essential parts from Scutellariae Radix raw Chinese medicine and wash the latter, soak it in cold water until softened and then take out, cut into thin slice and dry it.

5.2 Determination of baicalin in different processed products of Scutellariae Radix.

5.2.1 Chromatographic conditions and systematic adaptation test

Octadecyl silane bonded silica gel is used as filler. The mobile phase is methanol–water–phosphoric acid (47 ∶ 53 ∶ 0.2). The detection wavelength is 280nm.The theoretical plates number should not be less than 2500 according to the baicalin peak.

5.2.2 Preparation of reference sample solution

After decompression and drying at 60 degrees Celsius for 4 hours, an appropriate amount of baicalin reference sample is weighed accurately and methanol is added to make a solution containing 60μg/ml.

5.2.3 Preparation of test sample solution

Powder in different processed products of Scutellariae Radix in middle size is taken to be about 0.3g, weighed accurately, then 40ml of 70% ethanol is added. After heated reflux for 3 hours, allow to cool and filtered, subsequently, the filtrate is placed in a 100ml measuring bottle, the container and residue are washed with a small amount of 70% ethanol in separate times, then the washing liquid is filtered into the same measuring bottle, and 70% ethanol is added to the scale, then shaken well. Accurately, measure 3ml of the filtrate, place it in a 10ml volumetric flask, add methanol to the mark, and shake to obtain.

5.2.4 Measurement

The reference sample solution and the test sample solution are accurately pipetted with 10μl each and injected into the liquid chromatograph for determination. The contents of baicalin in different processed products of Scutellariae Radix are measured and calculated on the basis of dried product.

Results

Table 3-16 Determination of content of baicalin in different processed products of Scutellariae Radix

Sample	Sample Weight/g	Content of Baicalin/%
Scutellariae Radix		
Scutellariae Radix soaked in cold water		

Notes

7.1 Scutellariae Radix raw Chinese medicine should be classified processed according to different sizes.

7.2 During the experiment, the sample and the reference sample should be carried out in parallel, otherwise the experiment effect will be affected.

Questions

8.1 What softening method can improve the quality of Scutellariae Radix Yinpian (decoction pieces/processed Chinese medicine)?

8.2 Briefly describe the difference in baicalin content in Scutellariae Radix before and after steaming.

PPT

实验十一　煮制川乌质量评价实验

实验目的

1. **掌握**　煮制法及对药物的影响。

2. 通过川乌煮制前后质量评价实验，说明川乌炮制的意义。

实验原理

1. 煮制是通过加热水或加辅料煮制药物的方法改变毒性药物的成分及药性，以降低毒性或缓和药性等。采用煮法炮制生川乌，可以降低毒性，以供内服，用于风寒湿痹、关节疼痛、心腹冷痛、寒疝作痛及麻醉止痛。川乌的主要成分为生物碱，炮制后毒性降低的程度，主要取决于毒性强的双酯型生物碱的水解程度。生川乌所含的双酯型生物碱性质不稳定，遇水或加热容易被水解，使极毒的双酯型乌头碱 C_8 位上的乙酰基水解，生成苯甲酰单酯型生物碱，即苯甲酰乌头胺（乌头次碱）、苯甲酰中乌头胺、苯甲酰次乌头胺，其毒性为双酯型乌头碱的 1/500~1/200。再进一步水解，使 C_{14} 位上的苯甲酰基水解，生成醇胺型乌头原碱，即乌头胺（乌头原碱）、中乌头胺、次乌头胺。其毒性仅为双酯型乌头碱的 1/4000~1/2000。另一原因可能是炮制过程中脂肪酰基取代了 C_8 位上的乙酰基，生成酯碱，从而降低了毒性。川乌炮制后采用煮法或蒸法炮制乌头都能促进水解反应，从而达到降低毒性的目的。

2. 采用 HPLC 对川乌不同炮制品中双酯型乌头碱及苯甲酰单酯型生物碱的含量进行测定，分析比较川乌煮制对其主要成分生物碱的影响。

实验内容

1. 川乌的炮制。
2. 川乌不同炮制品中双酯型乌头碱的含量测定。
3. 川乌不同炮制品中苯甲酰单酯型生物碱的含量测定。

实验器具和材料

1. 实验器具　高效液相色谱仪、超声提取仪、旋转蒸发仪、水分测定仪、电热干燥箱、恒温水浴锅蒸锅、锅铲、煤气灶（或其他加热电器）、搪瓷盘、切药刀、三号筛等。

2. 实验材料　生川乌、乌头碱对照品、次乌头碱对照品、新乌头碱对照品、苯甲酰乌头原碱对照品、苯甲酰次乌头原碱对照品、苯甲酰新乌头原碱对照品；0.45μm 微孔滤膜、乙腈、四氢呋喃（均为色谱纯）、醋酸铵、乙醇、氨水、异丙醇、三氯甲烷、乙酸乙酯、冰醋酸（均为分析纯）、重蒸水等。

实验方法

1. 川乌的炮制　取净川乌，大小个分开，用水浸泡至内无干心，取出，加水煮沸 4~6 小时

（或蒸 6~8 小时）至取个大及实心者切开内无白心，口尝微有麻舌感时，取出，晾至六成干，切厚片，干燥，即得。

2. 川乌不同炮制品中双酯型乌头碱的含量测定

（1）色谱条件与系统适用性试验 以十八烷基硅烷键合硅胶为填充剂，以乙腈－四氢呋喃（25：15）为流动相 A，以 0.1mol/L 醋酸铵溶液（每 1000ml 加冰醋酸 0.5ml）为流动相 B，梯度洗脱，洗脱程序见表 3-17；检测波长为 235nm，理论塔板数按新乌头碱峰计算应不低于 2000。

表 3–17 梯度洗脱程序

时间（分钟）	流动相 A（%）	流动相 B（%）
0~48	15→26	85→74
48~49	26→35	74→65
49~58	35	65
58~65	35→15	65→85

（2）对照品溶液的制备 取乌头碱对照品、次乌头碱对照品、新乌头碱对照品适量，精密称定，加异丙醇－三氯甲烷（1：1）混合溶液分别制成每 1ml 含乌头碱 50μg、次乌头碱和新乌头碱各 0.15mg 的混合溶液，即得。

（3）供试品溶液的制备 取炮制品粉末（过三号筛）约 2g, 精密称定，置具塞锥形瓶中，加氨试液 3ml，精密加入异丙醇－乙酸乙酯（1：1）混合溶液 50ml，称定重量，超声处理（功率 300W，频率 40kHz；水温在 25℃以下）30 分钟，放冷，再称定重量，用异丙醇－乙酸乙酯（1：1）混合溶液补足减失的重量。摇匀，滤过。精密量取续滤液 25ml, 40℃以下减压回收溶剂至干，残渣精密加入异丙醇－三氯甲烷（1：1）混合溶液 3ml 溶解，滤过，取续滤液，即得。

（4）测定法 分别精密吸取对照品溶液与供试品溶液各 10μl，注入液相色谱仪，测定，即得。按干燥品计，分别计算川乌不同炮制品中含乌头碱、次乌头碱、新乌头碱的百分含量。

3. 川乌不同炮制品中苯甲酰单酯型生物碱的含量测定

（1）色谱条件与系统适用性试验 同“双酯型乌头碱的含量测定”方法。

（2）对照品溶液的制备 取苯甲酰乌头原碱对照品、苯甲酰次乌头原碱对照品、苯甲酰新乌头原碱对照品适量，精密称定，加异丙醇－三氯甲烷（1：1）混合溶液分别制成每 1ml 含苯甲酰乌头原碱和苯甲酰次乌头原碱 50μg、苯甲酰新乌头原碱 0. 3mg 的混合溶液，即得。

（3）供试品溶液的制备 同“双酯型乌头碱的含量测定”方法。

（4）测定法 同“双酯型乌头碱的含量测定”方法。按干燥品计，分别计算川乌不同炮制品中含苯甲酰乌头原碱、苯甲酰次乌头原碱、苯甲酰新乌头原碱的百分含量。

实验结果

表 3–18 川乌不同炮制品中生物碱的含量测定

样品组	取样量 /g	双酯型乌头碱含量 /%	苯甲酰单酯型生物碱含量 /%
生川乌			
制川乌			

注意事项

1. 生川乌属于毒性中药管理品种，毒性非常大，因此，在实验过程中应该严格进行管理，实验前领取药材及实验完毕交还制川乌时均需称重量并进行登记，严禁私自处理。

2. 炮制制川乌时，注意火候，至取个大及实心者切开内无白心、口尝微有麻舌感时，取出。

3. 生川乌及制川乌均应按干燥品计算含量。为了节约实验时间，可采用同一快速水分测定仪进行测定两种炮制品的水分。

思考题

1. 简述川乌煮制过程中双酯型乌头碱及苯甲酰单酯型生物碱的含量的变化。

2. 简述采用蒸制法代替煮制法炮制川乌，蒸制的压力、温度及时间等因素对双酯型乌头碱及苯甲酰单酯型生物碱的含量的影响。

Experiment 11 The quality evaluation experiment of Processed Aconiti Radix

Aims

1.1 To master boiling method and its effect on medicine.

1.2 To explain the significance of processing Aconiti Radix through the quality evaluation experiment before and after processing.

Principles

2.1 Boiling is a method to change the composition and property of toxic drugs by heating water or adding auxiliary materials to boil drugs, so as to reduce the toxicity or mitigate drug effect. Processing Aconiti Radix by boiling can reduce its toxicity and be used for oral administration, which can be used for the treatment of wind-cold-dampness caused pain or numbness, joint pain, cold pain in the heart and abdomen, pain caused by cold abdominal and pain, and it can be applied for anesthesia to relieve pain. The main components of Aconiti Radix are alkaloids. The degree of toxicity reduction after processing is mainly determined by the degree of hydrolysis of the highly toxic diester alkaloids. The properties of the diester alkaloids contained in Aconiti Radix are not stable and easily hydrolyzed in water and heat, so that the acetyl group at position C_8 of the extremely poisonous diester aconitine is hydrolyzed to form benzoyl monoester alkaloids, that are Benzoylaconine, Benzoylhypaconine, Benzoylmesaconin. The toxity of benzoyl monoester alkaloids is 1/500~1/200 that of diester aconitines. Further hydrolysis is carried out to hydrolyze benzoyl group at C_{14},which forms aconitine of amino alcohol type, that are Aconine, Mesaconine and Hypaconine, those are only 1/4000~1/2000 as toxic as diester aconitine. Another reason may be that fatty acyl groups replace acetyl groups at the C_8 position during processing to form ester bases, thereby reducing its toxicity. Processing Aconiti Radix by boiling or steaming can promote the hydrolysis reaction, so as to achieve the purpose of reducing toxicity.

2.2 HPLC is used to determine the content of diester aconitine and benzoyl monoester alkaloids in different processed products of Aconiti Radix.

Contents

3.1 The processing of Aconiti Radix.

3.2 Determination of the content of diester aconitine in different processed products of Aconiti Radix.

3.3 Determination of benzoyl monoester alkaloids in different processed products of Aconiti Radix.

Materials

4.1 Experimental apparatuses

High performance liquid chromatograph, ultrasonic extractor, rotary vaporizer, moisture tester, electric drying oven, constant temperature water bath steamer, truner, electric heater, enamel tray, herb cutting knife, No.3 sieve, etc.

4.2 Experimental materials

Aconiti Radix, Aconitine reference sample, Hypaconitine reference sample, Mesaconitine reference sample, Benzoylaconitine reference sample, Benzoylhypacoitine reference sample, Benzoylmesaconine reference sample, 0.45μm millipore filter, acetonitrile, tetrahydrofuran (all are chromatographic grade), ammonium acetate, ethanol, ammonia water, isopropanol, trichloromethane, ethyl acetate, glacial acetic acid. (all are analytical grade）, redistilled water, etc.

Methods

5.1 The processing of Aconiti Radix

Grade clean Aconiti Radix according to size, soak in water until there is no dry core. Take them out, boil in water for 4~6 hours (or steam for 6~8 hours)until there is no white core in the relatively large and solid root and the taste becomes slightly numb. After removal, dry in the air to 60% dryness, cut into thick slices and dry.

5.2 Determination of the content of diester aconitine in different processed products of Aconiti Radix.

5.2.1 Chromatographic system and systematic adaptation test

Use octadecylsilane bonded silica gel as the stationary phase, a mixture of acetonitrile and tetrahydrofuran (25 ∶ 15) as the mobile phase A and a 0.1mol/L solution of ammonium acetate (add 0.5ml glacial acetic acid in each 1000ml solution) as the mobile phase B, gradient elution procedures are shown in table 3-17. As detection wavelength set at 235nm, the number of theoretical plates of the column shall not less than 2000, calculated with reference to the peak of mesaconitine.

Table 3-17 Gradient elution procedures

Time（minutes）	Mobile phase A（%）	Mobile phase B（%）
0-48	15→26	85→74
48-49	26→35	74→65
49-58	35	65
58-65	35→15	65→85

5.2.2 Preparation of reference sample solution

Weigh accurately appropriate amount of aconitine, hypaconitine and mesaconitine reference sample, respectively, dissolve. Add isopropanol-chloroform (1 ∶ 1) mixture to produce a mixed solution containing 50μg of aconitine, 150μg each of hypaconitine and mesaconitine per 1ml.

5.2.3 Preparation of test sample solution

Weigh accurately 2g of processed product powder (passing sieve No.3), put into a conical flask with plug, add 3ml of ammonia test solution, accurately add 50ml of a mixture of isopropanol and ethyl acetate (1 : 1) and weigh. Ultrasonicate (power 300W, frequency 40kHz, keeping the water temperature below 25℃) for 30 minutes, allow to cool and weigh. again, replenish the weight loss of the solvent with the above mixture, mix well and filter. Measure accurately 25ml of the subsequent filtrate, recover the solvent to dryness in vacuum below 40℃, dissolve the residue in 3ml of the above mixture, filter and use the subsequent filtrate as the test sample solution.

5.2.4 Determination method

Accurately pipette 10μl of the reference sample solution and the test sample solution respectively into the column, and calculate the content. According to the dry products, the percentage contents of aconitine, hypaconitine and mesaconitine in different processed products of Aconiti Radix are calculated.

5.3 Determination of benzoyl monoester alkaloids in different processed products of Aconiti Radix.

5.3.1 Chromatographic system and systematic adaptation test

The same as the method of 5.2.1.

5.3.2 Preparation of reference sample solution

Weigh accurately appropriate amount of Benzoylaconine, Benzoylhypacoitine and Benzoylmesaconine, respectively, then dissolve. Add the mixture of isopropanol and chloroform (1 : 1) to produce a mixed solution containing 50μg each of Benzoylaconine and Benzoylhypacoitine, 300μg of Benzoylmesaconine per 1ml.

5.3.3 Preparation of test sample solution

The same as the method of 5.2.3.

5.3.4 Determination method

The same as the method of 5.2.4. According to the dry products, the percentage contents of Benzoylaconine, Benzoylhypacoitine and Benzoylmesaconine in different processed products of Aconiti Radix are calculated.

Results

Table 3-18 Determination of alkaloids in different processed products of Aconiti Radix

Sample group	Sampling quantity/g	Content of diester Aconitine/%	Content of benzoyl monoester alkaloids/%
Raw Aconiti Radix			
Processed Aconiti Radix			

Notes

7.1 Aconiti Radix is a kind of toxic traditional Chinese medicine, which is very toxic. Therefore, it should be strictly managed during the experiment. Before the experiment, when receiving the medicine and returning the processed Aconiti Radix raw Chinese medicine after the experiment, the weight should be weighed and registered. It is strictly prohibited to handle without permission.

7.2 When processing Aconiti Radix, pay attention to the Level of attainment, until the big and solid ones are cut without white core, and the taste slightly numb, take them out.

7.3 The content of Raw and processed Aconiti Radix should be calculated according to dried products. In order to save experimental time, the rapid moisture tester can be used to determine the moisture content of two processed products.

Question

8.1 Briefly describe the change of content of diester aconitine and benzoyl monoester alkaloids in the boiling process of Aconiti Radix.

8.2 If using steaming method instead of boiling method to process Aconiti Radix, what are the effects of pressure, temperature and time of steaming on the content of diester aconitine and benzoyl monoester alkaloids?

PPT

实验十二　制苦杏仁质量评价实验

实验目的

1. **掌握**　焯制法及对药物的影响。
2. 通过苦杏仁焯制前后质量评价实验，明确苦杏仁焯制目的及其炮制原理。

实验原理

焯制是在沸水中短时间浸煮的方法，主要在于破坏一些药物中的酶、毒蛋白，同时也有利于分离药用部分。苦杏仁，味苦，性微温，有小毒，归肺、大肠经。具有止咳平喘、润肠通便的功效，用于咳嗽痰多、肠燥便秘等。苦杏仁中的止咳平喘主要有效成分是苦杏仁苷，在一定的温度和湿度条件下，苦杏仁苷易被共存的苦杏仁苷酶水解，生成野樱苷，野樱苷在 野樱苷酶作用下生成杏仁腈，杏仁腈不稳定，遇热易分解为苯甲醛和氢氰酸，故剂量过大或使用不当易中毒。水解过程见图 3-2。

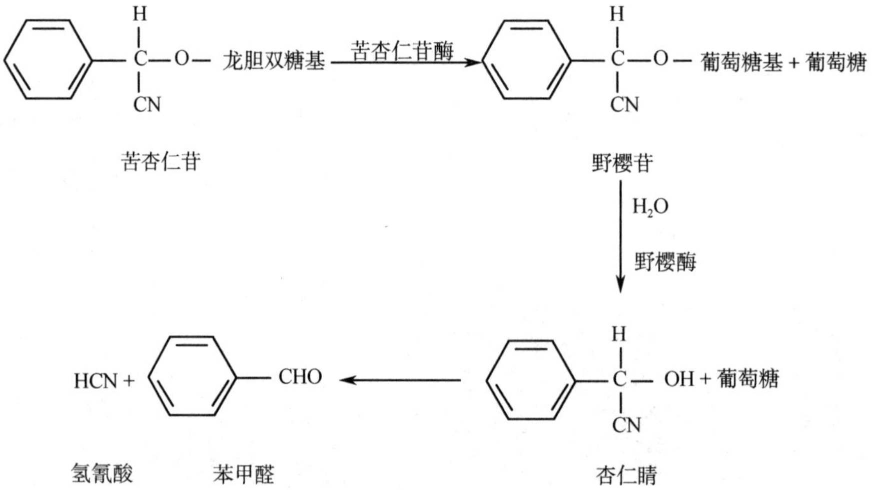

图 3-2　苦杏仁苷的水解示意图

焯法炮制能破坏苦杏仁酶的活性，增加了苦杏仁苷的稳定性，保证用药安全有效。本实验利用生品中苦杏仁苷被苦杏仁酶水解生成氰氢酸，接触苦味酸钠试纸，发生还原反应，生成异紫酸钠显砖红色（图 3-3），而制品则不显砖红色的苦味酸钠试验，定性检测苦杏仁中酶的活性。同时采用 HPLC 进行苦杏仁苷的含量测定。

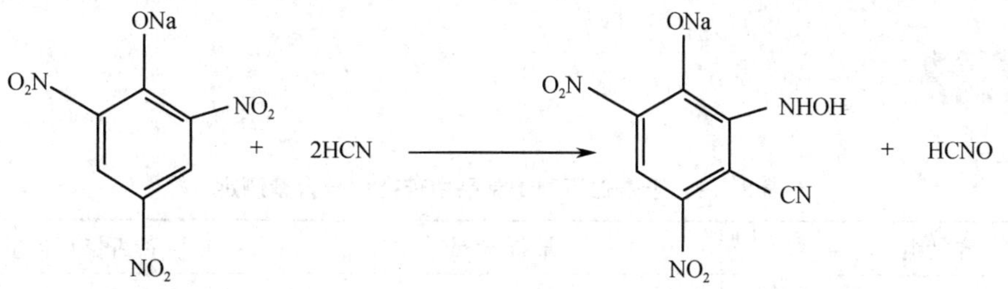

苦味酸钠　　异紫酸钠（砖红色）

图 3–3　苦味酸显色反应示意图

实验内容

1. 苦杏仁的炮制。
2. 苦杏仁不同炮制品中的酶活性检验。
3. 苦杏仁不同炮制品中苦杏仁苷含量测定。

实验器具和材料

1. 实验器具　高效液相色谱仪、电磁炉、不锈钢锅、托盘天平、筛子、烧杯、量筒、乳钵、具塞试管、恒温水浴锅、超声波清洗仪、电子天平（1/0000）等。

2. 实验材料　苦杏仁、苦味酸试纸、碳酸钠溶液、甲醇、乙腈、磷酸等。

实验方法

1. 苦杏仁的炮制　取净苦杏仁置 10 倍量沸水中略煮，加热约 5 分钟，至种皮微膨起即捞起，用凉水浸泡，取出，搓开种皮与种仁，干燥，筛去种皮。用时捣碎。

2. 苦杏仁不同炮制品中的酶活性检验

（1）取苦杏仁生品数粒，加水共研，有苯甲醛的特殊香气。

（2）取生、焯苦杏仁粗粉约 0.5g，分别放入两支试管中，加水数滴使之湿润，在试管口分别悬挂一条用碳酸钠试液润湿过的苦味酸试纸，用软木塞塞紧，将试管置 40~50℃的水浴中加热，观察生品和制品的颜色反应。

3. 苦杏仁不同炮制品中苦杏仁苷含量测定

（1）色谱条件与系统适用性试验　C_{18} 色谱柱（4.6mm × 250mm，5μm），流动相为乙腈 –0.1% 磷酸水（8 : 92），流速为 1.0ml/min，柱温为 35℃，检测波长为 207nm，进样体积为 10μl。

（2）对照品溶液的制备　精密取苦杏仁苷对照品适量，加甲醇配制成质量浓度 4.0mg/L 的苦杏仁苷对照品溶液。

（3）供试品溶液的制备　分别取生苦杏仁，焯苦杏仁粗粉（过二号筛）各 0.25g，精密称定，置具塞锥形瓶中，加入甲醇 25ml，称重。超声处理（功率 250W，频率 50kHz）30 分钟，放冷，再称重，用甲醇补足失重，摇匀，过滤，取续滤液 5ml 置 50ml 容量瓶中，加 50% 甲醇稀释至刻度，摇匀，过 0.45μm 滤膜，即得供试品溶液。

（4）测定法　取各供试品溶液各 10μl 进样分析，测定，即得。按干燥品计，分别计算出苦杏仁不同炮制品中苦杏仁苷的百分含量。

实验结果

表 3-19　苦杏仁不同炮制品中苦杏仁苷含量测定

样品组	取样量 /g	苦杏仁苷含量 /%
生苦杏仁		
焯苦杏仁		

注意事项

1. 焯制时温度要高，一定要水沸后投药。

2. 应控制适宜的水量和时间。水量为 10 倍以上；加热时间以 5~10 分钟为宜，时间短则不足以完全破坏酶，时间长则造成苦杏仁苷的损失。

3. 焯后宜当天晒干或低温烘干。

思考题

1. 简述苦杏仁苷酶活性检验原理。

2. 简述焯苦杏仁的炮制原理。

Experiment 12 The quality evaluation experiment of blanching Armeniacae Semen Amarum

Aims

1.1 To master the operation of the blanching and its influence on drugs.

1.2 To clarify the purpose and processing principle of blanching Armeniacae Semen Amarum through the quality evaluation before and after processing.

Principles

Blanching is a method of cooking in boiling water for a short time. The main purpose is to destroy the enzymes and toxic proteins in some drugs, and it is also beneficial to the separation of medicinal parts. Armeniacae Semen Amarum is bitter in flavor, mildly warm in property, small in toxicity, lung and large intestine in channel tropism, and it has the functions of relieving cough and asthma and relaxing bowel for cough phlegm, constipation due to intestinal dryness, etc. Amygdalin, the main active ingredient of cough and asthma in Armeniacae Semen Amarum, is easily hydrolyzed into prunasin by the coexisting amygdalase under the certain temperature and humidity conditions Prunasin is hydrolyzed into mandelonitrile under the Prunase. Due to its instability, mandelonitrile is easily decomposed into benzaldehyde and hydrocyanic acid when heated. Therefore, it is easy to be poisoned if the dosage is too large or improperly used. See Figure 3–2 for the hydrolysis process.

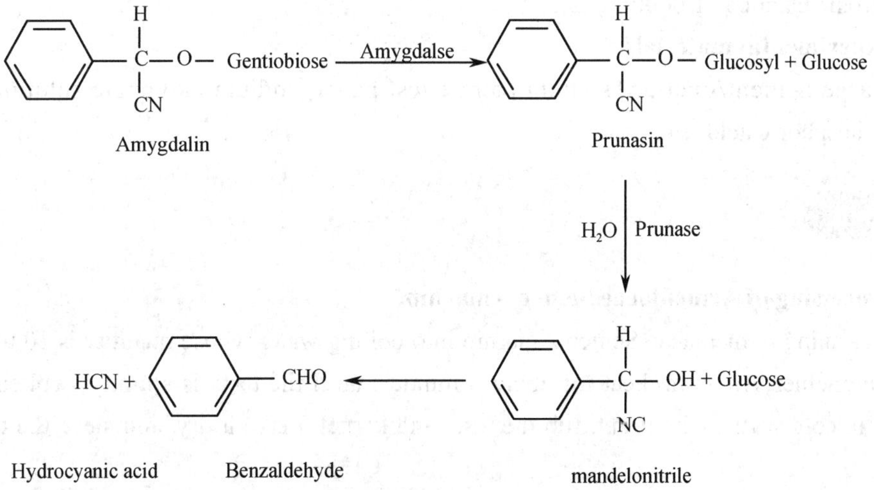

Figure 3–2 Hydrolysis of amygdalin

The activity of the amygdalase is destroyed by blanching processing and the stability of amygdalin is increased, safety and effectiveness of clinical application are guaranteed. In this experiment, the amygdalin in the Armeniacae Semen Amarum crude Chinese medicine is hydrolyzed by the amygdalase to generate hydrocyanic acid, which contacted with the sodium picrate test paper to produce sodium iso Violet (brick red color) (Figure 3–3) by a reduction reaction, while the processed Armeniacae Semen Amarum does not show a brick red. Therefore, the enzyme activity in Armeniacae Semen Amarum is qualitatively detected. At the same time, the content of amygdalin is determined by HPLC.

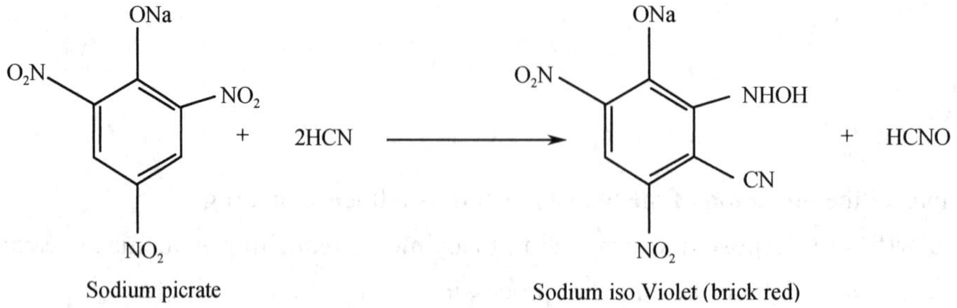

Figure 3–3 The color reaction of picric acid

Contents

3.1 The processing method of the Armeniacae Semen Amarum.

3.2 Testing of enzyme activity in different processed products of Armeniacae Semen Amarum.

3.3 Determination of amygdalin in different processed products of Armeniacae Semen Amarum.

Materials

4.1 Experimental apparatuses

High Performance Liquid Chromatography, induction cooker, stainless steel pot, counter balance, sieve, beaker, measuring cylinder, mortar, test tube with a stopper, thermostatic water bath, ultrasonic cleaner, electronic balance (1/0000) , etc.

4.2 Experimental materials

Armeniacae Semen Amarum, sodium picrate test paper, sodium carbonate solution, methanol, acetonitrile, phosphoric acid, etc.

Methods

5.1 Processing of Armeniacae Semen Amarum.

Put the cleaning Armeniacae Semen Amarum into boiling water whose quantity is 10 times as much as Armeniacae Semen Amarum, heat for about 5 minutes until the testa is slightly swollen, then scoop it up, soak it in cold water, take it out, rub the testa and kernel, make it dry, and sieve the testa. Mash it when used.

5.2 Tests of Enzyme Activity in Different Processed Armeniacae Semen Amarum.

5.2.1 Take a few crude Armeniacae Semen Amarum crude Chinese medicine and co-grind with water and the flavor of the Benzaldehyde will be given off.

5.2.2 Take the crude and processed Armeniacae Semen Amarum coarse powder about 0.5g each, put them into two test tubes, then add a few drops of water to moisten them, hang a piece of sodium picrate test paper moistened with sodium carbonate solution at the mouth of the test tube respectively, plug the test tube and heat the test tube in a water bath at 40~50℃ to observe the color reaction of the crude Chinese medicine and the processed.

5.3 Determination of amygdalin in different processed products of Armeniacae Semen Amarum.

5.3.1 Chromatographic conditions and systematic adaptation test.

Samples are analyzed on the C_{18} reversed phase chromatography column (4.6mm × 250mm,5μm) with the mobile phase consisted of acetonitrile –0.1% phosphoric acid (8 : 92). The flow rate of the mobile phase, column temperature, detection wavelength and the injection volume is set at 1.0ml/min, 35°C, 207nm and 10μl, respectively.

5.3.2 Preparation of reference sample solution.

Weigh an appropriate amount of amygdalin reference sample accurately and add methanol to prepare into an amygdalin reference substance sample solution with a mass concentration of 4.0mg/ml.

5.3.3 Preparation of test sample solution

Take the crude and processed Armeniacae Semen Amarum (passed through a No. 2 sieve) about 0.25g accurately, weight accurately placed in a conical flask with a plug, add 25ml of methanol and then weigh them. Ultrasonication (power 250W, frequency 50kHz) for 30 minutes, allow to cool, weigh again, replenish the weight loss with methanol, mix well, filter, take 5ml of the subsequent filtrate and pour it in a 50ml volumetric flask, add 50% methanol to the mark, mix well and filter with 0.45μm filter membrane to obtain the test sample solution.

5.3.4 Method of determination

Accurately pipette 10μl of each test sample solution for analysis, determination. Based on the dried product, calculate the percentage of amygdalin in different processed products of Armeniacae Semen Amarum.

Results

Table 3–19 Determination of amygdalin in different processed products of Armeniacae Semen Amarum

Sample set	Weight of sample/g	Content of Amygdalin/%
Crude Armeniacae Semen Amarum		
Blanching Armeniacae Semen Amarum		

Notes

7.1 The temperature must be high during the blanching and put the sample into the water after boiling.

7.2 Should control the appropriate amount of water and time, the amount of water is more than 10 times. The heating time is preferably about 5~10 minutes. A short time is not enough to destroy the enzyme, but the loss of amygdalin will be caused by long time processing.

7.3 It is better to dry in the sun or at a low-temperature intraday.

Questions

8.1 Briefly describe the principle of the amygdalase activity test.

8.2 Briefly describe the principle of processed Armeniacae Semen Amarum.

实验十三 清半夏炮制降低毒性的实验评价

PPT

实验目的

1. **掌握** 复制法及其对药物的影响。
2. 通过半夏用白矾炮制前后毒性评价实验，说明半夏炮制的意义。

实验原理

1. 清半夏的炮制 采用8%白矾水溶液浸泡半夏，可以降低半夏的刺激性、毒性；经过白矾溶液浸泡后的半夏，口尝稍有或无麻辣感，对家兔眼结膜刺激性急剧下降，其毒性也下降。

2. 半夏的刺激性毒性成分，是半夏中具有特殊针样晶形的针晶，存在于半夏的黏液细胞中。半夏的针晶显微镜下可以看到两种类型：短针晶和长针晶，以长针晶为主，极细长。电镜下（20000×）可以看到针晶表面有倒刺，两头尖锐，中间凹槽，直径0.5μm以下，长130μm左右。半夏的针晶是复合物，由草酸钙、蛋白和微量糖类成分组成。该针晶具有强烈的刺激性及毒性，产生的原因是由于针晶对机体黏膜组织细胞的物理刺激导致刺痛，加上针晶中蛋白的化学刺激导致肿胀麻木，共同作用形成半夏特殊的刺激性毒性。浸泡半夏的白矾溶液pH为3左右，白矾溶液中的Al^{3+}能够络合针晶含有的不溶性草酸钙的$C_2O_4^{2-}$，成为草酸铝络合物，使得支撑针晶刚性不溶性的草酸钙被溶解，针晶的针样晶形和倒刺等结构被破坏，产生物理性刺激的刚性载体被破坏；同时，白矾中的$KAl(SO_4)_2$可以使针晶中的蛋白变性，针晶的化学刺激消除。两方面的作用导致半夏的刺激性毒性成分破坏而降低刺激性毒性。

$$nC_2O_4^{2-}+Al^{3+}+mH_2O\rightarrow[Al(C_2O_4)n]^{(2n-3)}\cdot mH_2O$$

3. 利用家兔眼结膜刺激的模型，可以直接观察生半夏及半夏的刺激性毒性成分针晶对黏膜的刺激性作用。将半夏的粉末混悬液和半夏纯针晶混悬液直接滴入家兔眼中，由于半夏草酸钙针晶的尖锐针刺可以直接刺入家兔眼结膜的黏膜细胞，同时针晶中蛋白的化学刺激加重眼结膜水肿，分泌物增多，在30分钟到2小时之内可以清晰地观察到生半夏药材粉末和从半夏中提取获得的刺激性毒性成分（针晶）对家兔眼结膜的强烈刺激性作用，采用客观评分的方法进行打分可以评价刺激性的强弱。同时用清半夏粉末混悬液、淀粉混悬液进行对照比较刺激的强弱。

4. 由于半夏的针晶不溶于水及有机溶剂，通过对样品的预处理，先将样品中可溶性的草酸盐去除，再通过酸处理使针晶中草酸钙转化为草酸（$CaC_2O_4+2HCl=CaCl_2+H_2C_2O_4$），生成1mol草酸需要1mol草酸钙，据此利用RP-HPLC进行草酸钙含量测定。草酸在200~210nm具有末端吸收，选择210nm作为测定波长。以标准草酸作为对照品制备标准曲线，测定草酸的含量并换算成半夏药材中针晶的不溶性草酸钙的含量。

实验内容

1. 清半夏的炮制。
2. 半夏中刺激性毒针晶的提取与显微观察。
3. 半夏不同炮制品及毒性成分对家兔眼结膜刺激性实验。
4. 半夏不同炮制品毒针晶的含量测定。

实验器具和材料

1. 实验器具 高效液相色谱仪、超声波清洗机、光学显微镜、烘箱、真空干燥箱、减压泵、离心机（0~5000r/min）、恒温水浴锅、电子天平、C_{18}色谱柱，研钵、研锤、烧杯（250ml）、载玻片、抽滤瓶、酸度计、聚氟乙烯离心管（10ml）、40目筛、200目筛、兔盒、胶头滴管、垂熔玻璃滤器、微孔滤膜、具塞锥形瓶等。

2. 实验材料 生半夏、半夏鲜品、白矾；石油醚、纱布、蒸馏水、盐酸、磷酸、色谱纯甲醇、重蒸馏水、草酸基准试剂、10%四丁基氢氧化铵、磷酸二氢钾、生理盐水等。

3. 实验动物 健康大耳白家兔，体重1.5~2kg。

实验方法

1. 清半夏的炮制 取生半夏，大小分档，用清水浸泡，加水量以淹没药材为度，浸泡至内无干心。按照《中国药典》（2020年版）一部清半夏项下的炮制方法，加入8%白矾水溶液，继续浸泡至无干心，口尝无刺激麻舌感，取出，置烘箱中，80℃干燥。可将白矾溶液的温度提高至30℃，以缩短浸泡的时间。

2. 半夏中刺激性毒针晶的提取与显微观察

（1）针晶的提取 取半夏鲜品约80g，置研钵中，加入一定量的石油醚研磨，当石油醚变浑浊时，将上层石油醚混悬液转入具塞锥形瓶中加盖，重复上述过程约10次以上。上述混悬液，置载玻片上，光学显微镜（20×10，40×10）下观察，见大量的细长针晶，混悬液用有机微孔滤膜滤过（滤膜孔径0.45μm），石油醚少量多次洗涤，40℃以下真空干燥，得到纯白色针晶粉末，口尝具有强烈的刺痛感。

（2）针晶白矾溶液的制备 精密称取纯针晶50mg，加入8%白矾溶液2ml，配制成2.5%（mg/ml）的针晶混悬液，放置过夜。备用。

3. 半夏不同炮制品及毒性成分对家兔眼结膜刺激性实验

（1）供试品液的制备 ①半夏炮制前后的样品制备：分别称取生半夏和清半夏粉末（过200目筛）各1g，用生理盐水配制成20%的混悬液。②针晶混悬液的制备：精密称取纯针晶约50mg，加生理盐水配制成2.5%的针晶混悬液。③白矾炮制针晶溶液的制备：取上述以白矾溶液浸泡的针晶混悬液离心，取沉淀，以“针晶混悬液”同体积的生理盐水配制成混悬液，备用。④淀粉溶液的制备：取过200目筛的药用淀粉，以生理盐水配制成20%的混悬液，备用。

上述各样品均调节pH使溶液呈中性（pH=7.0）。

（2）口尝法比较半夏炮制前后刺激性 取半夏炮制前后的样品粉末（5~10mg）、纯针晶少量（1~2mg）以及白矾炮制针晶溶液中的沉淀少量，分别置于舌尖前1/3处，轻轻咀嚼约10秒，吐掉，30秒至1分钟后感觉并记录刺痛感和口舌肿胀麻木感。口尝实验按照清半夏、白矾溶液浸泡过的针晶的沉淀、生半夏、纯针晶顺序进行。生半夏、纯针晶因均会产生强烈的刺痛麻辣感，进行口尝实验时，需等到前一种样品麻辣感消失后，再进行另一种样品的口尝实验。

（3）半夏炮制品和针晶对家兔结膜的刺激性实验 将体重约1.5kg的健康家兔固定在兔笼，将各样品混悬液滴加到各兔左眼中，滴加20%的淀粉混悬液到兔右眼作为对照，每只眼2滴。轻轻闭合上下眼睑，注意不要使药液溢出，轻揉，使药液与眼结膜充分接触，3分钟后，用生理盐水30~40ml冲洗眼睛至眼中无任何异物。半小时后比较眼结膜的变化情况，并根据表3-20评分，无刺激0~2分，轻度刺激3~5分，中度刺激6~8分，重度刺激9~10分。

表 3-20 家兔眼结膜刺激程度评分标准

水肿程度	得分	充血	得分	分泌物	得分
无水肿	0	血管正常	0	无分泌物	0
轻微水肿	1	血管充血呈鲜红色	1	少量分泌物	1
明显水肿，伴部分眼睑外翻	2	血管充血呈深红色，血管不易分辨	2	分泌物使眼睑和睫毛潮湿或黏浊	2
水肿至眼睑近半闭合	3	弥漫性充血，呈紫红色	3	分泌物使整个眼区潮湿或黏浊	3
肿至眼睑超过半闭合	4				

4. 半夏不同炮制品毒针晶的含量测定

（1）色谱条件及系统适用性试验　以十八烷基硅烷键合硅胶为填充剂；流动相为 0.5%KH_2PO_4-0.5mmol/L TBA（四丁基铵盐）水溶液，以磷酸调节 pH 至 2.0；流速为 0.8ml/min；检测波长为 210nm；柱温为 28℃。理论板数以草酸峰计算不低于 3000。

（2）对照品溶液的制备　取水合草酸对照品约 14mg，精密称定，置于 50ml 容量瓶中，加蒸馏水，溶解并稀释至刻度，摇匀，使草酸浓度为 0.2mg/ml，作为对照品溶液。

（3）供试品溶液的制备　分别取生半夏和清半夏样品粉末（过 40 目筛）约 0.1g，精密称定，分别置玻璃容器中，各加入 3ml 蒸馏水混匀，震荡 5 分钟，然后置 60℃水浴加热并搅拌 10 分钟，3000r/min 离心 5 分钟，弃上清液。沉淀以热水洗涤 2 次，每次 2ml，离心，弃上清液。取沉淀，加盐酸溶液（1∶1）0.2ml，纯水 3ml，混匀。置 70℃水浴加热搅拌 10 分钟，离心，条件同上，分离沉淀与上清液，沉淀继续用 0.1mol/L 盐酸，同上法置“70℃水浴加热”起处理 2 次，每次 2ml，离心，合并上清液，置 10ml 容量瓶中，加纯水定容至刻度。

（4）测定法　每个样品进样 10μl，按上述色谱条件测定草酸的峰面积，根据标准曲线计算草酸含量并换算成草酸钙含量。草酸基准试剂分子量为 126.07，针晶以草酸钙计，草酸钙（$CaC_2O_4 \cdot H_2O$）的分子量为 146.12。

实验结果

表 3-21 半夏炮制前后毒性刺激性比较

样品组	口尝比较刺激性	家兔眼结膜刺激程度评分
清半夏		
针晶（白矾溶液浸泡）		
生半夏		
纯针晶		

表 3-22 半夏不同炮制品毒针晶的含量测定

样品组	取样量 /g	毒针晶含量 /%
生半夏		
清半夏		

注意事项

1. 半夏鲜品具有较强的刺激性，在提取针晶时要戴橡胶手套操作。因针晶中含有蛋白类成分，对针晶进行干燥时要低温操作，温度一般不要超过40℃。

2. 四丁基氢氧化铵为强碱性溶液，配制流动相时，注意防护。家兔眼结膜实验时，样品溶液应采用生理盐水配制，且要注意调节样品溶液的pH近中性；样品溶液在滴入兔眼前要充分振摇混匀，尤其是针晶混悬液、生半夏粉末混悬液、炮制品粉末混悬液要充分混悬。滴入的药液量以及冲洗时生理盐水的用量每个家兔的眼睛要保持一致，以便可以平行比较实验结果。

思考题

1. 结合半夏炮制前后针晶含量、家兔眼结膜刺激性实验及显微观察、口尝等结果，说明半夏炮制意义。

2. 简述为何测得的草酸钙含量可以代表半夏中针晶的含量。

3. 白矾能使半夏中的针晶含量下降，试分析其原因。

Experiment 13 Experimental evaluation on attenuating toxicity of Pinelliae Rhizoma processed into Pinelliae Rhizoma Praeparatum Cum alumenine

Aims

1.1 To master the repeated processing method which using specified auxiliary materials and processing to the specified degree, and its effects on drugs.

1.2 To explain the significance of crude Pinelliae Rhizoma processed with alumen by the toxicity evaluation experiment of crude Pinelliae Rhizoma and Pinelliae Rhizoma Praeparatum Cum alumenine.

Principles

2.1 Preparation of Pinelliae Rhizoma Praeparatum Cum alumenine. Immersing crude Pinelliae Rhizoma in the 8% alumen solution, it can reduce the irritation and toxicity of Pinelliae Rhizoma. Pinelliae Rhizoma's spicy taste would become very slight or disappeared after it is processed in the way of soaking in alumen solution. The irritation to conjunctiva of rabbits decreased sharply, and its toxicity also decreased.

2.2 The irritant and toxic component of crude Pinelliae Rhizoma is raphides with a special needle-like crystal form exists in the mucous cells of Pinelliae Rhizoma. There are two kinds of raphides observed through microscope, long and short raphides, most of them are long, which are extremely slender. Under an electron microscope (20000 ×), the crystal surface is covered with barbs, they are sharp at both ends, and with grooves in the middle of them, the diameter is less than 0.5μm, and the length is about 130μm. The raphides of crude Pinelliae Rhizoma is a complex composed of calcium oxalate, protein, and trace sugars. The raphides are strongly irritant and toxic, due to the physical stimulation of the raphides to the body's mucosal tissue cells causes tingling, the chemical stimulation of the protein in the raphides causes swelling and numbness, which together form the special irritant toxicity of crude Pinelliae Rhizoma. The pH value of the alumen solution which is used to process Pinelliae Rhizoma is about 3, and the Al^{3+} in the alumen solution can complex with the $C_2O_4^{2-}$ of the insoluble calcium oxalate contained in the raphides. After that the Al^{3+} becomes an aluminum oxalate complex, which causes the rigidity of the raphides that is supported by the calcium oxalate to be dissolved, and the shapes as well as the barbs of the raphides are damaged, the rigid carriers that produce the physical stimulus are destroyed, at the same time, $KAl(SO_4)_2$ in alumen can denature protein molecules, and eliminate the chemical stimulation of raphides. These two effects lead to the destruction of the irritant toxic components of crude Pinelliae Rhizoma and the irritant toxicity reduction.

$$nC_2O_4^{2-}+Al^{3+}+mH_2O \rightarrow [Al(C_2O_4)n]^{(2n-3)} \cdot mH_2O$$

2.3 The irritant effect of Pinelliae Rhizoma and the irritant toxic component on mucous membrane can be observed directly by using the model of eyes conjunctival stimulation in rabbits. The powder suspension of crude Pinelliae Rhizoma and the pure raphides suspension are directly instilled into the rabbits eyes, because the sharp raphides which are made up of calcium oxalate can directly penetrate the mucosal cells of rabbits' eye conjunctiva, meanwhile, the chemical irritation of the protein in the raphides aggravates the edema of the conjunctiva as well as the increase of secretions, within 30 minutes to 2 hours the strong irritant effect on the conjunctiva of rabbits' eyes can be clearly observed, which is caused by the crude Pinelliae Rhizoma powder and the irritant toxic ingredients (raphides) which are extracted from crude Pinelliae Rhizoma. The irritation can be evaluated by scoring using an objective scoring method. The Pinelliae Rhizoma Praeparatum Cum alumenine and starch suspension are used to compare the strength of irritation.

2.4 Because the raphides of Pinelliae Rhizoma are insoluble in water and organic solvents, so the samples of Pinelliae Rhizoma can be pre-treated to remove the soluble oxalate, and then the calcium oxalate in the raphides is converted into oxalic acid that formed from CaC_2O_4 by suffering hydrochloric acid treatment ($CaC_2O_4+2HCl = CaCl_2+H_2C_2O_4$), 1mol of oxalic acid is generated from 1mol of calcium oxalate, according to the principle, the content of calcium oxalate is determined by RP-HPLC. The oxalic acid has terminal absorption at 200 ~ 210nm, 210nm is selected as the UV detection wavelength. The standard curve are prepared with oxalic acid standard as reference, and then calculate oxalic acid content, finally, convert oxalic acid content into the insoluble calcium oxalate content in raphides of Pinelliae Rhizoma.

Contents

3.1 Processing of Pinelliae Rhizoma Praeparatum Cum alumenine.

3.2 Extraction and microscopic observation of raphides with irritation and toxicity in Pinelliae Rhizoma.

3.3 The irritation experiment of different processed products and toxic raphides of Pinelliae Rhizoma on the conjunctiva of rabbits.

3.4 Assay of the toxic raphides content in different processed products of Pinelliae Rhizoma.

Materials

4.1 Experimental apparatuses

HPLC, ultrasonic cleaner, optical microscope, oven, vacuum drying box, decompression pump, centrifuge(0~5000r/min), thermostatic water bath, electronic scales, C_{18} chromatography column, mortar, hammer for grinding, beaker (250ml), glass slide, suction filter bottle, acidiometer, polyvinyl fluoride centrifuge tube (10ml), 40-mesh sieve, 200-mesh sieve, rabbit box, plastic tip dropper, vertical melting glass filter, millipore filter, conical flasks with plug, etc.

4.2 Experimental materials

Crude Pinelliae Rhizoma, fresh Pinelliae Rhizoma, alumen, petroleum ether, gauze, distilled water, hydrochloric acid, phosphoric acid, chromatographically pure methanol, redistilled water, oxalic acid reference reagen, tetrabutylammonium hydroxide 10%, potassium dihydrogen phosphate, physiological saline, etc.

4.3 Experimental animals

Healthy big-eared white rabbits, weighing 1.5~2kg.

Methods

5.1 Preparation of Pinelliae Rhizoma Praeparatum Cum alumenine.

Take some crude Pinelliae Rhizoma, grade in size, soak in clear water, add water to submerge all drugs, and soak them in the water until there is no dry core. According to the processing method of Pinelliae Rhizoma Praeparatum Cum alumenine which is record in the Chinese Pharmacopoeia (2020 Edition): soak in 8% alumen solution until the centre of the cut surface without a dry core and with no a slight numbing taste, take out, put in an oven, and dry at 80℃. During the procedure, the temperature of the alumen solution can be raised to 30℃ to shorten the soaking time.

5.2 Extraction and microscopic observation of raphides with irritation and toxicity in Pinelliae Rhizoma.

5.2.1 Extraction of raphides

Take about 80g fresh Pinelliae Rhizoma, put them in a mortar, grind them with a certain amount of petroleum ether, and when the petroleum ether becomes turbid, transfer the upper petroleum ether suspension into a capped conical flask and cap it. Repeat the above operation about 10 times or more. After that, put the suspension on a glass slide and observe under an optical microscope (20 × 10, 40 × 10), and a large number of slender needle-like crystals are seen. Filter the suspension with an organic microporous membrane (pore size of filter membrane is 0.45μm), wash the filtered crystals several times with a small amount of petroleum ether, then dry it in a vacuum oven below 40℃. Pure white raphides powder is obtained after that, which can cause strong tingling sensation in the mouth after tasting.

5.2.2 Suspension preparation of raphides processed with alumen solution

Weigh 50mg of pure raphides accurately, add 2ml of 8 % alumen solution, and prepared 2.5%(mg/ml) raphide-alumen suspension, leave it to stand overnight for use.

5.3 The irritation experiment of different processed products and toxic components of Pinelliae Rhizoma on the conjunctiva of rabbits.

5.3.1 Preparation of test solution.

A. Pinelliae Rhizoma and Pinelliae Rhizoma Praeparatum Cum alumenine suspension: Weigh 1g crude Pinelliae Rhizoma and Pinelliae Rhizoma Praeparatum Cum alumenine powder (passed through a 200-mesh sieve), respectively, add physiological saline to prepare 20% suspension of the two samples. B. Raphides suspension. Accurately weigh about 50mg of pure raphides, add saline to prepare 2.5% suspension. C. Raphide-alumen suspension. Take the above-mentioned suspension of raphide processed with alumen solution, centrifuge it, the precipitate is added physiological saline to prepare suspension for use, the saline volume is the same as the "raphides suspension" preparation method. D. Starch solution. Take medicinal starch sifted by a 200-mesh sieve, add physiological saline to prepare 20% starch suspension for use.

The pH of above samples solution should be adjusted to be neutral (pH = 7.0).

5.3.2 The irritation comparison of Pinellia Rhizoma before and after processing by tasting method.

Take the samples (5~10mg) of Pinellia Rhizoma and Pinelliae Rhizoma Praeparatum Cum alumenine powder, a small amount of pure raphides (1~2mg) and sediment of raphide-alumen suspension, respectively place them on the front 1/3 of the tongue tip, chew gently for about 10 seconds, then spit out. From 30 seconds to 1 minute, the sensation of tingling, swelling and numbness of tongue and mouth is felt and record. The experimental sequence of tasting samples is Pinelliae Rhizoma Praeparatum Cum alumenine, sediment of raphide-alumen suspension, crude Pinelliae Rhizoma and pure raphides. The crude Pinelliae Rhizoma and pure raphides have strong tingling and spicy sensation, so the taste of later sample need to wait for experiment until the former sample's taste disappear.

5.3.3 The irritation experiment of different processed products and toxic raphides of Pinelliae Rhizoma on the conjunctiva of rabbits.

1.5kg healthy rabbits are weighed and fixed in rabbit cages, the sample suspension is added dropwise to the left eye of each rabbit, 20% starch suspension is added dropwise to the right eye of each rabbit as control, 2 drops sample per eye. Gently close the upper and lower eyelids, pay attention not to overflow the liquid medicine, gently rub eyes to make the liquid fully contact with the conjunctiva. After 3 minutes, rinse the eyes with 30~40ml of physiological saline until there is no foreign matter in the eyes. After half an hour, compare and evaluate the changes of the conjunctiva according to the Table 3–20, record the scores, 0~2 points for no irritation, 3~5 points for mild irritation, 6~8 points for moderate irritation and 9~10 points for severe irritation.

Table 3–20 Scoring criteria for the irritation degree of conjunctiva in rabbits' eyes

Degree of edema	Score	Hyperemia	Score	Secretions	Score
No edema	0	Normal blood vessels	0	No secretions	0
Slight edema	1	Vascular congestion is bright red	1	Small amount of secretion	1
Significant edema with eversion of some eyelids	2	Vascular congestion is dark red, blood vessels are not easy to distinguish	2	Secretions make the eyelids and eyelashes moist or cloudy	2
Edema to nearly half-closed eyelids	3	Diffuse hyperemia, purplish red	3	Secretions make the entire eye area moist or Cloudy	3
Swelling to more than half closed eyelids	4				

5.4 Assay of the toxic raphides content in different processed products of Pinelliae Rhizoma.

5.4.1 Chromatographic conditions and systemetic adaptation

Use octadecylsilane bonded silica as the stationary phase, the mobile phase is 0.5% KH_2PO_4–0.5mmol/L TBA (tetrabutylammonium salt) aqueous solution, pH is adjusted to 2.0 with phosphoric acid, the flow rate is 0.8ml/min, the detection wavelength is set at 210nm, the column temperature is 28℃. The theoretical plate number of the column calculated with reference to the oxalic acid peak is not less than 3000.

5.4.2 Preparation of reference sample solution

Take about 14mg of hydrated oxalic acid reference, weigh it accurately, place it in a 50ml volumetric flask, add distilled water to dissolve, and dilute to scale, shake well, obtain the 0.2mg/ml oxalic acid as the reference solution.

5.4.3 Preparation of test solution.

Accurately weigh about 0.1g of crude Pinelliae Rhizoma and Pinelliae Rhizoma Praeparatum Cum alumenine powder (passed through a 40-mesh sieve), place them in glass containers, add 3ml of distilled water, blend the powder and the distilled water, shake for 5 minutes. After that, put the glass containers into the water bath, heat and stir the solution for 10 minutes, centrifuge it at 3000r/min for 5 minutes, discard the supernatant liquid. Wash the sediments twice with hot water, 2ml each time, centrifuge, and discard the supernatant liquid. Take the sediments, add 0.2ml hydrochloric acid solution (1 : 1) and 3ml pure water, mix well. Place it in a 70℃ water bath and stir for 10 minutes. Centrifuge under the same conditions as above. Separate the sediments from the supernatant liquid, add 2ml 0.1mol/L hydrochloric acid to deal with the sediments, the following steps is same as above method beginning from "place it in a 70℃ water", repeat this round two times, use hydrochloric acid 2ml each time, combine the supernate, place in a 10ml volumetric flask, add pure water to scale volume.

5.4.4 Assay method

Inject accurately 10μl of each of the reference solution and the test solution, respectively, into the column, measure the oxalic acid peak area and obtain the standard curve, calculate the oxalic acid content and convert into the calcium oxalate content. The molecular weight of the oxalic acid reference reagent is 126.07, and the raphides content are calculated as calcium oxalate ($CaC_2O_4 \cdot H_2O$) with molecular weight of 146.12.

Results

Table 3–21 Comparison of toxicity and irritation of Pinelliae Rhizoma before and after processing

Sample group	Irritation comparsion by taste	Irritation score of rabbit' eyes conjunctival
Pinelliae Rhizoma Praeparatum cum alumenine		
Raphides (soaked in alumen solution)		
Crude Pinelliae Rhizoma		
Pure raphides		

Table 3–22 Content determination of toxic raphides in different processed products of Pinelliae Rhizoma

Sample group	Sampling amount/g	Toxic raphides content/%
Crude Pinelliae Rhizoma		
Pinelliae Rhizoma Praeparatum cum alumenine		

Notes

7.1 Fresh Pinelliae Rhizoma is highly irritating, so the rubber gloves are needed to wear when extracting the raphides. Because the raphides contain protein components, the raphides should be dried at a low temperature, and the temperature should not exceed 40℃.

7.2 Tetrabutylammonium hydroxide is a strong alkaline solution, pay attention to protect operators when preparing the mobile phase. In rabbits' eyes conjunctival experiments, the sample solution should be prepared with physiological saline, and the pH of the sample solution should be adjusted to be nearly neutral; the test solution which is used to drop into the rabbits' eyes should be fully shaken and mixed, especially the raphides suspension, the crude Pinelliae Rhizoma powder suspension, and the processed product powder suspension should be suspended enough. The quantity of each sample that dropped in the eyes of rabbits and physiological saline that used to rinse the eyes of rabbits should be consistent, so that the experimental results can be compared in parallel.

Questions

8.1 Explain the significance of crude Pinelliae Rhizoma processed with alum, combining with the results of raphides content, rabbits' eyes conjunctival irritation experiment, microscopic observation and taste experiment of Pinelliae Rhizoma before and after processing.

8.2 Why can use the measured calcium oxalate content represent the raphides content in Pinelliae Rhizoma.

8.3 Try to analyze the reason that alumen can reduce the raphides content in Pinelliae Rhizoma.

实验十四　制霜对巴豆成分的影响实验

PPT

实验目的

1. **掌握**　制霜的炮制方法及对药物的影响。

2. 通过巴豆制霜前后脂肪油的含量测定实验，说明巴豆炮制的意义。

实验原理

某些种子类药物经过适当加热、压榨去油等处理，制成松散的粉末，以缓和药性或降低毒性。巴豆有大毒，生巴豆毒性强烈，仅供外用蚀疮。巴豆去油制霜后，能降低毒性、缓和泻下作用。巴豆毒性成分是其所含的毒性蛋白及脂肪油，巴豆制霜可以去除一部分脂肪油，加热可以破坏毒性蛋白，从而使其毒性降低。另外，对其有效成分巴豆苷进行含量控制，以保证巴豆霜临床使用安全有效。

实验内容

1. 巴豆霜的炮制。

2. 巴豆制霜前后脂肪油及巴豆苷的含量测定。

实验器具和材料

1. **实验器具**　高效液相色谱仪、C_{18}色谱柱、超声波清洗器、电子天平、水浴锅、蒸制工具、压榨工具、研钵、纱布、索氏提取器、蒸发皿、具塞锥形瓶、滤纸、脱脂棉等。

2. **实验材料**　巴豆，巴豆苷对照品；乙醚等。

实验方法

1. **巴豆霜的炮制**　取巴豆，去壳。取净巴豆仁，碾成泥状，布包严，蒸至上大量蒸汽30分钟。取出，压榨去油，再蒸再压。如此反复几次，至药物松散成粉末，不再粘结成饼为度。或取净巴豆仁碾细，测定脂肪油含量，加适量淀粉稀释，使脂肪油含量符合规定，混匀，即得。

2. **巴豆制霜前后脂肪油及巴豆苷的含量测定**

（1）脂肪油的含量测定　取本品约5g，精密称定，置索氏提取器中，加乙醚100ml，加热回流提取（6~8小时）至脂肪油提尽，收集提取液，置已干燥至恒温的蒸发皿中，在水浴上低温蒸干，在100℃干燥1小时，置于干燥器中，冷却30分钟，精密称定，计算，即得。以干燥品计，巴豆制霜前后含脂肪油的百分含量。

（2）巴豆苷的含量测定　①色谱条件与系统适用性试验：以十八烷基硅烷键合硅胶为填充剂；以乙腈－甲醇－水（1∶4∶95）为流动相；检测波长为292nm。理论板数按巴豆苷峰计算应为不低于5000。②对照品溶液的制备：取巴豆苷对照品适量，精密称定，加水制成每1ml含60μg的溶液，即得。③供试品溶液的制备：取本品约0.15g精密称定，置索氏提取器中，加乙醚

5ml，加热回流 3 小时，弃去乙醚液，药渣挥干溶剂，连同滤纸筒移入具塞锥形瓶中，精密加入水 50ml，称定重量，超声处理（功率 300W，频率 24kHz）20 分钟，放冷，再称定重量，用水补足减失的重量，摇匀，滤过，即得。④测定法：分别精密吸取对照品溶液与供试品溶液各 10μl，注入液相色谱仪，测定，即得。以干燥品计，巴豆制霜前后含巴豆苷的百分含量。

实验结果

表 3-23　巴豆制霜前后脂肪油及巴豆苷的含量测定

样品组	样品取样量 /g	脂肪油含量 /%	巴豆苷含量 /%
生巴豆			
巴豆霜			

注意事项

1. 制备巴豆霜要注意劳动保护，应戴口罩、手套，实验用具应及时洗刷干净。

2. 加入乙醚量不得超过烧瓶的 2/3。挥发乙醚时，水浴温度以 40℃为宜，温度太高，易溢出。蒸发皿必须将乙醚在水浴上完全挥尽后，才能放入烘箱内。

思考题

1. 简述巴豆制霜方法及如何进一步改进。
2. 简述控制巴豆霜的质量方法。

Experiment 14 The effect of making frost-like powder on the composition of Crotonis Fructus

Aims

1.1 To master the processing method of making frost-like powder and its effect on medicine.

1.2 To signify the processing Crotonis Fructus illustrated by the content determination experiment of fatty oil and crotonoside before and after Crotonis Fructus making frost-like powder.

Principles

Some seed medicines are heated properly, pressed to remove oil, etc., and made into loose powders to mitigate drug effect or reduce their toxicity. Crotonis Fructus has seriously poison, crude Crotonis Fructus toxicity is strong, for external use only for corrosion of sores. Crotonis Fructus can reduce its toxicity and relieve its diarrhea after removing oil by making frost-like powder. The toxic components of Crotonis Fructus are the toxic proteins and fatty oils contained in it. Making frost-like powder processing can remove some of the fatty oils, and heating can destroy the toxic proteins, thus making him less toxic. In addition, the content control of crotonin, the active composition of Crotonis Fructus, ensure the safety and effectiveness of Crotonis Fructus making frost-like powder of the active ingredient of Crotonis Fructus is controlled to ensure the safety and effectiveness of Crotonis Fructus Cream.

Contents

3.1 Processing of Crotonis Fructus Cream.

3.2 Determination of fatty oil and crotonoside before and after Crotonis Fructus making frost-like powder.

Materials

4.1 Experimental apparatuses

High performance liquid chromatograph, C_{18} chromatographic column, ultrasonic cleaner, electronic scale/balance, water bath, steaming tool, pressing tool, mortar, gauze, Soxhlet extractor, evaporating dish, conical flask with plug, filter paper, absorbent cotton, etc.

4.2 Experimental materials

Crotonis Fructus, Crotonoside reference sample, ether, etc.

Methods

5.1 For the processing of Crotonis Fructus Cream.

Take Crotonis Fructus, remove the shell, take the clean Crotonis Fructus kernel, grind it into a mud shape, wrap it tightly, steam it for 30 minutes. Remove, press to remove oil, steam and press again. Repeat above procedure several times, until the drug loose into powder, no longer bonded into the cake for degree. Or take the net Crotonis Fructus kernel grinding fine, determine the content of fatty oil, add appropriate amount of starch dilution, make the content of fatty oil in accordance with the provisions, mix.

5.2 Determination of fatty oil and Crotonoside before and after Crotonis Fructus making frost-like powder.

5.2.1 Determination of the content of fatty oil

Take this product for about 5g, weight accurately, soxhlet extractor, add 100ml ether, Heated reflux (6~8 hours) until the fatty oil was exhausted and collect extract to evaporating dish which was dried to constant temperature, evaporate to dry at low temperature in the bath, dry at 100℃ for 1 hour, put in desiccator, After cooling for 30 minutes , weigh accurately and calculate. In terms of dry products, calculate the percentage of fatty oil before and after Crotonis Fructus making frost-like powder.

5.2.2 Determination of Crotonoside content

A. Chromatographic conditions and systemetic adaptation test. Octadecyl silane bonded silica gel as the filler, acetonitrile–methanol–water (1 ∶ 4 ∶ 95) as the mobile phase, The detection wavelength is 292nm. The theoretical plates should be no less than 5000 based on the Crotonoside peak. B. Preparation of the reference sample solution. Take the appropriate amount of the reference sample weighing accurately and add water to make a solution containing 60μg/ml, for later use. C. The preparation of test sample solution: take this product about 0.15 grams, weighing accurately, to soxhlet extractor, and add ether 5ml. Heat reflux for 3 hours and discard the ether liquid. Drugs are evaporated the solvent and moved to conical flask with plug with filter paper. Add accurately 50ml of water, weigh and ultrasonicate (power 300W, frequency 24kHz) for 20 minutes, allow to cool, weigh, and replenish the lost weight with water, shake and filter. D. Determination method: accurately pipette reference sample solution and test solution. Accurately inject 10μl of the reference solution and test sample solution into the column respectively and determination. The content of Crotonis Fructus before and after Crotonis Fructus making frost-like powder was measured by dry products.

Results

Table 3–23 Content determination of fatty oil and crotonoside before and after Crotonis Fructus making frost-like powder

Sample	Size of sample group/g	Fatty oil content/%	Crotonoside content/%
Raw Crotonis Fructus			
Crotonis Fructus Cream			

Notes

7.1 The preparation of Crotonis Fructus Cream should pay attention to labor protection, Workers should wear masks, gloves, laboratory equipment should be promptly brushed clean.

7.2 The amount of ether added shall not exceed 2/3 of the flask. When volatilize ether, water bath temperature to 40 degrees Celsius is appropriate, the temperature is too high that lead ether easy to overflow. Evaporating dish can be put inside oven after ether being volatilized completely on water bath.

Questions

8.1 What are the Crotonis Fructus Cream methods and how to improve?

8.2 How to control the quality of Crotonis Fructus Cream.

第四章 中药炮制设计性实验

传统中药炮制实验模式的实验内容多为理论教学的验证。教学方法主要是由教师将实验器具准备齐全，根据“实验指导”详细讲解实验目的、实验原理、操作步骤、注意事项等，学生依据“实验指导”中的步骤进行操作，观察实验现象，记录实验过程，最后按要求将实验中观察的各种数据进行处理，得出结论，撰写实验报告。验证性实验的教学目的是通过实验检验已学过的理论知识，加深对理论知识的理解和掌握。

综合设计性实验有别于传统的中药炮制实验模式。综合性体现在实验内容不局限于中药炮制本身，已扩展到中药学各专业知识、实验基础知识和实验基本技能，因而具有实验内容的复合性、实验手段与方法的多样性的特点，设计性体现在该实验是由教师指定实验项目的范围、实验目的和实验要求，由学生自行设计实验方案、确定实验条件、选择实验器材、加以实施并对结果进行综合分析处理，中药炮制设计性实验不仅要求学生综合多学科知识和多种实验原理、方法、手段来设计实验方案，还要求学生运用已有的专业知识去发现、分析和解决问题，其目的在于培养学生掌握科研设计实验的方法和步骤，激发学生学习的主动性、创造性，提高学生自主学习能力、认识能力，开拓学生的创新意识。

设计性实验开展的关键在于实验规定项目中具体实验课题的选择，对于中药炮制学设计性实验而言，其选题内容广泛，涉及不同炮制方法的比较研究、炮制工艺的优选研究、饮片质量的评价方法研究、饮片质量标准的研究、炮制前后化学成分的比较研究、传统炮制经验的科学内涵研究、炮制程度对饮片质量的影响研究、饮片的指纹图谱研究、炮制前后毒性的比较研究、炮制前后药效的比较研究、炮制前后成分变化与毒性和药效的相关性研究等，需要遵循中医药理论知识，综合中药炮制、化学、药理、数理统计分析等多学科知识，进行实验设计，充分体现其科学性、创新性及可行性，选择的实验项目要充分考虑所在实验室能提供的实验材料、仪器设备及其他相关的实验条件是否具备，不能好高骛远，防止出现因条件所限而使实验设计不能完成的窘境。

实验设计是实验研究所涉及的各项基本问题的合理安排，严密合理的实验设计是顺利进行研究工作的保证，同时也能最大限度地减少实验误差以获得精确可靠的实验结论，实验设计涉及的各方面内容，都要从科学研究的角度认真思考确定。

例如：①对于选用什么样的药材进行炮制品的制备的问题，要考虑是否为药典规定品种，并且应符合药典规定的质量要求？在设计时需考虑是否鉴定品种，如何鉴定？是否需要考察药材的质量？按照什么方法检测？按照什么标准评价其质量？②对于炮制样品的制备问题，首先要确定中药的炮制方法，在制备炮制品时是否需要控制炮制条件，如何控制？如何确保实验结果的重复性和准确度？③对于饮片质量的评价，既要考虑传统质量要求，又要考虑现代质量评价指标的选择，确定所选择指标的具体的实验方法与步骤，供试液制备及检测批次是否进行方法学考察，如何计算含量，如何进行数据处理等，均应在实验设计时考虑周全，以保证实验结果的科学性和可靠性。④对于毒性和药效实验，除基本要求外，还应考虑所选用的供试液的制备方法是否使中药饮片的成分产生变化，该变化是否影响结果的准确性和可靠性。如做川乌的毒性实验时，选择常规水煎煮的方法制备供试液，则可能因煎煮过程中生川乌的毒性成分双酯型生物碱已经发生了水解，使毒性显著降低，而测不出 LD_{50}，得出生川乌无毒的错误结论。

Chapter 4 Design Experiments of Chinese Medicine Processing

The experimental content of Traditional Chinese medicine processing experiment is mostly the verification of theoretical teaching.Before the experiment, the teacher prepares all the equipment for the students. They explain the experimental purpose, principle, operation steps, notes and so on according to the "experimental guidance". Students operate the experiment according to the steps in the "experimental guidance" , observe the phenomena, record the experimental process, and draw conclusions after processing the various data observed in the experiment, and finally write an experimental report. The purpose of confirmatory experiments is to test the theoretical knowledge that the students have been learned through experiments, and deepen the understanding and mastery of theoretical knowledge.

The comprehensive design experiment is different from the traditional Chinese medicine processing experiment. The comprehensiveness is reflected in that the experiment content is not limited to the traditional Chinese medicine processing, but has been extended to various professional knowledge, basic experimental knowledge and skills of Chinese materia medica. Therefore, it has the characteristics of complex experimental content and diverse experimental methods. The design is reflected in that the teacher specifies the scope, the purpose and the requirements of the experiment, while the students design the experimental scheme, determine the experimental conditions, select the equipments, implement it, and comprehensively analyze and process the results. The design experiments not only require students to use multi-disciplinary knowledge and multiple experimental principles, methods, and means to design experimental solutions, but also require students to discover, analyze, and solve problems by their professional knowledge. The purpose is to train students to master the methods and steps of scientific research and design experiments, stimulate students' initiative and creativity, improve students' autonomous learning and cognitive ability, as well as develop their innovative consciousness.

The key to carrying out design experiments lies in the selection of specific experimental topics in the experimental stipulated projects. For the design experiments of Chinese medicine processing, the topic is extensive, involving the comparative study among different processing methods, processing technology of Chinese medicine, quality evaluation, chemical composition before and after processing, the scientific connotation of the traditional processing experience, the influence on the quality of processing degree, the fingerprints, toxicity, efficacy before and after processing, correlation studies of changes in ingredients before and after processing, toxicity and efficacy and so on. It is necessary to follow the theoretical knowledge of Chinese materia medica, integrate multidisciplinary knowledge of Chinese medicine processing, chemistry, pharmacology, and statistical analysis of mathematics, with conducting experimental design to fully reflect its scientificity, innovation and feasibility. The choice of experimental items must fully consider whether the experimental materials, instruments, and other relevant experimental conditions that can be provided by the laboratory are available. They should not be high and remote to prevent the dilemma that the experimental design cannot be completed due to conditions.

The design of experiments is a reasonable arrangement for the basic issues involved in experimental research. A rigorous and reasonable experimental design is a guarantee for successful research, and it can also minimize experimental errors and obtain accurate and reliable experimental conclusions. All aspects involved in experimental design must be carefully considered and determined from the perspective of scientific research.

For example: A. What kinds of medicinal materials are used for the preparation of processed products, it is necessary to consider whether the variety is prescribed by the Pharmacopoeia, and it should conform the quality requirements that prescribed by the Pharmacopoeia. When designing, it is necessary to consider whether the students should identify the variety, and how to identify it? Is it necessary to inspect the quality of medicinal materials, What method is used for testing? What standards are used to evaluate its quality? B. For the preparation of processed samples, first, the students should determine the processing method. When preparing processed products, the processing conditions whether the students should control, and how to do? How to ensure the repeatability and accuracy of experimental results? C. For the quality evaluation, it is necessary to consider both the traditional quality requirements and the selection of modern quality evaluation indicators. Determine the specific experimental methods and steps for the selected indicators for test solution preparation and testing batches. The aspects refer to a methodological inspection, how to calculate the content, how to perform data processing, etc., should be considered in the design of the experiment to ensure the scientificity and reliability of the results. D. For the toxicity and efficacy experiments, in addition to the basic requirements, it should also consider whether the preparation method of the test solution used changes the composition of Chinese herbal medicine, and whether the changes affect the accuracy and reliability of the results. For example, in the toxicity test of Aconitum carmichaelii, the conventional water decoction method is used to prepare the test solution. The diester alkaloid, which is the toxic component of unprocessed Aconitum carmichaelii in the boiling process, may have been hydrolyzed, which significantly reduced the toxicity. LD_{50} is not detected, and draw a wrong conclusion that unprocessed Aconitum carmichaelii was non-toxic.

PPT

实验一　制何首乌饮片综合设计性实验

实验目的

1. **掌握**　中药炮制综合设计性实验的目的、要求与思路；文献查阅的方法、文献综述和科研论文的撰写方法。

2. 通过实验掌握何首乌的炮制方法、原理及意义。

3. 提高学生对中药知识的综合应用能力，分析和解决问题的能力。

4. 通过分组开展各项实验设计和研究工作，培养学生的团队合作精神及协作意识。

实验设计指导

一、《中国药典》2020年版收载制何首乌内容概述

何首乌为蓼科植物何首乌的干燥块根。秋、冬二季叶枯萎时采挖，削去两端，洗净，个大的切成块，干燥。

1. 何首乌饮片　为何首乌的炮制加工品。

【炮制】除去杂质，洗净，稍浸，润透，切厚片或块，干燥。

【性状】本品呈不规则的厚片或块。外表皮红棕色或红褐色，皱缩不平，有浅沟，并有横长皮孔样突起及细根痕。切面浅黄棕色或浅红棕色，显粉性；横切面有的皮部可见云锦状花纹，中央木部较大，有的呈木心。气微，味微苦而甘涩。

【性味与归经】苦、甘、涩，微温。归肝、心、肾经。

【功能与主治】解毒，消痈，截疟，润肠通便。用于疮痈，瘰疬，风疹瘙痒，久疟体虚，肠燥便秘。

【含量测定】

（1）二苯乙烯苷　避光操作。照高效液相色谱法（药典通则Ⅵ D）测定。

1）色谱条件与系统适用性试验　以十八烷基硅烷键合硅胶为填充剂；以乙腈-水（25：75）为流动相；检测波长为320nm。理论板数按2,3,5,4'-四羟基二苯乙烯-2-O-β-D-葡萄糖苷峰计算应不低于2000。

2）对照品溶液的制备　取2,3,5,4'-四羟基二苯乙烯-2-O-β-D-葡萄糖苷对照品适量，精密称定，加稀乙醇制成每1ml含0.2mg的溶液，即得。

3）供试品溶液的制备　取本品粉末（过四号筛）约0.2g，精密称定，置具塞锥形瓶中，精密加入稀乙醇25ml，称定重量，加热回流30分钟，放冷，再称定重量，用稀乙醇补足减失的重量，摇匀，静置，上清液滤过，取续滤液，即得。

4）测定法　分别精密吸取对照品溶液与供试品溶液各10μl，注入液相色谱仪，测定，即得。

本品按干燥品计算，含2,3,5,4'-四羟基二苯乙烯-2-O-β-D-葡萄糖苷（$C_{20}H_{22}O_9$）不得少于1.0%。

（2）结合蒽醌　照高效液相色谱法（药典通则Ⅵ D）测定。

1）色谱条件与系统适用性试验　以十八烷基硅烷键合硅胶为填充剂；以甲醇-0.1%磷酸溶液（80：20）为流动相；检测波长为254nm。理论板数按大黄素峰计算应不低于3000。

2）对照品溶液的制备　取大黄素对照品、大黄素甲醚对照品适量，精密称定，加甲醇分别

制成每1ml含大黄素80μg，大黄素甲醚40μg的溶液，即得。

3）供试品溶液的制备　取本品粉末（过四号筛）约1g，精密称定，置具塞锥形瓶中，精密加入甲醇50ml，称定重量，加热回流1小时，取出，放冷，再称定重量，用甲醇补足减失的重量，摇匀，滤过，取续滤液5ml作为供试品溶液A（测游离蒽醌用）。另精密量取续滤液25ml，置具塞锥形瓶中，水浴蒸干，精密加8%盐酸溶液20ml，超声处理（功率100W，频率40kHz）5分钟，加三氯甲烷20ml，水浴中加热回流1小时，取出，立即冷却，置分液漏斗中，用少量三氯甲烷洗涤容器，洗液并入分液漏斗中，分取三氯甲烷液，酸液再用三氯甲烷振摇提取3次，每次15ml，合并三氯甲烷液，回收溶剂至干，残渣加甲醇使溶解，转移至10ml量瓶中，加甲醇至刻度，摇匀，滤过，取续滤液，作为供试品溶液B（测总蒽醌用）。

4）测定法　分别精密吸取对照品溶液与上述两种供试品溶液各10μl，注入液相色谱仪，测定，即得。

结合蒽醌含量＝总蒽醌含量－游离蒽醌含量。

本品按干燥品计算，含结合蒽醌以大黄素（$C_{15}H_{10}O_5$）和大黄素甲醚（$C_{16}H_{12}O_5$）的总量计，不得少于0.10%。

2. 制何首乌饮片　为何首乌的炮制加工品。

【制法】取何首乌片或块，照炖法（药典通则Ⅱ D）用黑豆汁拌匀，置非铁质的适宜容器内，炖至汁液吸尽；或照蒸法（药典通则Ⅱ D），清蒸或用黑豆汁拌匀后蒸，蒸至内外均呈棕褐色，或晒至半干，切片，干燥。

每100kg何首乌片（块），用黑豆10kg。

黑豆汁制法　取黑豆10kg，加水适量，煮约4小时，熬汁约15kg，豆渣再加水煮约3小时，熬汁约10kg，合并得黑豆汁约25kg。

【性状】本品呈不规则皱缩状的块片，厚约1cm。表面黑褐色或棕褐色，凹凸不平。质坚硬，断面角质样，棕褐色或黑色。气微，味微甘而苦涩。

【性味与归经】苦、甘、涩，微温。归肝、心、肾经。

【功能与主治】补肝肾，益精血，乌须发，强筋骨，化浊降脂。用于血虚萎黄，眩晕耳鸣，须发早白，腰膝酸软，肢体麻木，崩漏带下，高脂血症。

【含量测定】

（1）二苯乙烯苷　避光操作。

取本品粉末（过四号筛）约0.2g，精密称定，照何首乌药材[含量测定]项下的方法测定。

本品按干燥品计算，含2,3,5,4'－四羟基二苯乙烯－2－O－β－D－葡萄糖苷（$C_{20}H_{22}O_9$）不得少于0.70%。

（2）游离蒽醌　照高效液相色谱法（药典通则Ⅵ D）测定。

1）色谱条件与系统适用性试验　以十八烷基硅烷键合硅胶为填充剂；以甲醇－0.1%磷酸溶液（80：20）为流动相；检测波长为254nm。理论板数按大黄素峰计算应不低于3000。

2）对照品溶液的制备　取大黄素对照品、大黄素甲醚对照品适量，精密称定，加甲醇分别制成每1ml含大黄素80μg、大黄素甲醚40μg的溶液，即得。

3）供试品溶液的制备　取本品粉末（过四号筛）约1g，精密称定，置具塞锥形瓶中，精密加入甲醇50ml，称定重量，加热回流1小时，取出，放冷，再称定重量，用甲醇补足减失的重量，摇匀，滤过，取续滤液，即得。

4）测定法　分别精密吸取对照品溶液与供试品溶液各10μl，注入液相色谱仪，测定，即得。

本品按干燥品计算，含游离蒽醌以大黄素（$C_{15}H_{10}O_5$）和大黄素甲醚（$C_{16}H_{12}O_5$）的总量计，不得少于0.10%。

二、何首乌综合设计性实验选题思路

1. 何首乌的炮制方法 何首乌饮片的炮制方法中未见水处理软化的工艺参数，切制规格包括厚片和块。文献报道制何首乌的炮制方法有清蒸和黑豆汁蒸两种蒸制方法、常压蒸和加压蒸两种加热方式，各方法有无差别？何首乌蒸制时要求使用非铁质容器，有无实验证实其原因？

2. 何首乌生、制品的质量评价 饮片外观性状与其内在质量之间是否存在关联性？二苯乙烯苷、蒽醌类成分能否表明其有效性？有无更科学的何首乌饮片质量评价方法？

3. 何首乌生、制品的药效评价 文献资料表明，何首乌的炮制原理不仅仅体现在增效上，还体现在减轻毒副作用，主要指对胃肠道的刺激引起腹泻等副作用。已采用的实验方法有哪些？如何设计才能体现在中医药理论指导下开展实验研究？

4. 何首乌生、制品的药性评价 中药炮生为熟引起的药性改变与其内在物质基础的变化有关。内在物质基础的变化包括量变和质变，单纯一种成分的变化并不能全面解释整个单味中药饮片功效的改变。在查阅文献时需注意采用什么方法研究炮制前后物质基础的变化能够基本表明炮制前后的物质基础变化情况，如何选择药效指标研究生品、制品的功效改变阐明其炮制程度与药性改变的关系，寻找其药性改变的物质基础，进一步探讨其炮制原理。

实验要求

1. 通过对何首乌炮制方法及工艺研究的设计，掌握中药炮制方法及工艺优选的基本方法与思路。
2. 通过对制何首乌饮片质量研究的设计，掌握传统及现代中药饮片质量评价方法与思路。
3. 通过对何首乌生品和制品功效比较研究的设计，掌握何首乌饮片的主要药效评价方法与思路。

实验内容

1. 何首乌炮制相关文献查阅及实验项目综述的撰写 通过查阅《中国药典》、各地《炮制规范》、查阅何首乌的文献资料，撰写何首乌饮片炮制研究进展综述，分析何首乌的炮制工艺、饮片质量评价、炮制化学和药理、炮制缓性、增效原理、临床应用的现状及发展趋势，找出存在的问题，明确研究目标，为实验方案设计奠定基础。

2. 分组制订何首乌炮制的设计性实验方案 在综合整理何首乌炮制相关文献的基础上，对何首乌相同问题感兴趣的学生 3~5 人自由组合，根据设计实验的要求及查阅资料的情况，并应用所学习的中药学专业知识围绕实验目标拟定和完善实验方案，论证方案的可行性，分析实验中可能出现的各种问题，形成实验方案（初稿）；以小组方式汇报实验方案，教师组织学生听取汇报，并针对方案设计的科学性、可行性、合理性、完整性、操作性等相关问题进行引导性的评价；学生根据教师的评价对方案进行修订，完成实验研究方案（修订稿）。此项工作以学生为主体，指导教师参与共同确定方案。各小组根据选定的实验课题研读相关文献资料，复习相关基础知识和实验技能，设计实验方案，然后各小组与指导教师共同讨论，确定合理可行的实验方案，作为实验研究的依据。

各组撰写的设计性实验方案报告应包括：①课题名称，每个小组依据本小组需要解决何首乌炮制的问题及采用的方法提炼题目。②立题依据，包括何首乌炮制理论依据和实验依据两部分内容，主要说明做该实验研究的原因，采用该方法能达到实验目标的原因。③实验目的，即本次实验安排解决何首乌炮制的问题或应达到的目的，任何一个实验都要求有明确实验目的，但应注意目的不能过多，以 1~3 个实验目的为宜，并且通过选择的实验方法能够达到目标。④实验原理，主要简述所何首乌炮制采用方法的科学依据。⑤实验材料，包括何首乌药材来源、实验动物、试剂、试药、仪器、材料、对照品和对照物质等。⑥实验方法及操作步骤，为设计方案中的重点。如选择的题目为制首乌炮制工艺的优选，则应包括对何首乌的哪种炮制方法进行优选，炮制方法的依据，采用单因素还是多因素考察，采用正交实验法还是其他方法，各炮制工艺条件的因素和水平如何选择，确定关键工艺技术参数的因素及水平。若选择适宜的传统性状及化学成分为主要评价指标时，对传统性状如何评价，对选定的化学成分如何测定，是否需要进行方法学考察，供试液的制备方法，样品制备及检测批次以保证实验结果的准确。⑦数据处理，对检测的结果进行必要的数据处理，如含量计算、方差分析、综合评分等。⑧注意事项，为保证实验结果的准确、可靠，实验过程中需要注意的事项均在这里列出。⑨参考文献，主要列出本实验设计用到的文献，需要给出电子版便于查证。

3. 实验实施

（1）准备　学生依据实验方案（修订稿），向教学实验室管理部门提交所需试药和实验物品的清单，预订使用实验室和大型仪器的时间。

（2）实验　学生按照实验方案进行实验，并作好原始记录。根据实验的实际情况及出现的问题，及时与教师沟通，调整优化实验方案（终稿）。

（3）注意　①实验中应按照设计要求进行全程认真的观察，并及时准确全面地记进行录。②如发现预期之外的情况，可按原设计进行必要调整。③对实验结果必须进行全面的整理分析，对实验数据必须按统计学要求进行准确地处理。

4. 总结实验结果，完成实验报告　学生根据原始记录，分析、归纳、整理实验数据，讨论实验结果、实验中遇到的主要问题及自己认为的解决办法，并撰写实验报告。实验报告撰写要求：①检查设计性实验应按设计要求完成，如未完成，应客观地、实事求是地找出原因。共同讨论实验结果的可信度。②实验结论应符合逻辑，是由实验结果推导而来，不能轻易下结论，以养成科学严谨的科研素质。认真讨论实验的经验教训，心得体会。③实验结果无论是符合预期还是与预期不符甚至相反，均需实事求是地分析讨论。

5. 实验分析与总结　同组同学对实验整个过程进行自我评价；指导教师从学生的实验原始记录、实验报告中找出普遍存在的问题进行集中分析，并对实验方案的合理性、实验操作的正确性及论文的写作情况等进行评价总结。

实验注意事项

1. 每组同学可选定本实验项下的单一研究方向进行实验设计。所设计的实验方案需合理可行，注意细节性及可操作性，需附有相应的文献资料作为支撑材料。

2. 实验方案中的工艺、质量、药效等评价指标，应充分体现与何首乌生制品的功能主治相一致的原则。

思考题

1. 请简述中药炮制研究的方法与思路。

2. 请阐述实验过程中的注意事项。

Experiment 1 Comprehensive experiment design for decoction pieces of Polygoni Multiflori Radix

Experimental purposes

1.1 To master the purpose, requirements, and ideas of comprehensively designing experiments for traditional Chinese medicine (TCM) processing. To master the methods for searching and collecting related references in literature, writing reviews and scientific papers.

1.2 To master the processing methods, principles and significance of Polygoni Multiflori Radix through performing the experiment. To train and promote team spirit and cooperative consciousness through designing related experiments.

1.3 To improve students' comprehensive abilities in TCM and the abilities to analyze and solve problems.

Guidances for experimental design

2.1 The contents of the processed Polygoni Multiflori Radix collected in the Pharmacopoeia of People's Republic of China (2020 edition).

Polygoni Multiflori Radix is the dried root tuber of Polygonum multiflorum Thunb. The drug is collected when the leaves fall off in autumn and winter, two ends are removed, washed cleanly. The large one is cut into small pieces, and then dried.

2.1.1 Polygoni Multiflori Radix

It is a processed product of Polygonum multiflorum thunb.

[Processing] Remove non-essential parts, wash, macerate and soften thoroughly. Cut it into thick slices or pieces, and finally dried.

[Characters] Polygoni Multiflori Radix is irregular thick slices or pieces, and shows reddish brown externally, shrunken and uneven, shallowly grooved, with transverse elongated lenticels and fine rootlet scars. Fracture pale yellowish-brown or reddish-brown, starchy, bark exhibiting brocaded patterns, wood in central part, relatively large, some having a woody core. Odourless, taste bitterish, sweetish and astringent.

[Property and flavor and meridian tropism] It is bitter, sweet, astringent, and warm in nature. Its functions are superior and used to invigorate the liver, heart, and kidney.

[Functions] The crude drug can counteract toxicity, cure carbuncles and relax bowels. Thus, it is used in treatments for constipation, carbuncles, hyperlipemia and tuberculosis of lymphathic glands.

[Content determination]

2.1.1.1 2,3,5,4′-tetrahydroxystilbene-2-O-β-D-glucoside

Operate protected from light. Carry out the method for high performance liquid chromatography (Pharmacopoeia General Rules 0512).

Chromatographic conditions and systemetic adaptation

Octadecylsilane bonded silica gel is used as the stationary phase and a mixture of acetonitrile and water (25 ∶ 75) is used as the mobile phase. The detection wavelength is 320nm. The theoretical plates is more than 2000 calculated with the reference to the peak of 2, 3, 5, 4′–tetrahydroxystilbene–2–O–β–D–glucoside.

Preparation of reference sample solution

The quantity of 2,3,5,4′–tetrahydroxystilbene–2–O–β–D– glucoside needs to be appropriate amount and dissolved in dilute ethanol to produce a solution containing 0.2mg/ml as the reference solution.

Preparation of test solution

0.2g of the powder (through No.4 sieve) is weighted accurately and put into a conical flask with plug, 25ml of dilute ethanol is accurately measured and added into the flask and weighted. Reflux for 30 minutes, then allowed to cool, weighed again, the loss of the solvent is replenished and mixed well, subsequent filtrate is finally filtered through Millipore filter.

Procedure

10μl of each of the reference sample solution and the test solution is accurately pipette, and eaccurately injected into the liquid chromatograph, respectively, the content is determined and calculated. It contains more than 1.0% of 2,3,5,4′–tetrahydroxystilbene–2–O–β–D–glucoside ($C_{20}H_{20}O_9$) calculated based on the dried product.

2.1.1.2 Conjugated anthraquinone

High performance liquid chromatography (HPLC) is carried out according to the method described in Pharmacopoeia General Rules 0512.

Chromatographic conditions and systematic adaptation

Octadecylsilane bonded silica gel is used as the stationary phase and a mixture of methanol and 0.1% phosphoric acid solution (80 ∶ 20) is used as the mobile phase. The detection wavelength is 254nm. The theoretical plates is not less than 3000 calculated with the reference to the peak of rhubarb.

Preparation of reference sample solution

The needed quantities of emodin and emodin methyl ether are appropriate amount, dissolved in methanol to produce a solution containing 80μg of emodin and 40μg of emodin methyl ether per 1ml.

Preparation of test solution

1g of the powder (filtered through No.4 sieve) is weighted accurately and put into a conical flask with plug, and 50ml of methanol is added accurately and weighted, under reflux is heated reflux for 1 hour, allowed to cool, weighed again, the loss of the solvent is replenished and mixed well, and then filtered. 5ml of subsequent filtrate is used as the test solution A for the determination of free anthraquinone. In addition, 25ml of subsequent filtrate is measured accurately and poured into a conical flask with plug, evaporated to dry, 20ml of 8% hydrochloric acid solution is added precisely, extracted with ultrasonication (100W, 40kHz) for 5 minutes, 20ml of chloroform is added, heated reflux for 1 hour, cooled, and then transfered to the separating funnel, the container is washed with a small amount of chloroform to separate the chloroform layer. The acid solution is extracted with 15ml of chloroform 3 times, combine the chloroform extractions are combined and recover solvents to dryness were recovered and the residues are dissolved in methanol, transfered to a 10ml volumetric flask, methanol is added to up to the mark, allowed to shake and filtered. The subsequent filtrate is used as the test solution B for determination of total anthraquinone.

Procedure

10μl of each of the reference sample solution and the test solutions is accurately pipetted and injected into the liquid chromatograph, respectively, the content is determined and calculated.

Combined anthraquinone content = Total Anthraquinone content–Free anthraquinone content.

It contains not less than 0.1% of conjugated anthraquinone. The total amount of emodin ($C_{15}H_{10}O_5$) and emodin methyl ether ($C_{16}H_{12}O_5$) is calculated.

2.1.2 Polygoni Multiflori Radix Preparata

It is the processed product of Polygoni Multiflori Radix.

[Processing] Slices or pieces of Polygoni Multiflori Radix are mixed with black bean juice. According to method described in Pharmacopoeia General Rule 0213 Strewing is carried out in a suitable non-ferrous container until the juice is exhausted or carry out pieces of Polygoni Multiflori Radix is steamed alone or after being mixed with black bean juice to a brown color, dried under the sun to partial dryness, and then cut into slices and dried.

For each 100kg of slices or pieces of Polygoni Multiflori Radix, 10kg of black beans is used.

Preparation of black bean juice

10kg of black beans in a appropriate amount of water is boiled for about 4 hours and stewed to obtain about 15kg of black bean juice. The bean residue is boiled again in water for about 3 hours and stewed to obtain about 10kg of black bean juice andcombined to obtain about 25kg of the black bean juice.

[Characters] Irregular piece, about 1cm thick, show dark brown or tan externally, shrunken and uneven. Texture is heavy compact,. fracture horny and tan or black. It is odourless and tastes sweetish and bitter.

[Property and flavor and meridian tropism] It is sweet and bitter in taste, and warm in nature. It is used to converge liver, heart and kidney channel.

[Functions] Polygoni Multiflori Radix Preparata can be used to invigorate the liver and the kidney, replenish vital essence and blood, blacken the hair, and strengthen the tendon and bones. It can also be used to treat dizziness and tinnitus, premature graying at the hair and beard, soreness and weakness of the loins and the knees, numbness of the extremities, neurasthenia and hyperlipemia.

[Content determination]

2.1.2.1 2,3,5,4′-tetrahydroxystilbene-2-O-β-D-glucoside

It needs to be protected from light. 0.2 g of the powder (filtered through No.4 sieve) is weighed accurately, assay is carried out with the method described according to the above part of “2.1.1 Polygoni Multiflori Radix” .

It contains not less than 0.70% of 2,3,5,4′–tetrahydroxystilbene–2–O–β–D–glucoside ($C_{20}H_{20}O_9$), calculated on the base of dry weight of the sample.

2.1.2.2 Free anthraquinones

Assay for free anthraquinones is carried out with high performance liquid chromatography according to the method described in Pharmacopoeia General Rules 0512.

Chromatographic conditions and system suitability

Octadecylsilane bonded silica gel is used as the stationary phase and a mixture of methanol and 0.1% phosphoric acid solution (80 ∶ 20) is used as the mobile phase. The detection wavelength is 254nm. The number of theoretical plates of the column is not less than 3000 calculated with the reference to the peak of rhubarb.

Preparation of reference solution

A quantity of emodin, emodin methyl ether is weighted accurately, dissolved in methanol to produce a solution containing 80μg of emodin and 40μg of emodin methyl ether per 1ml.

Preparation of test solution

1g of the powder (filterded through No.4 sieve) is weighted accurately and put into a conical flask with a stopper, 50ml of methanol is measured accurately and added and weighted, under reflux is heated on a water bath for 1 hour, cooled and weighed again, the loss of the solvent is replenished and mixed well, and filtered finally.

Procedure

10μl of each of the reference solution and the test solution is injected accurately inject into the liquid chromatograph, respectively, the content is determineed and calculated.

It contains not less than 0.10% of free anthraquinone, calculated based on the total amount of emodin ($C_{15}H_{10}O_5$)and emodin methyl ether ($C_{16}H_{12}O_5$).

2.2 The topic basis of comprehensively designing experiment of Polygoni Multiflori Radix.

2.2.1 The methods for processing Polygoni Multiflori Radix

The parameters of processing with water are not seen in the processing methods. They are usually cut into thick slices or blocks. There are two processing methods available in the literature, (a) steam it alone or steam it after being mixed with black bean juice and (b) normal pressure steaming or high pressure steaming. Questions: A. Are there any differences among these methods? B. Non-ferrous container is required in the process. C. Are there any experiment(s) which can confirm it?

2.2.2 Quality evaluation of Raw and Processed Polygoni Multiflori Radix

Questions: A. Is there a correlation between the appearance characters and their intrinsic quality? B. Can stilbene glycosides and anthraquinones indicate their effectiveness? C. Is there a more scientific quality evaluation method for Polygoni Multiflori Radix?

2.3 Efficacy evaluation of Raw and Processed Polygoni Multiflori Radix.

It has been shown in the literature that the processing principle of Polygoni Multiflori Radix is not only to increase efficacy, it also can reduce the side effects, such as diarrhea caused by the stimulation of gastrointestinal tract. Questions: A. Which experiments have been done? B. How to design the experiment under the guidance of TCM theory?

2.4 The evaluation of medicinal properties of raw and processed Polygoni Multiflori Radix.

The changes in the medicinal properties caused by the processing of traditional Chinese medicine, are related to its internal material basis. The changes in the internal material basis include both quantitative and qualitative changes. The efficacy changes of the single Chinese herb could not be fully explained by the single compound. Thus, when we review the literature, it is necessary for us to pay specific attention to what methods can be used to monitor the changes in the material basis before and after processing, and how to select the appropriate pharmacodynamics indexes to evaluate the relation between processing degree and efficacy. Search the material basis which can change efficacy, and explore further its processing mechanism.

Experimental requirements

3.1 To master the processing method and the basic ideas and to oprimize methods of technology through designing the processing method and technology of Polygoni Multiflori Radix.

3.2 To master the methods and ideas of quality evaluation of traditional and modern Chinese herbal pieces through the study on the quality of Polygoni Multiflori Radix Preparata.

3.3 To master the methods and ideas for evaluating the efficacy of Polygoni Multiflori Radix through the study on the efficacy of raw and processed Polygoni Multiflori Radix.

Experimental contents

4.1 Retrieval of related literatures and review writing

By referring Pharmacopoeia of People's Republic of China and the specifications of Chinese material medica processing in different provinces in China, and medical literatures related to Polygoni Multiflori Radix, the students should summarize the current research status. They should analyze the processing technology and quality standards of of Polygoni Multiflori Radix, study the processing chemistry and pharmacology, explore mechanism of relieving drug nature and reinforce therapeutic effect of the processed Polygoni Multiflori Radix, and summarize clinical application and development of Raw and Processed Polygoni Multiflori Radix. Then, they can find out the existing problems, identify research objectives and establish a foundation for designing experimental protocol.

4.2 Grouping design experiment program

On the basis of reviewing the related literatures of Polygoni Multiflori Radix, the teacher should encourage 3~5 students who are interested in the same issues of Polygoni Multiflori Radix to combine freely in groups. The students should draft and improve the experiment program according to experimental demands and the literature. The students demonstrate the feasibility of the experimental scheme, analyze various problems that may occur during the experiment an formulate an experimental scheme (draft), and then report the scheme in groups. Teachers will organize students to listen to the report, and evaluate its science, feasibility, rationality, and completeness etc. Students revise the plan based on the teacher's evaluation, revise and complete the experimental research plan. This work takes students as major part, and teachers should participate in designing experiment program together. Each group review relevant literature and understand the relevant basic knowledge and acquire the experimental skills, and final design experimental plans. Then each group discuss with the instructor/teacher to determine the reasonable and feasible experimental schemes.

The experiment report will be written by each group and should include the following aspects.

A. Project title: Each group refines the topic based on the methods and problems that need to be resolved.

B. Research basis: Including the theoretical basis and experimental basis of Polygoni Multiflori Radix processing. Each group should mainly explain why they do this experiment, and why and how the method can achieve objectives.

C. The purpose: This experiment is designed to solve the problem in Polygoni Multiflori Radix processing. Any experiment requires a definite purpose, but it should be noted that the purposes should not be too many, and 1~3 aims or so are appropriate, and what experimental methods can be applied to achieve its aim.

D. Principles: Mainly provide the descriptions of scientific basis for processing Polygoni Multiflori Radix.

E. Materials: Including the origins, experimental animals, reagents, instruments, materials, reference materials and reference materials, etc.

F. Methods and Procedures: This is the focus of design program. If the topic is the optimization of the processing technology of Polygoni Multiflori Radix, it should include the optimization of processing methods and the basis of the processing methods. Whether single factor or multi-factor, orthogonal experiment or other method is used, how to choose the factors and levels of each processing condition, and how to determine the factors and levels of the key technological parameters. If we choose suitable traditional traits and chemical components as the main evaluation indexes, we need to know how to evaluate the traditional traits, how to determine the selected chemical components, and whether we need to carry out methodological investigation. Preparation method of test solution, sample preparation and test batch must ensure the accuracy of results.

G. Data analysis: We need to carry out necessary data processing, such as content calculation, analysis of variance, synthesis grade and so on.

H. Notes: In order to ensure the accuracy and reliability of the experimental results, during the experimental process, we needs to pay attention to the items listed.

I. References: Mainly list the documents used in the experiment design, the cited references need to be given in an electronic version for easy to check.

4.3 Experimental implementation

4.3.1 Preparation

According to the revised experimental plan, students submit the list of the required drugs and materials to the Teaching Laboratory Management, and reserve and schedule the date/time of using the laboratory and large-scale instruments.

4.3.2 Experiment

The students carry out the experiment according to the experiment plan, and make the original record, communicate with the teacher in time, adjust and optimize the final draft of the experiment plan according to the actual situation and problems of the experiment.

4.3.3 Cautions

A. You should observe carefully and record accurately and comprehensively during the entire experimental process.

B. If unexpected circumstances are found, necessary adjustments/changes may need to be made according to the original design.

C. The results must be analyzed comprehensively and the experimental data must be processed accurately according to the statistical requirements.

4.4 Summarize the results and write the experimental report.

According to the original record, students should analyze, summarize and process the experimental data, discuss the results, the main problems encountered during the experiment, and write the final experiment report. The demands for writing are as follows. A. To ensure whether the design experiment is completed according to requirements, if not, students should find out the reasons objectively and realistic, and discuss the credibility of the results. B. To achieve scientificity and rigour in research accomplishment, the conclusions should derived and drawn logically from the experiment results, should not be reached readily. Please discuss the experiences and lesson learned from the experiment. C. The results, whether in line with or against expectations, need to be analyzed and discussed in a matter-of-fact way.

4.5 Analysise and summaries.

The students in the same group should make self-evaluation throughout the experiment. The instructor/teacher should find out the common problems from the students' original records and experiment reports, evaluate the rationality of scheme, check-up of the operations and the writing of the paper.

Notes

5.1 Students in every group can choose a single research to design experiment. The experimental design should be reasonable and feasible, pay attention to the details and operability, with the corresponding literature as supporting materials.

5.2 The evaluation indexes of technology, quality and pharmacodynamics in the experiment design should be consistent with the function and symptom of the raw and processed Polygoni Multiflori Radix.

Question

6.1 Please briefly describe the research methods and ideas of processing Chinese materia medica.

6.2 Please state the points requiring the attention during the process of experiment.

PPT

实验二　制草乌饮片综合设计性实验

实验目的

1. **掌握**　中药炮制综合设计性实验的目的、要求与思路；文献查阅的方法，文献综述和科研论文的撰写方法。

2. 通过实验掌握草乌的炮制方法、原理及意义。

3. 提高学生对中药知识的综合应用能力，分析和解决问题的能力。

4. 通过分组开展各项实验设计和研究工作，培养学生的团队合作精神及协作意识。

实验设计指导

一、《中国药典》2020 年版收载制草乌内容概述

草乌为毛茛科植物北乌头的干燥块根。

1. 草乌饮片　为草乌的炮制加工品。

【炮制】除去杂质，洗净，干燥。本品呈不规则长圆锥形，略弯曲，长2~7cm，直径0.6~1.8cm。顶端常有残茎和少数不定根残基，有的顶端一侧有一枯萎的芽，一侧有一圆形或扁圆形不定根残基。表面灰褐色或黑棕褐色，皱缩，有纵皱纹、点状须根痕及数个瘤状侧根。质硬，断面灰白色或暗灰色，有裂隙，形成层环纹多角形或类圆形，髓部较大或中空。气微，味辛辣、麻舌。

【性味与归经】辛、苦，热；有大毒。归心、肝、肾、脾经。

【功能与主治】祛风除湿，温经止痛。用于风寒湿痹，关节疼痛，心腹冷痛，寒疝作痛及麻醉止痛。

【用法与用量】一般炮制后用。

【注意】生品内服宜慎；孕妇禁用；不宜与半夏、瓜蒌、瓜蒌子、瓜蒌皮、天花粉、川贝母、浙贝母、平贝母、伊贝母、湖北贝母、白蔹、白及同用。

【含量测定】照高效液相色谱法（药典通则Ⅵ D）测定。

（1）色谱条件与系统适用性试验　以十八烷基硅烷键合硅胶为填充剂；以乙腈－四氢呋喃（25：15）为流动相A，以0.11mol/L醋酸铵溶液（每1000ml加冰醋酸0.5ml）为流动相B，按表4-1中的规定进行梯度洗脱；检测波长为235nm。理论板数按新乌头碱峰计算应不低于2000。

表4-1　草乌饮片含量测定

时间（分钟）	流动相A（%）	流动相B（%）
0~48	15→26	85→74
48~48.1	26→35	74→65
48.1~58	35	65
58~65	35→15	65→85

（2）对照品溶液的制备　取乌头碱对照品、次乌头碱对照品、新乌头碱对照品适量，精密称定，加异丙醇－三氯甲烷（1：1）混合溶液分别制成每1ml含乌头碱0.3mg、次乌头碱0.18mg、

新乌头碱 1mg 的混合溶液，即得。

（3）供试品溶液的制备　取本品粉末（过三号筛）约 2g，精密称定，置具塞锥形瓶中，加氨试液 3ml，精密加入异丙醇－乙酸乙酯（1∶1）混合溶液 50ml，称定重量，超声处理（功率 300W，频率 40kHz；水温在 25℃以下）30 分钟，放冷，再称定重量，用异丙醇－乙酸乙酯（1∶1）混合溶液补足减失的重量，摇匀，滤过。精密量取续滤液 25ml，40℃以下减压回收溶剂至干，残渣精密加入异丙醇－三氯甲烷（1∶1）混合溶液 3ml 溶解，密塞，摇匀，滤过，取续滤液，即得。

（4）测定法　分别精密吸取对照品溶液与供试品溶液各 10μl，注入液相色谱仪，测定，即得。

本品按干燥品计算，含乌头碱（$C_{34}H_{47}NO_{11}$）、次乌头碱（$C_{33}H_{45}NO_{10}$）和新乌头碱（$C_{33}H_{45}NO_{11}$）的总量应为 0.10%~0.50%。

2. 制草乌　为草乌的炮制加工品。

【制法】取草乌，大小个分开，用水浸泡至内无干心，取出，加水煮至取大个切开内无白心、口尝微有麻舌感时，取出，晾至六成干后切薄片，干燥。

【性状】本品呈不规则圆形或近三角形的片。表面黑褐色，有灰白色多角形形成层环和点状维管束，并有空隙，周边皱缩或弯曲。质脆。气微，味微辛辣，稍有麻舌感。

【性味与归经】辛、苦，热；有毒。归心、肝、肾、脾经。

【功能与主治】同草乌。

【用法与用量】1.5~3g，宜先煎、久煎。

【含量测定】照高效液相色谱法（药典通则Ⅵ D）测定。

（1）色谱条件与系统适用性试验　以十八烷基硅烷键合硅胶为填充剂，以乙腈－四氢呋喃（25∶15）为流动相 A，以 0.1mol/L 醋酸铵溶液（每 1000ml 加冰醋酸 0.5ml）为流动相 B，按表 4-1 中的规定进行梯度洗脱；检测波长为 235nm。理论板数按苯甲酰新乌头原碱峰计算应不低于 2000。

（2）对照品溶液的制备　取苯甲酰乌头原碱对照品、苯甲酰次乌头原碱对照品、苯甲酰新乌头原碱对照品适量，精密称定，加异丙醇－三氯甲烷（1∶1）混合溶液分别制成每 1ml 含苯甲酰乌头原碱 20μg、苯甲酰次乌头原碱 0.1mg、苯甲酰新乌头原碱 80μg 的混合溶液，即得。

（3）供试品溶液的制备　取本品粉末（过三号筛）约 2g，精密称定，置具塞锥形瓶中，加氨试液 3ml，精密加入异丙醇－乙酸乙酯（1∶1）混合溶液 50ml，称定重量，超声处理（功率 300W，频率 40kHz；水温在 25℃以下）30 分钟，放冷，再称定重量，用异丙醇－乙酸乙酯（1∶1）混合溶液补足减失的重量，摇匀，滤过。精密量取续滤液 25ml，40℃以下减压回收溶剂至干，残渣精密加入异丙醇－三氯甲烷（1∶1）混合溶液 3ml 溶解，滤过，取续滤液，即得。

（4）测定法　分别精密吸取对照品溶液与供试品溶液各 10μl，注入液相色谱仪，测定，即得。

本品按干燥品计算，含苯甲酰乌头原碱（$C_{32}H_{45}NO_{10}$）、苯甲酰次乌头原碱（$C_{31}H_{43}NO_9$）及苯甲酰新乌头原碱（$C_{31}H_{43}NO_{10}$）的总量应为 0.020%~0.070%。

二、草乌综合设计性实验选题思路

1. 草乌的炮制方法　草乌饮片的炮制方法中未见具体的水处理软化及加热煎煮的工艺参数。草乌水浸泡要求“至内无干心”，煮制要求“内无白心，口尝微有麻舌感”，如何用现代科学实验证明草乌炮制要求的合理性。

2. 草乌生、制品的质量评价　饮片外观性状与其内在质量之间是否存在关联性？在草乌饮片中只以乌头碱、次乌头碱和新乌头碱作为考察指标，制草乌除此以外，还以苯甲酰乌头原碱、苯甲酰次乌头原碱及苯甲酰新乌头原碱作为指标，其科学依据是什么？

3. 草乌生、制品的药效及毒性评价 文献资料表明，草乌的炮制原理主要体现在经炮制后减轻毒副作用，可采用哪些实验方法验证炮制或使其毒性降低且仍保留其药效作用。

实验要求

1. 通过对草乌炮制方法及工艺研究的设计，掌握中药炮制方法及工艺优选的基本方法与思路。

2. 通过对生、制草乌饮片质量研究的设计，掌握传统及现代中药饮片质量评价方法与思路。

3. 通过对生草乌及制草乌功效、毒性比较研究的设计，掌握草乌饮片的主要药效、毒性评价方法。

实验内容

1. 草乌炮制相关文献查阅及实验项目综述的撰写 通过查阅《中国药典》、各地《炮制规范》、查阅草乌的文献资料，撰写草乌饮片炮制研究进展综述，分析草乌的炮制工艺、饮片质量评价、炮制化学和药理、炮制减毒原理、临床应用的现状及发展趋势，找出存在的问题，明确研究目标，为实验方案设计奠定基础。

2. 分组制订草乌炮制的设计性实验方案 在综合整理草乌相关炮制文献的基础上，对草乌相同问题感兴趣的学生3~5人自由组合，根据设计实验的要求及查阅资料的情况，并应用所学习的中药学专业知识围绕实验目标拟定和完善实验方案，论证方案的可行性，分析实验中可能出现的各种问题，形成实验方案（初稿）；以小组方式汇报实验方案，教师组织学生听取汇报，并针对方案设计的科学性、可行性、合理性、完整性、操作性等相关问题进行引导性的评价；学生根据教师的评价对方案进行修订，完成实验研究方案（修订稿）。此项工作以学生为主体，指导教师参与共同确定方案。各小组根据选定的实验课题研读相关文献资料，复习相关基础知识和实验技能，设计实验方案，然后各小组与指导教师共同讨论，确定合理可行的实验方案，作为实验研究的依据。

各组撰写的设计性实验方案报告应包括：①课题名称，每个小组依据本小组需要解决草乌炮制的问题及采用的方法提炼题目。②立题依据，包括草乌炮制理论依据和实验依据两部分内容，主要说明做该实验研究的原因，采用该方法能达到实验目标的原因。③实验目的，即本次实验安排解决草乌炮制的问题或应达到的目的，任何一个实验都要求有明确实验目的，但应注意目的不能过多，以1~3个实验目的为宜，并且通过选择的实验方法能够达到目标。④实验原理，主要简述所草乌炮制采用方法的科学依据。⑤实验材料，包括草乌药材来源、实验动物、试剂、试药、仪器、材料、对照品和对照物质等。⑥实验方法及操作步骤，为设计方案中的重点。如选择的题目为制首乌炮制工艺的优选，则应包括对草乌的哪种炮制方法进行优选，炮制方法的依据，采用单因素还是多因素考察，采用正交实验法还是其他方法，各炮制工艺条件的因素和水平如何选择，确定关键工艺技术参数的因素及水平。若选择适宜的传统性状及化学成分为主要评价指标时，对传统性状如何评价，对选定的化学成分如何测定，是否需要进行方法学考察，供试液的制备方法，样品制备及检测批次以保证实验结果的准确。⑦数据处理，对检测的结果进行必要的数据处理，如含量计算、方差分析、综合评分等。⑧注意事项，为保证实验结果的准确、可靠，实验过程中需要注意的事项均在这里列出。⑨参考文献，主要列出本实验设计用到的文献，需要给出电子版便于查证。

3. 实验实施

（1）准备 学生依据实验方案（修订稿），向教学实验室管理部门提交所需试药和实验物品的清单，预订使用实验室和大型仪器的时间。

（2）实验 学生按照实验方案进行实验，并作好原始记录。根据实验的实际情况及出现的问题，及时与教师沟通，调整优化实验方案（终稿）。

（3）注意 ①实验中应按照设计要求进行全程认真的观察，并及时准确全面地记进行录。②如发现预期之外的情况，可按原设计进行必要调整。③对实验结果必须进行全面的整理分析，对实验数据必须按统计学要求进行准确地处理。

4. 总结实验结果，完成实验报告

学生根据原始记录，分析、归纳、整理实验数据，讨论实验结果、实验中遇到的主要问题及自己认为的解决办法，并撰写实验报告。实验报告撰写要求：①检查设计性实验应设计要求完成，如没有完成，应客观地、实事求是地找出原因。共同讨论实验结果的可信度。②实验结论应符合逻辑，是由实验结果推导而来，不能轻易下结论，以养成科学严谨的科研素质。认真讨论实验的经验教训，心得体会。③实验结果无论是符合预期还是与预期不符甚至相反，均需实事求是地分析讨论。

5. 实验分析与总结

同组同学对实验整个过程进行自我评价；指导教师从学生的实验原始记录、实验报告中找出普遍存在的问题进行集中分析，并对实验方案的合理性、实验操作的正确性及论文的写作情况等进行评价总结。

实验注意事项

1. 各组设计的实验方案需合理可行，注意细节性及可操作性，需附有相应的文献资料作为支撑材料。

2. 实验方案中的工艺、质量、药效等评价指标，应充分体现与草乌不同炮制品的功能主治相一致的原则。

思考题

1. 请简述毒性中药炮制研究的方法与思路。
2. 请阐述实验过程中的注意事项。

Experiment 2 Comprehensive experiment design for decoction pieces of Aconiti Kusnezoffii Radix Cocta

Experimental purposes

1.1 To master the aim, requirement and topic ideas of comprehensive design experiment.

1.2 To master methods of searching and reviewing related references and writing research paper.

1.3 To master the processing methods, principle and significance of Aconiti Kusnezoffii Radix.

1.4 To improve students' comprehensive application ability in Traditional Chinese Medicine and the abilities to analyze and solve problems.

1.5 To develop students' team spirit and cooperative consciousness by designing related experiments.

Guidance of the experimental design

2.1 The contents of the Aconiti Kusnezoffii Radix Cocta recorded in the Chinese Pharmacopoeia (2020 edition).

Aconiti Kusnezoffii Radix is the dried root tuber of Aconitum kusnezoffii Reichb.

2.1.1 Decoction pieces of Aconiti Kusnezoffii Radix

It is the processed Aconiti Kusnezoffii Radix.

[Processing] Aconiti Kusnezoffii Radix (unprepared) Eliminate foreign matter, wash cleanly, and dry. Irregularly long-conical, slightly curved, 2~7cm long, 0.6~1.8cm in diameter. Apex usually with remains of stem and a few adventitious root bases, sometimes apex bearing a withered bud at one side and a circular or oblate base of adventitious root at the other side. Externally greyish-brown or blackish-brown, shrivelled, with longitudinal wrinkles, dotted rootlet scars and several tubercular lateral roots. Texture hard, fracture greyish-white or dark grey, with fissure, cambium ring polygonal or subrounded, pith relatively large or hollowed. Odour is slight. Taste is pungent and numb.

[Property and flavor and meridian tropism] It is hot, pungent and bitter, highly toxic. It used to converge heart, live, kidney and spleen meridians.

[Functions] To dispel wind, remove dampness, warm the meridians and relieve pain. Wind cold dampness *bi* disorder, joint pain, cold pain in the heart and abdomen, pain in cold abdominal colic, and it can be applied for anesthesia to relieve pain.

[Administration and dosage] Generally it is prepared before application.

[Precautions and Warnings] Unprepared one should be used cautiously for oral administration. Contraindicated for pregnant woman. Incompatible with Pinelliae Rhizoma, Trichosanthis Fructus, Trichosanthis Semen, Trichosanthis Pericarpium, Trichosanthis Radix, Fritillariae Cirrhosae Bulbus, Fritillariae Thunbergii Bulbus, Fritillariae Ussuriensis Bulbus, Fritillariae Pallidiflorae Bulbus, Fritillariae Hupehensis Bulbus, Ampelopsis Radix, and Bletillae Rhizoma.

[Assay] Carry out the method for high performance liquid chromatography (0512).

Chromatographic system and system suitability

Use octadecylsilane bonded silica gel as the stationary phase, a mixture of acetonitrile and tetrahydrofuran (25 : 15) as the mobile phase A and a 0.1mol/L solution of ammonium acetate (add 0.5ml of glacial acetic acid per 1000ml) as the mobile phase B, elute in gradient as the following.

Table 4-1 Assay of Aconiti Kusnezoftii Radix

Time（minutes）	mobile phase A（%）	mobile phase B（%）
0~48	15→26	85→74
48~48.1	26→35	74→65
48.1~58	35	65
58~65	35→15	65→85

As detector a spectrophotometer set at 235nm. The number of theoretical plates of the column is not less than 2000, calculated with reference to the peak of mesaconine.

Reference solution Dissolve a quantity of aconitine CRS, hypaconitine CRS and mesaconine CRS in a mixture of isopropanol and chloroform (1 : 1) to produce a mixture containing 0.3mg, 0.18mg and 0.1mg of each per ml as the reference solution.

Test solution Weigh accurately 2g of the powder (through No.3 sieve) to a conical flask with plug, accurately add 3ml of ammonia TS and 50ml of a mixture of isopropanol and ethyl acetate (1 : 1) and weigh. Ultrasonicate (power 300W, frequency 40kHz, water temperature below 25°C) for 30 minutes, cool and weigh again, replenish the loss of solvent with the mixture of isopropanol and ethyl acetate (1 : 1), mix well and filter. Measure accurately 25ml of the subsequent filtrate and evaporate to dryness under reduced pressure below 40℃. Dissolve exactly the residue in 3ml of the mixture of isopropanol and chloroform (1 : 1), mix well, filter and use the subsequent filtrate as the test solution.

Procedure Inject accurately 10μl of each of the reference solution and the test solution, respectively, into the column, and calculate the content.

It should be contain 0.10%~0.50% of the total amount of aconitine ($C_{34}H_{47}NO_{11}$), hypaconitine ($C_{33}H_{45}NO_{10}$) and mesaconine ($C_{33}H_{45}NO_{11}$), calculated with reference to the dried drug.

2.1.2 Aconiti Kusnezoffii Radix Cocta

Prepared Kusnezoff Monkshood Root. The drug is the processed Aconiti Kusnezoffii Radix.

[Processing] Grade Aconiti Kusnezoffii Radix according to size, soak it in water until there is no dry core. Take it out, boil in water until there is no white core in the larger root and the taste becomes slightly numb. After removal, allow it to dry in air appropriately, cut into slices, and dry.

[Characters] Irregularly rounded or nearly triangular slices. Externally dark brown, with a greyish-white polyangular cambium ring, dotted vascular bundles and clefts; the edges wrinkled or curved. Texture fragile. Odour, slight, Taste, slightly pungent and numb.

[Property and flavor and meridian tropism] It is hot, pungent and bitter, toxic.

It used to converge heart, liver, kidney and spleen meridian.

[Functions] To dispel wind, remove dampness, warm the meridians and relieve pain. Wind cold dampness *bi* disorder, joint pain, cold pain in the heart and abdomen, pain in cold abdominal colic, and it can be applied for anesthesia to relieve pain.

[Administration and dosage] 1.5~3g. It should be decocted first for a long time.

[Assay] Carry out the method for high performance liquid chromatography (0512).

Chromatographic system and system suitability

Use octadecylsilane bonded silica gel as the stationary phase and a mixture of acetonitrile and tetrahydrofuran (25 ∶ 15) as the mobile phase A and a 0.1 mol/L solution of ammonium acetate (add 0.5 ml of glacial acetic acid per 1000ml) as the mobile phase B, elute in gradient as the Table 4-1.

As detector a spectrophotometer set at 235nm. The number of theoretical plates of the column is not less than 2000, calculated with reference to the peak of benzoylmesaconine.

Reference solution

Dissolve benzoylaconitine CRS, benzoylhypaconitine CRS and benzoylmesaconine CRS, weighed accurately, in a mixture of isopropanol and chloroform (1 ∶ 1) to produce a mixture containing 20μg, 0.1mg and 80μg of each per ml as the reference solution.

Test solution

Weigh accurately 2g of the powder (through No.3 sieve) to a stoppered conical flask, accurately add 3ml of ammonia TS and 50ml of a mixture of isopropanol and ethyl acetate (1 ∶ 1) and weigh. Ultrasonicate (power 300W, frequency 40kHz, water temperature below 25°C) for 30 minutes, cool and weigh again, replenish the loss of solvent with the mixture of isopropanol and ethyl acetate (1 ∶ 1) , mix well and filter. Measure accurately 25ml of the subsequent filtrate, evaporate to dryness under reduce pressure below 40°C. Dissolve the residue in a mixture of isopropanol and chloroform (1 ∶ 1), mix well, filter and use the subsequent filtrate as the test solution.

Procedure

Inject accurately 10μl of each of the reference solution and the test solution, respectively, into the column, and calculate the content.

It should be contain 0. 020%~0.070% of the total amount of benzoylaconitine ($C_{32}H_{45}NO_{10}$), benzoylhypaconitine ($C_{31}H_{43}NO_9$) and benzoylmesaconine($C_{31}H_{43}NO_{10}$), calculated with reference to the dried drug.

2.2 The topic ideas of comprehensive designing experiment about Aconiti Kusnezoffii Radix

2.2.1 Processing method of Aconiti Kusnezoffii Radix.

There are no specific technological parameters about softening and decoction in processing method of Aconiti Kusnezoffii Radix. How to explain the reasonableness of the requirements, including soaking in water "until there is no dry core", and the requirement of boiling in water "until there is no white core and the taste becomes slightly numb", by modern scientific experiments?

2.2.2 Quality evaluation of Aconiti Kusnezoffii Radix and Aconiti Kusnezoffii Radix Cocta.

Is there any correlation between the outward properties and inner quality of processed Chinese medicine? Quality of Aconiti Kusnezoffii Radix should be evaluated with aconitine ($C_{34}H_{47}NO_{11}$), hypaconitine ($C_{33}H_{45}NO_{10}$) and mesaconine ($C_{33}H_{45}NO_{11}$). While benzoylaconitine ($C_{32}H_{45}NO_{10}$), benzoylhypaconitine ($C_{31}H_{43}NO_9$) and benzoylmesaconine($C_{31}H_{43}NO_{10}$) have been taken as indicator of quality evaluation of Aconiti Kusnezoffii Radix Cocta. What is the scientific basis of this difference?

2.2.3 Efficacy and toxicity evaluation of Aconiti Kusnezoffii Radix and Aconiti Kusnezoffii Radix Cocta.

According to the reported references, processing mechanism of Aconiti Kusnezoffii Radix is that the toxicity of Aconiti Kusnezoffii Radix could be reduced after processed. Which experiments could approve the reduction of toxicity and the reservation of efficacy.

Experiment requirements

3.1 To grasp the basic method and thought of processing method and process optimization of Traditional Chinese Medicine through the design of processing method and preparation technical study of Aconiti Kusnezoffii Radix.

3.2 To grasp the quality evaluation method and thought of traditional and modern processed Chinese medicine through the design of the quality research of Aconiti Kusnezoffii Radix and Aconiti Kusnezoffii Radix Cocta.

3.3 To grasp the evaluation methods of efficacy and toxicity evaluation of Aconiti Kusnezoffii Radix, through the design of comparative study on toxicity and efficacy of Aconiti Kusnezoffii Radix and Aconiti Kusnezoffii Radix Cocta.

Experiment Contents

4.1 Retrieval of Related literatures and review writing

Write reviews about advances in processing of Aconiti Kusnezoffii Radix according to Chinese Pharmacopoeia, the specifications of Chinese material medica processing in different provinces in China and related literatures. Analyze current situation and development trend of processing technology, quality evaluation, chemical and pharmacological mechanism of reduction of toxicity, and clinical application of Aconiti Kusnezoffii Radix.

4.2 Develop a program for experiment design in groups

Based on the literature work, 3~5 students interested in the same problem should be freely grouped. And then, protocol and complete preliminary experimental plan based on specialized knowledge of TCM and the aim of the experiment, feasibility analysis and presupposition of problems that could happen during the experiment. Present preliminary experimental scheme as a group, teacher assess the preliminary experimental plan on scientificity, feasibility, rationality, integrity and operability. Students revise the plan according to the teachers' evaluation and complete the experimental research plan (revised version). Students should be the main body of the work and teachers should participate in confirmation of the plan. According to the selected experimental subject, each group study relevant references, review relevant basic knowledge and experimental skills, and design experimental plan. Then, each group discuss with teacher to ensure a reasonable and feasible experimental plan which would be used as the basis of experimental research.

The experimental plan of each group should contains the following points.

A. Project title: Each group abstracts the title according to the problem to be solved and the method to be used.

B. Research basis: Include theoretical basis of processing of Aconiti Kusnezoffii Radix and experimental basis, which can explain the reason for doing the experimental research and the reason for choosing this method to achieve the experimental aim.

C. Aims of the experiment: Aims should be the problem which would be solved or the aim which would be achieved by this experiment. Any experiment requires clear aims. It should be noted that the aims should not be too many, 1~3 aims should be appropriate, and should not be achieved by this chosen experiment methods.

D. Experiment principles: Mainly describe the scientific basis of the processing method of Aconiti Kusnezoffii Radix.

E. Material: Including the source of Aconiti Kusnezoffii Radix, experimental animals, reagents, apparatus, material, reference standards and substances.

F. Experimental methods and operating procedures: The emphasis is experimental plan. For example, if the title is optimization of processing technology of Aconiti Kusnezoffii Radix, experimental plan should contain the following points: specific processing method, basis of this processing method, single factor or multi-factor, orthogonal test or other design, factors and levels of each processing technology, and etc. If the title is evaluation indicator of traditional characteristics or chemical compositions questions including how to use traditional characteristics as indicators, determination of the chosen chemical compositions, necessity of methodology investigation, preparation method of samples, and batches of samples should be considered to ensure the accuracy of the experimental results.

G. Data analysis: Analyze the results data as necessary, such as content calculation, variance analysis, comprehensive evaluation, etc.

H. Matters need attention: List he matters need attention during the experiment, to ensure the accuracy and reliability of the experimental results.

I. References: List references used in the design of this experiment, and provide electronic version for verification.

4.3 Practice of the experiment

4.3.1 Preparation

According to the experiment plan (revised version), students submit the application of necessary reagent, materials, laboratory and apparatus to management department of teaching laboratory.

4.3.2 Practice

Students carry out experiments according to the experimental plan, and make original records. Connect teachers timely with the actual problems of the experiment, adjust and complete the experiment plan (final version).

4.3.3 Cautions

A. Observe carefully during the experiment in accordance with the design, and original record should be timely, accurate and comprehensive.

B. Adjust the original design if there is unexpected situation.

C. The experimental results must be analyzed comprehensively, and the experimental data must be processed accurately according to the statistical requirements.

4.4 Summarize experimental results and complete experimental report.

Students organize and analyze the experimental data based on the original record. Summarize the problem encountered in the experiment and their solution. And then complete the report after discussion.

Reports should be composed of followings.

A. Inspect whether the experiment is completed in accordance with experimental plan. If not, find out the reason objectively and realistically. Discuss the reliability of the results.

B. Conclusion should be logically deduced from the results. Realize the basis of a serious science. Discuss the experiences and lessons.

C. Analyze and discuss realistically, no matter whether the experimental results are consisting with the expectation, or even contrary to the expectation

4.5 Summarize and analyze.

Self-evaluated the whole process of the experiment in group. Teachers analyze the common problems from the students' original records and experimental reports, and evaluates rationality of the experimental plans, correctness of the experimental operation and quality of the papers.

Notes

5.1 The experimental plan designed by each group should be reasonable, feasible and detailed, and be supported by relevant literature.

5.2 Evaluation indicators of processing technology, quality and efficacy should reflect the principle that the actions of different processed products of Aconiti Kusnezoffii Radix is consistent.

Consider questions

6.1 Sketch methods and thoughts of the study on processing toxic Chinese Materia Medica.

6.2 State matters need attention in the experiments

第五章 中药饮片企业见习

PPT

一、见习目的

通过中药饮片企业见习（实习），使学生掌握中药饮片生产的工艺设计、生产、包装、储存过程，增强学生对中药饮片企业在生产、质量控制、仓储等方面的感性认识；要求学生掌握常见中药饮片的炮制产业化生产过程以及中药饮片质量标准判定，熟悉中药库房管理相关要求，进一步深化课堂理论教学内容，培养学生理论联系实践的能力和实际工作能力。

二、见习内容

1. 参观见习生产区

（1）了解中药饮片厂的厂区设计（例如厂区的选择、厂房的设计和要求、车间设计和要求等）、厂房车间布局以及厂房的安全卫生和环境保护设计要求。根据《药品生产质量管理规范》（GMP）要求而制定的生产工艺流程和岗位操作规程和《中药饮片 GMP 认证检查项目》的基本要求，了解《危险化学品安全管理条例》等规定对饮片厂的消防、安全、电力配备、污水处理等相关的理论知识。

（2）了解中药饮片的生产过程。了解毒性中药饮片和直接口服中药饮片生产控制情况。

（3）重点了解各岗位的生产前准备、生产操作、质量控制及物料平衡等内容，包括中药净制、切制、炒制、炙制、煅制与蒸、煮、燀制等关键岗位单元操作技术，各种炮制方法的主要工艺流程与岗位操作规程，相关中药饮片生产的常用设备构造、性能以及操作规程、要点和注意事项。

（4）了解中药饮片厂饮片自然干燥及人工干燥方式。

2. 参观见习仓储区 了解中药饮片厂的仓储区分类、物料管理、仓库管理、中药材及中药饮片的养护等知识。了解中药材或中药饮片的入库检验和成品出库检验方法。

3. 参观见习质控中心 了解企业质控中心的情况。熟悉企业质量标准制订和检验操作规程内容，检品的取样及留样观察制度，相关仪器分析设备，检验报告的格式和正确填写方法。掌握对检品进行的杂质检查、水分测定、灰分测定、浸出物测定、有效成分测定、有毒成分测定、有害成分测定等方法，包括原料药的品种鉴定、成品和半成品检验操作，按照国家中药饮片标准或企业的内控标准对原料药和中药饮片的质量进行判定。

三、见习方案

见习指导教师负责拟定见习计划，选择有一定条件或具有代表性的中药饮片加工企业作为见习（实习）单位。见习内容由各院校可根据教学计划并结合实际条件，选取必要的见习（实习）项目进行训练。见习结束后，撰写见习小结，并组织一次班级交流。

1. 见习方式 集中到通过 GMP 认证的中药饮片企业见习。

2. 见习时间 中药炮制课程授课期间段或假期，时间为 1~2 周；有条件者可安排 1 个月。

参观见习后及时就体会、意见或建议写出报告。

Chapter 5 Noviciate in enterprises of decoction pieces

1. Purpose of noviciate

Noviciate in enterprises of Yinpian (decoction pieces/processed Chinese medicine) can help students master the technological design, production, packaging, storage of Yinpian (decoction pieces/processed Chinese medicine) and enhance perceptual understanding of enterprise in production, quality control and storage. Students are required to master industrial production process and quality standard of Yinpian (decoction pieces/processed Chinese medicine) as well as be familiar with requirements for management of Chinese medicine warehouse. Teachers are required to further deepen the content of theory, cultivate students' ability of linking up theory with practice and practical work ability.

2. Content of noviciate

2.1 Visiting production district.

2.1.1 To understand the requirements of plant design (such as plant site selection, the design and requirements of factory building and workshop, etc.), layout, safety, sanitation and environmental protection design of the workshop. Based on requirements of *Good Manufacturing Practice for Medicines, Production Technical Processes*, *Operating Procedures and Inspection for TCM Decoction Pieces GMP Certification* are formulated. To understand relevant theoretical knowledge of fire protection, safety, electrical equipment, sewage treatment in plant of Yinpian (decoction pieces/processed Chinese medicine) stipulated by *Regulations on Safety Management of Hazardous Chemicals*.

2.1.2 To understand production process of Yinpian (decoction pieces/processed Chinese medicine). To understand production control of toxic and direct oral taken Yinpian (decoction pieces/processed Chinese medicine).

2.1.3 To focus on pre-production preparation, production operation, quality control and material balance of each position. To focus on the operation techniques of key positions including cleansing, cutting, stir-frying, stir-frying with liquid adjuvants, calcining, steaming, boiling, blanching and so on. To focus on the main technological process and operation procedures of various processing methods. To focus on the common equipment construction, performance, operating procedures, points and notes used in the production of Yinpian (decoction pieces/processed Chinese medicine).

2.1.4 To understand natural drying and artificial drying methods in the factory of Yinpian (decoction pieces/processed Chinese medicine).

2.2 Visiting warehouse district.

To understand classification, material management, storage management and maintenance of raw Chinese medicine and Yinpian (decoction pieces/processed Chinese medicine) in storage district in the factory. To understand the methods of going in and out storage inspection of raw Chinese medicine and Yinpian (decoction pieces/processed Chinese medicine).

2.3 Visiting quality control center.

To understand the profile of quality control center in enterprises of Yinpian (decoction pieces/processed Chinese medicine). To be familiar with formulation of quality standard and inspection procedures. To be familiar with regulations for sampling and reserving samples for observation. To be familiar with analysis equipment. To be familiar with the format of inspection report. To grasp the determination method for impurities, moisture, ash, extract, active components, toxic components, harmful components and so on. To grasp the testing operation including species identification of raw Chinese medicines, semi-finished and finished products. To assess the quality of raw Chinese medicines and Yinpian (decoction pieces/processed Chinese medicine) according to the national standards for Yinpian (decoction pieces/processed Chinese medicine) or the control standards of the enterprise.

3. Project of noviciate.

The guidance counselor is responsible for drawing up the noviciate plan. Qualified or representative enterprises of Yinpian (decoction pieces/processed Chinese medicine) should be selected as the noviciate (practice) base. Each university/institution may select the necessary internship program for training according to the teaching plan and the actual conditions. After the noviciate, students should be required to write the summary of the noviciate and a class communication should also be organized.

3.1 Noviciate mode

To gather in GMP certified enterprises of Yinpian (decoction pieces/processed Chinese medicine) for noviciate.

3.2 Noviciate duration

1~2 weeks during the course of Chinese medicine processing or vacation. One month can be arranged if possible.

Write a report on experience, comments or suggestions when the noviciate is finished.

附　录

PPT

附录一　中药饮片生产质量管理规范

根据《药品生产质量管理规范（2010年修订）》（国家食品药品监督管理局令第32号，2014年）公告，中药饮片生产管理和质量控制的全过程需符合相关原则，在人员、厂房与设施、设备、物料和产品、确认与验证、文件管理、生产管理、质量管理及术语等方面应符合以下要求。

第一章　范　围

第一条　本附录适用于中药饮片生产管理和质量控制的全过程。

第二条　产地趁鲜加工中药饮片的，按照本附录执行。

第三条　民族药参照本附录执行。

第二章　原　则

第四条　中药饮片的质量与中药材质量、炮制工艺密切相关，应当对中药材质量、炮制工艺严格控制；在炮制、贮存和运输过程中，应当采取措施控制污染，防止变质，避免交叉污染、混淆、差错；生产直接口服中药饮片的，应对生产环境及产品微生物进行控制。

第五条　中药材的来源应符合标准，产地应相对稳定。

第六条　中药饮片必须按照国家药品标准炮制；国家药品标准没有规定的，必须按照省、自治区、直辖市食品药品监督管理部门制定的炮制规范或审批的标准炮制。

第七条　中药饮片应按照品种工艺规程生产。中药饮片生产条件应与生产许可范围相适应，不得外购中药饮片的中间产品或成品进行分包装或改换包装标签。

第三章　人　员

第八条　企业的生产管理负责人应具有药学或相关专业大专以上学历（或中级专业技术职称或执业药师资格）、三年以上从事中药饮片生产管理的实践经验，或药学或相关专业中专以上学历、八年以上从事中药饮片生产管理的实践经验。

第九条　企业的质量管理负责人、质量受权人应当具备药学或相关专业大专以上学历（或中级专业技术职称或执业药师资格），并有中药饮片生产或质量管理五年以上的实践经验，其中至少有一年的质量管理经验。

第十条　企业的关键人员以及质量保证、质量控制等人员均应为企业的全职在岗人员。

第十一条　质量保证和质量控制人员应具备中药材和中药饮片质量控制的实际能力，具备鉴别中药材和中药饮片真伪优劣的能力。

第十二条　从事中药材炮制操作人员应具有中药炮制专业知识和实际操作技能；从事毒性中药材等有特殊要求的生产操作人员，应具有相关专业知识和技能，并熟知相关的劳动保护要求。

第十三条　负责中药材采购及验收的人员应具备鉴别中药材真伪优劣的能力。

第十四条　从事养护、仓储保管人员应掌握中药材、中药饮片贮存养护知识与技能。

第十五条　企业应由专人负责培训管理工作，培训的内容应包括中药专业知识、岗位技能和药品 GMP 相关法规知识等。

第十六条　进入生产区的人员应进行更衣、洗手；进入洁净区的工作服的选材、式样及穿戴方式应符合通则的要求；从事对人体有毒、有害操作的人员应按规定着装防护，其专用工作服与其他操作人员的工作服应分别洗涤、整理，并避免交叉污染。

第四章　厂房与设施

第十七条　生产区应与生活区严格分开，不得设在同一建筑物内。

第十八条　厂房与设施应按生产工艺流程合理布局，并设置与其生产规模相适应的净制、切制、炮炙等操作间。同一厂房内的生产操作之间和相邻厂房之间的生产操作不得互相妨碍。

第十九条　直接口服饮片的粉碎、过筛、内包装等生产区域应按照 D 级洁净区的要求设置，企业应根据产品的标准和特性对该区域采取适当的微生物监控措施。

第二十条　毒性中药材加工、炮制应使用专用设施和设备，并与其他饮片生产区严格分开，生产的废弃物应经过处理并符合要求。

第二十一条　厂房地面、墙壁、天棚等内表面应平整，易于清洁，不易产生脱落物，不易滋生霉菌；应有防止昆虫或其他动物等进入的设施，灭鼠药、杀虫剂、烟熏剂等不得对设备、物料、产品造成污染。

第二十二条　中药材净选应设拣选工作台，工作台表面应平整，不易产生脱落物。

第二十三条　中药饮片炮制过程中产热产汽的工序，应设置必要的通风、除烟、排湿、降温等设施；拣选、筛选、切制、粉碎等易产尘的工序，应当采取有效措施，以控制粉尘扩散，避免污染和交叉污染，如安装捕尘设备、排风设施等。

第二十四条　仓库应有足够空间，面积与生产规模相适应。中药材与中药饮片应分库存放；毒性中药材和饮片等有特殊要求的中药材和中药饮片应当设置专库存放，并有相应的防盗及监控设施。

第二十五条　仓库内应当配备适当的设施，并采取有效措施，对温、湿度进行监控，保证中药材和中药饮片按照规定条件贮存；贮存易串味、鲜活中药材应当有适当的设施（如专库、冷藏设施）。

第五章　设　　备

第二十六条　应根据中药材、中药饮片的不同特性及炮制工艺的需要，选用能满足生产工艺要求的设备。

第二十七条　与中药材、中药饮片直接接触的设备、工具、容器应易清洁消毒，不易产生脱落物，不对中药材、中药饮片质量产生不良影响。

第二十八条　中药饮片生产用水至少应为饮用水，企业定期监测生产用水的质量，饮用水每年至少一次送相关检测部门进行检测。

第六章　物料和产品

第二十九条　生产所用原辅料、与药品直接接触的包装材料应当符合相应的质量标准，分别编制批号并管理；所用物料不得对中药饮片质量产生不良影响。

第三十条　质量管理部门应当对生产用物料的供应商进行质量评估，并建立质量档案；直接从农户购入中药材应收集农户的身份证明材料，评估所购入中药材质量，并建立质量档案。

第三十一条　对每次接收的中药材均应当按产地、供应商、采收时间、药材规格等进行分类，分别编制批号并管理。

第三十二条　购入的中药材，每件包装上应有明显标签，注明品名、规格、数量、产地、采收（初加工）时间等信息，毒性中药材等有特殊要求的中药材外包装上应有明显的标志。

第三十三条　中药饮片应选用能保证其贮存和运输期间质量的包装材料或容器。包装必须印有或者贴有标签，注明品名、规格、产地、生产企业、产品批号、生产日期、执行标准，实施批准文号管理的中药饮片还必须注明药品批准文号。

第三十四条　直接接触中药饮片的包装材料应至少符合食品包装材料标准。

第三十五条　中药材、中药饮片应按质量要求贮存、养护，贮存期间各种养护操作应当建立养护记录；养护方法应当安全有效，以免造成污染和交叉污染。

第三十六条　中药材、中药饮片应制定复验期，并按期复验，遇影响质量的异常情况须及时复验。

第三十七条　中药材和中药饮片的运输应不影响其质量，并采取有效可靠的措施，防止中药材和中药饮片发生变质。

第三十八条　进口药材应有国家食品药品监督管理部门批准的证明文件，以及按有关规定办理进口手续的证明文件。

第七章　确认与验证

第三十九条　净制、切制可按制法进行工艺验证，炮炙应按品种进行工艺验证，关键工艺参数应在工艺验证中体现。

第四十条　关键生产设备和仪器应进行确认，关键设备应进行清洁验证。直接口服饮片生产车间的空气净化系统应进行确认。

第四十一条　生产一定周期后应进行再验证。

第四十二条　验证文件应包括验证总计划、验证方案、验证报告以及记录，确保验证的真实性。

第八章　文 件 管 理

第四十三条　中药材和中药饮片质量管理文件至少应包含以下内容。

（一）制定物料的购进、验收、贮存、养护制度，并分类制定中药材和中药饮片的养护操作规程。

（二）制定每种中药饮片的生产工艺规程，各关键工艺参数必须明确，如中药材投料量、辅料用量、浸润时间、片型、炒制温度和时间（火候）、蒸煮压力和时间等要求。

（三）根据中药材的质量、投料量、生产工艺等因素，制定每种中药饮片的收率限度范围，关键工序应制定物料平衡参数。

（四）制定每种中药材、中药饮片的质量标准及相应的检验操作规程，制定中间产品、待包装产品的质量控制指标。

第四十四条　应当对从中药饮片生产和包装的全过程的生产管理和质量控制情况进行记录，批记录至少包括以下内容。

（一）批生产和包装指令。

（二）中药材以及辅料的名称、批号、投料量及投料记录。

（三）净制、切制、炮炙工艺的设备编号。

（四）生产前的检查和核对的记录。

（五）各工序的生产操作记录，包括各关键工序的技术参数。

（六）清场记录。

（七）关键控制点及工艺执行情况检查审核记录。

（八）产品标签的实样。

（九）不同工序的产量，必要环节物料平衡的计算。

（十）对特殊问题和异常事件的记录，包括偏离生产工艺规程等偏差情况的说明和调查，并经签字批准。

（十一）中药材、中间产品、待包装产品中药饮片的检验记录和审核放行记录。

第九章 生 产 管 理

第四十五条 净制后的中药材和中药饮片不得直接接触地面。中药材、中药饮片晾晒应有有效的防虫、防雨等防污染措施。

第四十六条 应当使用流动的饮用水清洗中药材，用过的水不得用于清洗其他中药材。不同的中药材不得同时在同一容器中清洗、浸润。

第四十七条 毒性中药材和毒性中药饮片的生产操作应当有防止污染和交叉污染的措施，并对中药材炮制的全过程进行有效监控。

第四十八条 中药饮片以中药材投料日期作为生产日期。

第四十九条 中药饮片应以同一批中药材在同一连续生产周期生产的一定数量相对均质的成品为一批。

第五十条 在同一操作间内同时进行不同品种、规格的中药饮片生产操作应有防止交叉污染的隔离措施。

第十章 质 量 管 理

第五十一条 中药材和中药饮片应按法定标准进行检验。如中药材、中间产品、待包装产品的检验结果用于中药饮片的质量评价，应经过评估，并制定与中药饮片质量标准相适应的中药材、中间产品质量标准，引用的检验结果应在中药饮片检验报告中注明。

第五十二条 企业应配备必要的检验仪器，并有相应标准操作规程和使用记录；检验仪器应能满足实际生产品种要求，除重金属及有害元素、农药残留、黄曲霉毒素等特殊检验项目和使用频次较少的大型仪器外，原则上不允许委托检验。

第五十三条 每批中药材和中药饮片应当留样。中药材留样量至少能满足鉴别的需要，中药饮片留样量至少应为两倍检验量，毒性药材及毒性饮片的留样应符合医疗用毒性药品的管理规定。留样时间应当有规定，中药饮片留样时间至少为放行后一年。

第五十四条 企业应设置中药标本室（柜），标本品种至少包括生产所用的中药材和中药饮片。

第五十五条 企业可选取产量较大及质量不稳定的品种进行年度质量回顾分析，其他品种也应定期进行产品质量回顾分析，回顾的品种应涵盖企业的所有炮制范围。

第十一章 术 语

第五十六条 下列术语含义。

（一）直接口服中药饮片

指标准中明确使用过程无需经过煎煮，可直接口服或冲服的中药饮片。

（二）产地趁鲜加工中药饮片

指在产地用鲜活中药材进行切制等加工中药饮片。不包括中药材的产地初加工。

Appendix

Appendix I Good Manufacturing Practice for Chinese medicine decoction pieces

According to the *Good Manufacturing Practice for Pharmaceutical Products (Revised in 2010)* (State Food and Drug Administration Order No. 32 in 2014) announcement, the entire process of Chinese medicine decoction pieces production management and quality control must comply with relevant principles. Personnel, workshop and establishment, equipment, material and product, confirmation and validation, document management, manufacturing management, quality management and terminology shall be in accordance with the following requirements.

Chapter 1 Scope

Article 1 This appendix applies to the entire process of production management and quality control of Chinese medicine decoction pieces.

Article 2 Chinese medicine decoction pieces freshly processed in the place of origin shall be implemented in accordance with this appendix.

Article 3 Ethnic medicine is implemented with reference to this appendix.

Chapter 2 Principle

Article 4 The quality of Chinese medicine decoction pieces is closely related to the quality of raw Chinese medicine and processing technology. The quality of raw Chinese medicine and processing technology shall be strictly controlled. In the process of processing, storage and delivery, measures shall be taken to control pollution, prevent deterioration, and avoid cross-pollution, confusion and mistake. In the production of direct oral Chinese medicine decoction pieces, the production environment and product microorganisms shall be controlled.

Article 5 The source of raw Chinese medicine shall be in accordance the standards and the place of origin shall be relatively stable.

Article 6 Chinese medicine decoction pieces must be processed in accordance with national drug standards. If there are no national drug standards, they must be processed according to processing standards or approval standards formulated by the Food and Drug Administration departments of provinces, autonomous regions and municipalities.

Article 7 Chinese medicine decoction pieces shall be produced according to the variety process regulations. The production conditions of Chinese medicine decoction pieces shall be compatible with the scope of production permits. The semifinished products or finished products of outsourced Chinese medicine decoction pieces must not be sub-packaged or the packaging labels changed.

Chapter 3 Personnel

Article 8 Director of manufacturing management shall at least have pharmacology or related specialty college degree background (or secondary professional technical title or licensed pharmacist qualification), have at least three years' Chinese medicine decoction pieces' manufacturing and quality management experience, or pharmacology or related specialty junior degree college background, have at least eight years' Chinese medicine decoction pieces' manufacturing and quality management experience.

Article 9 Director of quality management shall at least have pharmacology or related specialty junior degree college background (or secondary professional technical title or licensed pharmacist qualification), have at least five years' Chinese medicine decoction pieces' manufacturing and quality management experience, including at least one year's pharmaceutical goods' quality management experience.

Article 10 The important personnel, the quality guarantee personnel and the quality control, etc. personnel of the enterprise shall be the full-time job person.

Article 11 The quality guarantee and quality control personnel shall have the practical ability to control the quality of raw Chinese medicine and Chinese medicine decoction pieces, and have the ability to distinguish the authenticity of raw Chinese medicine and Chinese medicine decoction pieces.

Article 12 The operate personnel engaged in the processing of raw Chinese medicine shall have the expertise and practical skills of Chinese medicine processing. The operate person engaged in production with special requirements such as toxic raw Chinese medicine shall have the relevant professional knowledge and skills, and be familiar with related labor protection requirements.

Article 13 The personnel responsible for the ordering, checking and accepting of raw Chinese medicine shall have the ability to identify the authenticity of raw Chinese medicine.

Article 14 The Personnel engaged in conservation and storage shall have knowledge and skills in the conservation and storage of raw Chinese medicine and Chinese medicine decoction pieces.

Article 15 The enterprise shall designate department or person to take responsible for training management work, and the training content shall include the knowledge of traditional Chinese medicine, post skills and knowledge of pharmaceutical GMP regulations.

Article 16 The personnel enters into manufacturing area shall change clothes, wash hands. The material, style and dressing method of work clothes enters into clean manufacturing area shall be in accordance with the requirements of the general rules. Personnel engaged in toxic and harmful operations to the human body shall wear protective clothing in accordance with regulations. Their special work clothes and other operator's work clothes shall be washed and sorted separately to avoid cross pollution.

Chapter 4 Workshop and Establishment

Article 17 The manufacturing area shall be strictly separated from the living area and shall not be located in the same building.

Article 18 Workshop and establishment shall reasonable designed according to the technique process, and cleaning, cutting, stir-baking and other operation rooms suitable for the production scale shall be set up. Manufacture operations in the same factory building and between adjacent factory buildings must not interfere with each other.

Article 19 Manufacturing areas for crushing, sieving, and inner packaging of direct oral decoction pieces shall be set in accordance with the requirements of Class D clean areas. Enterprises shall take appropriate microbiological monitoring measures for the areas according to the standards and characteristics of products.

Article 20 The processing and manufacturing of toxic raw Chinese medicine shall use special establishment and equipment, and be strictly separated from other decoction pieces manufacturing areas. The waste produced shall be processed and in accordance with the related requirements.

Article 21 The internal surfaces of the factory floor, walls, ceiling, etc. shall be flat, easy to clean, not easy to produce falling objects, not easy to breed molds; Establishment shall be provided to prevent insects or other animals from entering, and rodenticides, insecticides, fumigants, etc. shall not cause pollution to equipment, materials and products.

Article 22 A sorting workbench shall be set for the cleaning and selection of raw Chinese medicine, and the surface of the workbench shall be flat and not easy to produce falling objects.

Article 23 During the process of producing Chinese medicine decoction pieces, the processes of heat generation and steam generation shall be provided with necessary equipment for ventilation, smoke removal, dehumidification, temperature reduction, etc. And processes of dust-producing such as selection, screening, cutting, and crushing shall take effective measures to control dust and avoid pollution and cross-pollution, such as installation of dust collection equipment, ventilation facilities, etc.

Article 24 The warehouse shall have sufficient space and the area shall be suitable for the scale of manufactory. The raw Chinese medicine and Chinese medicine decoction pieces shall be stored separately. The raw Chinese medicine and Chinese medicine decoction pieces with special requirements such as toxic raw Chinese medicine and Chinese medicine decoction pieces shall be stored in a special stock with corresponding anti-theft and monitoring facilities.

Article 25 The warehouse shall be equipped with appropriate facilities, and effective measures shall be taken to monitor temperature and humidity to ensure that raw Chinese medicine and Chinese medicine decoction pieces are stored in accordance with the prescribed conditions. Appropriate facilities (such as special warehouses and refrigeration storage) shall be provided for the storage of raw Chinese medicine which are easy to cross-taste and fresh.

Chapter 5 Equipment

Article 26 According to the different characteristics of raw Chinese medicine and Chinese medicine decoction pieces and the needs of processing technology, the equipment shall be selected in accordance with requirements of production technology.

Article 27 Equipment, tools and containers in direct contact with raw Chinese medicine and Chinese medicine decoction pieces shall be easy to clean and disinfect, not easy to produce falling objects, and not have adverse effects on the quality of raw Chinese medicine and Chinese medicine decoction pieces.

Article 28 The water used for the production of Chinese medicine decoction pieces shall be drinking water at least. The quality of the production water shall be regularly monitored by the enterprise. Drinking water shall be sent to relevant testing departments at least once a year for detection.

Chapter 6 Material and Product

Article 29 The raw material used for pharmaceutical goods' manufacturing, wrapper material direct contact with pharmaceutical goods shall be in accordance with the quality standard, and batch numbers shall be prepared and managed separately. The materials used must not take bad influence to the quality of the Chinese medicine decoction pieces.

Article 30 The quality management department shall conduct quality evaluation on the suppliers of production materials and establish quality files. When purchasing raw Chinese medicine directly from farmers, it shall collect the identification materials of the farmers, evaluate the quality of the purchased raw Chinese medicine and establish the quality files.

Article 31 The raw Chinese medicine received each time shall be classified according to the place of origin, supplier, collection time, herbal medicines specifications, etc., and batch numbers shall be prepared and managed separately.

Article 32 Each package of purchased raw Chinese medicine shall be clearly labeled with products' name, specification, quantity, place of origin, collection (initial processing) time , etc., and the external package of toxic raw Chinese medicine with special requirements shall be clearly marked.

Article 33 Chinese medicine decoction pieces shall be packaging materials or containers that can ensure their quality during storage and transportation. The package must be printed or labeled with the product name, specifications, origin, manufacturer, batch number, date of production, implementation standards, and the drug approval number must also be indicated for the Chinese medicine decoction pieces under the approval number management.

Article 34 The packaging materials that are in direct contact with the Chinese medicine decoction pieces shall at least be in accordance with the standards of food packaging materials.

Article 35 The raw Chinese medicine and Chinese medicine decoction pieces shall be stored and conserved in accordance with quality requirements, and maintenance records shall be established for various maintenance operations during the storage period. The maintenance methods shall be safe and effective to avoid pollution and cross-pollution.

Article 36 Period of double examination shall be established for raw Chinese medicine and Chinese medicine decoction pieces, and the double examination shall be scheduled on a regular basis. In the case of abnormal conditions affecting quality, the double examination shall be conducted in time.

Article 37 The transportation of raw Chinese medicine and Chinese medicine decoction pieces shall not affect their quality, and effective and reliable measures shall be taken to prevent the Chinese medicine decoction pieces from deteriorating.

Article 38 The imported medicinal materials shall have the certification documents approved by the State Food and Drug Administration and the certification documents for handling import procedures in accordance with relevant regulations.

Chapter 7 Confirmation and Validation

Article 39 The process of the cleaning and the cutting can be verified by the manufacturing method. The process of the the stir-baking shall be verified by the variety. The important process parameters shall be reflected in the process verification.

Article 40 Critical production equipment and instruments shall be confirmed, and critical equipment shall be cleaned and verified. The air purification system of the workshop for direct oral Chinese medicine decoction pieces production shall be confirmed.

Article 41 Revalidation shall be performed after a certain period of production.

Article 42 The validation documents shall include the validation master plan, validation scheme, validation report and records to ensure the authenticity of the validation.

Chapter 8 Document Management

Article 43 The quality management documents of raw Chinese medicine and Chinese medicine decoction pieces shall at least include the following.

Ⅰ. Formulate the purchase, check, acceptance, storage and conservation system of materials, and formulate the classification and conservation operation procedures for raw Chinese medicine and Chinese medicine decoction pieces.

Ⅱ. Formulate the production process specification of each kind of Chinese medicine decoction pieces, and the key process parameters must be clear, such as the amount of raw Chinese medicine input, the amount of auxiliary materials, infiltration time, tablet type, processing temperature and time (heating), pressure and time requirements of steaming and boiling process, etc.

Ⅲ. According to factors such as the quality of raw Chinese medicine, the amount of input, the manufactory process, etc., the yield limit range of each Chinese medicine decoction pieces shall be formulated, and the material balance parameters shall be formulated for key processes.

Ⅳ. Formulate the quality standards and corresponding examination operating procedures for each raw Chinese medicine and Chinese medicine decoction pieces, and formulate quality control indicators for semifinished products and products to be packaged.

Article 44 The production management and quality control of the entire process of the production and packaging of Chinese medicine decoction pieces shall be recorded, and the batch record shall at least include the following contents.

Ⅰ. Batch production and packaging instructions.

Ⅱ. The name, batch number, input amount and input record of raw Chinese medicine and auxiliary materials.

Ⅲ. Equipment numbers for cleaning, cutting, and stir-baking.

Ⅳ. Pre-production inspection and verification records.

Ⅴ. Production operation records of each process, including technical parameters of each key process.

Ⅵ. Clearance record.

Ⅶ. Inspection records of critical control points and process implementation.

Ⅷ. Sample of product label.

Ⅸ. The output of different processes and the calculation of necessary material balance.

Ⅹ. Records of special problems and abnormal events, including descriptions and investigations of deviations from production process regulations, etc., and signed for approval.

Ⅺ. Inspection records and audit release records of raw Chinese medicine, semifinished products, and Chinese medicine decoction pieces to be packaged.

Chapter 9 Manufacturing Management

Article 45 The cleaned raw Chinese medicine and Chinese medicine decoction pieces shall not directly contact the ground. There shall be effective measures to prevent pollution such as insect and rain.

Article 46 The raw Chinese medicine shall be cleaned with flowing drinking water, and the used water shall not be used for cleaning other raw Chinese medicine. Different raw Chinese medicine must not be washed and infiltrated in the same container at the same time.

Article 47 The production and operation of toxic raw Chinese medicine and toxic Chinese medicine decoction pieces shall have measures to prevent pollution and cross-pollution, and the entire process of processing raw Chinese medicine shall be effectively monitored.

Article 48 The production date of Chinese medicine decoction pieces is based on the date when the raw Chinese medicine are feeding.

Article 49 Chinese medicine decoction pieces shall be a batch of relatively homogeneous finished products produced in the same batch of raw Chinese medicine in the same continuous production cycle.

Article 50 There shall be isolation measures to prevent cross-pollution in the production of different varieties and specifications of Chinese medicine decoction pieces in the same operation room.

Chapter 10 Quality management

Article 51 The raw Chinese medicine and Chinese medicine decoction pieces shall be inspected according to legal standards. If the test results of raw Chinese medicine, semifinished products, and products to be packaged are used for the quality evaluation of Chinese medicine decoction pieces, they shall be evaluated and the quality standards of raw Chinese medicine and semifinished products compatible with the quality standards of Chinese medicine decoction pieces shall be formulated, and indicated in the inspection report of the decoction pieces.

Article 52 The enterprise shall be equipped with necessary inspection instruments, and have corresponding standard operating procedures and use records. The inspection instruments shall be able to be in accordance with the requirements of the actual production variety, except for special inspection items such as heavy metal and harmful elements, pesticide residues, aflatoxin and large-scale instruments with less frequency, the entrusted inspection is not allowed in principle.

Article 53 Samples of each batch of raw Chinese medicine and Chinese medicine decoction pieces shall be retained. The amount of sample retention of raw Chinese medicine can at least meet the needs of identification. The amount of sample retention of Chinese medicine decoction pieces shall be at least twice the inspection amount. The retention of toxic raw Chinese medicine and toxic Chinese medicine decoction pieces shall meet the management regulations of toxic drugs for medical use. Sample retention time shall be specified, and the sample retention time of Chinese medicine decoction pieces shall be at least one year after release.

Article 54 The enterprise shall set up a Chinese medicine specimen room (cabinet) and the specimens shall include at least the raw Chinese medicine and Chinese medicine decoction pieces used in the production.

Article 55 The enterprise can select varieties with large output and unstable quality for annual quality review and analysis. Other varieties shall also conduct regular product quality review and analysis.

The reviewed varieties shall cover all the processing scope of the enterprise.

Chapter 11 Terminology

Article 56 The following terms mean.

Ⅰ. Direct oral Chinese medicine decoction pieces

Refers to the Chinese medicine decoction pieces that can be taken orally without decoction in the standard.

Ⅱ. Chinese medicine decoction pieces processed freshly at the place of origin

Refers to the processing of Chinese medicine decoction pieces by cutting freshly raw Chinese medicine in the production area. It does not include the primary processing at the place of origin.

附录二　中药饮片 GMP 认证检查项目

为加强中药饮片生产监督管理，2003 年 6 月，国家食品药品监督管理总局开始了中药饮片 GMP 认证试点工作。根据《药品管理法》及国家食品药品监督管理总局发布关于推进中药饮片等类别药品监督实施 GMP 工作的通知规定（国食药监安〔2004〕514 号），总局决定推进中药饮片等药品监督实施 GMP 工作。明确要求自 2008 年 1 月 1 日起，所有中药饮片生产企业必须在符合 GMP 的条件下生产。为规范中药饮片的生产管理，在企业申报中药饮片认证和核发中药饮片《药品 GMP 证书》时，其认证范围应注明含毒性饮片、含直接服用饮片及相应的炮制范围，包括净制、切制、炒制、炙制、煅制、蒸制等。中药饮片 GMP 认证检查项目的具体要求如下：

1. 中药饮片 GMP 认证检查项目共 111 项，其中关键项目（条款号前加“*”）18 项，一般项目 93 项。

2. 结果评定：

项　目		结　果
严重缺陷	一般缺陷	通过 GMP 认证
0	≤18	
0	19-37	限期 6 个月整改后追踪检查
≤3	≤18	
≤3	>18	不通过 GMP 认证
>3		

条款	检查内容
*0301	中药饮片生产企业是否建立与质量保证体系相适应的组织机构，明确各级机构和人员的职责。
0302	是否配备与中药饮片生产相适应的管理人员和技术人员，并具有相应的专业知识。
0401	主管生产和质量的企业负责人是否具有大专以上学历或中级以上技术职称，并具有中药专业知识。
0501	生产和质量管理部门负责人是否具有中医药大专以上学历，3 年以上实际工作经验或中医药中专学历，5 年以上实际工作经验。
*0502	生产管理和质量管理部门负责人是否互相兼任。
0601	从事药材炮制操作人员是否进行中药炮制专业知识的培训，具有中药炮制专业知识和实际操作技能。
0604	从事质量检验的人员是否具有检验理论知识，是否掌握相关质量标准和实际检验操作技能，并具有经验鉴别能力。
0605	从事毒性药材（含按麻醉药品管理的药材）等有特殊要求的生产操作人员，是否具有相关专业知识和实际操作技能，并熟知相关的劳动保护要求。
0606	从事仓库保管、养护人员是否具有掌握中药材、中药饮片贮存养护知识与技能。
0701	从事中药饮片生产的各级人员是否按照本规范要求进行培训和考核。
0801	中药饮片生产环境是否整洁，厂区地面、路面及运输等是否对生产造成污染，生产、行政、生活和辅助区总体布局是否合理，相互妨碍。

续表

条款	检查内容
0901	厂房设施是否按工艺流程合理布局，并设置与其生产规模相适应的净制、切制、炮炙等操作间。
0902	同一厂房内的生产操作之间和相邻厂房之间的生产操作是否相互妨碍。
1001	厂房是否有防止昆虫和其他动物进入的设施（生产操作间不应使用灭鼠药）。
1104	厂房地面、墙壁、天棚等内表面是否平整，易于清洁，不易产生脱落物，不易滋生霉菌。
1105	净选是否设拣选工作台，工作台表面是否平整、不易产生脱落物。
1201	生产区是否有与生产规模相适应的面积和空间。
1202	中药材、中药饮片的蒸、炒、炙、煅等厂房是否与其生产规模相适应。
1204	储存区是否有与生产规模相适应的面积和空间。
1205	储存区物料、中间产品、待验品的存放是否有能够防止差错和交叉污染的措施。
1604	直接口服的中药饮片的粉碎、过筛、内包装等生产厂房应符合洁净区要求。
2302	净制、切制、炮炙等操作间是否有相应的通风、除尘、除烟、排湿、降温等设施。
2304	筛选、切制、粉碎等易产尘的操作间是否安装捕吸尘等设施。
2305	生产过程中产生的废气、废水、粉尘等是否经处理后排放并符合国家环保要求。并由当地具有环境检验、监测资质的单位出具符合要求的相关证明文件。
2601	仓储区是否保持清洁和干燥，是否安装照明和通风设施。仓储区的温度、湿度控制是否符合储存要求，按规定定期监测。
2801	实验室、中药标本室、留样观察室是否与生产区分开。
2901	对有特殊要求的仪器、仪表是否安放在专门的仪器室内，有防止静电、震动、潮湿或其他外界因素影响的设施。
3104	是否根据中药材、中药饮片的不同特性及炮制工艺的需要，选用能满足工艺参数要求的设备。
3201	与中药材、中药饮片直接接触的设备、工具、容器表面是否易清洗消毒、不易产生脱落物，并不与中药材、中药饮片发生化学反应，不吸附中药材、中药饮片。
3206	设备所用的润滑剂、冷却剂等是否对中药饮片或容器造成污染。
*3207	毒性药材（含按麻醉药品管理的药材）等有特殊要求的饮片生产是否符合国家有关规定。毒性药材生产应有专用设备及生产线。
3301	与设备连接的主要固定管道是否标明管内物料名称、流向。
3501	生产和检验用仪器、仪表、量具、衡器等适用范围、精密度是否符合生产和检验要求，是否有明显的合格标志，是否定期校验。
3601	生产设备是否有明显的状态标志。
3602	生产设备是否定期维修、保养。设备安装、维修、保养的操作是否影响产品的质量。
3701	生产、检验设备是否有使用、维修、保养记录，并由专人管理。
3801	物料的购入、储存、发放、使用等是否制定管理制度。
3802	原料、辅料是否按品种、规格、批号分别存放。
*3901	物料是否符合药品标准、包装材料标准和其他有关标准，不得对中药饮片质量产生不良影响。
*3903	进口药材是否有国家药品监督管理部门批准的证明文件。
4001	生产使用的中药材，是否按质量标准购入，其产地是否保持相对稳定。
4002	购入的中药材是否有详细的记录，包装上是否有明显标签，注明品名、规格、数量、产地、来源、采收（初加工）日期。实施批准文号的中药材是否注明药品的批准文号。

续表

条款	检查内容
4101	物料是否从符合规定的单位购进，是否按规定入库。
4201	待验、合格、不合格物料是否严格管理。
*4202	不合格的物料是否专区存放，是否有易于识别的明显标志，并按有关规定及时处理。
4301	有特殊要求的物料、中间产品和成品是否按规定条件储存。阴凉库温度是否不高于 25℃。
4302	挥发性物料是否避免污染其他物料，炮制、整理加工后是否使用清洁容器或包装，净药材是否与未加工、炮制的药材严格分开。
4303	中药材、中药饮片是否分别设库，是否按要求储存、养护。
*4401	毒性药材（含按麻醉药品管理的药材）等有特殊要求的药材是否按规定验收、储存、保管，是否设置专库或专柜。
*4411	毒性药材（含按麻醉药品管理的药材）等有特殊要求的药材外包装上是否有明显的规定标志。
4501	物料是否按规定的使用期限储存，期满后是否按规定复验；储存期内如有特殊情况是否及时复验。
4601	中药饮片是否选用能保证其贮存和运输期间质量的包装材料和容器。
4602	标签是否经质量管理部门校对无误后印制、发放、使用。
4603	包装是否印有或者贴有标签，注明品名、规格、产地、生产企业、产品批号、生产日期。实施批准文号管理的中药饮片是否注明药品批准文号。
4701	标签是否由专人保管、领用。
4702	标签是否按品种、规格专柜存放，是否按照实际需要量领取。
4703	标签是否记数发放，由领用人核对、签名。标签使用数、残损数及剩余数之和是否与领用数相符。
4704	印有批号的残损标签或剩余标签是否由专人销毁，是否有记数，发放、使用、销毁记录。
4801	是否有防止污染的卫生措施和各项卫生管理制度，并由专人负责。
4904	是否制定厂房、设备、容器的清洁规程，内容是否包括：清洁方法、程序、间隔时间，使用的清洁剂或消毒剂，清洁工具的清洁方法和存放地点。
5001	生产区是否存放非生产物品和个人杂物，生产中的废弃物是否及时处理。
5201	从事对人体有毒、有害操作的人员是否按规定着装防护。其专用工作服与其他操作人员的工作服是否分别洗涤、整理，并避免交叉污染。
5402	进入生产区的人员是否按规定更衣、洗手。
5601	生产人员是否有健康档案，直接接触中药饮片的生产人员是否每年至少体检一次。传染病、皮肤病患者和体表有伤口者是否从事直接接触中药饮片的生产。
5701	是否进行中药饮片生产验证，是否根据验证对象建立验证小组，提出验证项目、制定验证方案，并组织实施。
*5704	生产过程中关键工序是否进行设备验证和工艺验证。
5801	生产一定周期后是否进行再验证。
5901	验证工作完成后是否写出验证报告，由验证工作负责人审核、批准。
6001	验证过程中的数据和分析内容是否以文件形式归档保存，验证文件是否包括验证方案、验证报告、评价和建议、批准人等。
6401	是否建立文件的起草、修订、审查、批准、撤销、印制及保管的管理制度。
6402	分发、使用的文件是否为批准的现行文本。已撤销和过时的文件除留档备查外，是否在工作现场出现。
6501	文件的制定是否符合规定。

续表

条款	检查内容
*6601	是否有生产工艺规程、岗位操作法或标准操作规程，是否任意更改，如需更改时是否按规定程序执行。
6602	生产工艺规程内容是否包括名称、规格、炮制工艺的操作要求和技术参数，物料、中间成品、成品的质量标准及贮存注意事项，物料平衡的计算方法，包装规格等要求。
*6603	中药饮片是否按照国家药品标准炮制。国家药品标准没有规定的，是否按照省、自治区、直辖市人民政府药品监督管理部门制定的炮制规范炮制。
6701	产品是否进行物料平衡检查。物料平衡超出规定限度，应查明原因，在得出合理解释、确认无潜在质量事故后，方可按正常产品处理。
6801	是否按工艺规程编写标准操作规程和批生产记录。批生产记录是否及时填写、字迹清晰、内容真实、数据完整，并由操作人及复核人签字。
6802	批生产记录是否保持整洁、不得撕毁和任意涂改。批生产记录填写错误时，是否按规定更改。批生产记录是否按批号归档，是否保存三年。
*6901	中药饮片批号是否以同一批中药材在同一连续生产周期生产一定数量的相对均质的中药饮片为一批。
7001	生产前是否确认无上次生产遗留物。
7003	不同产品品种、规格的生产操作在同一操作间同时进行时，是否有隔离措施或其他有效防止污染和混淆的设施。
7009	每一生产操作间或生产用设备、容器是否有所生产的产品或物料名称、批号、数量等状态标志。
7015	中药材经净选后是否直接接触地面。
7016	毒性药材（含按麻醉药品管理的药材）等有特殊要求的药材生产操作是否有防止交叉污染的特殊措施。
7017	拣选后药材的洗涤是否使用流动水，用过的水是否用于洗涤其他药材。
7018	不同的中药材不得在一起洗涤。炮制后的中药饮片不可露天干燥。
7021	中药材的浸润是否做到药透水尽。
*7101	生产用水的质量标准是否低于饮用水标准。
7202	中药饮片零头包装是否只限两个批号为一个合箱。合箱外是否标明全部批号，并建立合箱记录。
7301	中药饮片的每一生产阶段完成后是否由生产操作人员清场，填写清场记录内容。清场记录内容是否完整，是否纳入批生产记录。
7401	质量管理部门是否受企业负责人直接领导。
7402	质量管理和检验人员的数量是否与中药饮片生产规模相适应。
7403	质量管理部门是否设置与中药饮片生产规模、种类、质量检验要求相适应的仪器设备。
7406	质量部门是否对毒性药材（含按麻醉药品管理的药材）等有特殊要求的药材炮制全过程进行有效监控。
*7501	质量文件中是否有中药材、辅料、包装材料、中间产品、中药饮片的质量标准及其检验操作规程。
7502	质量管理部门是否履行制定取样和留样制度的职责。
7503	质量管理部门是否履行制定检验用设备、仪器、试剂、试液、标准品（或对照品）、滴定液等管理办法的职责。
*7504	质量管理部门是否履行决定物料和中间产品使用的职责。
*7505	中药饮片放行前是否由质量管理部门对有关记录进行审核，并由审核人员签字。审核内容是否包括：配重、称重过程中的复核情况；各生产工序检查记录；清场记录；中间产品质量检验结果；偏差处理；成品检验结果等。

续表

条款	检查内容
*7506	质量管理部门是否履行审核不合格品处理程序的职责。
*7507	质量管理部门是否履行对物料、中间产品和成品进行取样、检验、留样，并出具检验报告的职责。
7511	质量管理部门是否履行制定质量管理和检验人员职责的职责。
7601	质量管理部门是否会同有关部门对主要物料供应商进行评估。
7701	每批中药饮片是否有销售记录。根据销售记录能追查每批中药饮片的售出情况，必要时是否能及时全部追回。销售记录内容是否包括品名、批号、规格、数量、收货单位和地址和发货日期等。
7801	销售记录是否保存三年。
7901	是否建立药品退货和收回的书面程序，并有记录。药品退货和收回记录内容是否包括品名、批号、规格、数量、退货和收回单位及地址、退货和收回原因及日期、处理意见。
7902	因质量原因退货和收回的中药饮片，是否在质量管理部门监督下销毁，涉及其他批号时，是否同时处理。
8101	对用户的中药饮片质量投诉是否有详细记录和调查处理。
8201	中药饮片生产出现重大质量问题时，是否及时向当地药品监督管理部门报告。
8301	企业是否定期组织自检。自检是否按预定的程序对企业进行全面检查。
8401	自检是否有记录。自检报告是否符合规定的内容。

Appendix II GMP certification inspection items for Chinese medicine decoction pieces

In order to strengthen the supervision and management of the production of Chinese medicine decoction pieces, the State Food and Drug Administration started the pilot project of GMP certification of Chinese medicine decoction pieces in June 2003. According to the "*Pharmaceutical Administration Law of the People's Republic of China*" and the provisions of the notice on Promoting the Implementation of GMP in the Supervision in Chinese medicine decoction pieces and other categories drug issued by the State Food and Drug Administration (SFDA〔2004〕No. 514), the State Food and Drug Administration decided to promote the supervision and implementation of GMP for Traditional Chinese Medicine and Other Categories. It is clearly required that from January 1, 2008, all manufacturers of Chinese medicine decoction pieces must produce under the conditions of GMP. In order to standardize the production management of Chinese medicine decoction pieces, when the enterprise applies for the certification of Chinese medicine decoction pieces and issues the GMP certificate of Chinese medicine decoction pieces, its certification scope shall indicate the toxic decoction pieces, direct orally decoction pieces and corresponding processing scope, including cleaning, cutting, stir-baking, stir-baking with liquid excipient, calcining, steaming, etc., and the specific requirements for the GMP certification inspection items of Chinese medicine decoction pieces are as follows.

1. There are 111 GMP certification inspection items for Chinese medicine decoction pieces, including 18 key items (with "*" before the clause number), and 93 general items.

2. Evaluation of results

items		Evaluation of results
serious defects	general defects	
0	≤18	GMP certified
0	19~37	6 months follow-up inspection after rectification
≤3	≤18	
≤3	≤18	Not GMP certified
≥3		

clause	Inspection contents
*0301	Whether the Chinese medicine decoction pieces manufacturing enterprises have established an organization that is compatible with the quality assurance system, and clarify the responsibilities of institutions and personnel at all levels.
0302	Whether there are management and technical personnel suitable for the production of Chinese medicine decoction pieces, with corresponding professional knowledge.

continued

clause	Inspection contents
0401	Whether the person in charge of production and quality has college degree at least or above intermediate technical title, and has professional knowledge of Chinese medicine decoction pieces.
0501	Whether the person in charge of production and quality management department has college degree or above in traditional Chinese medicine, more than 3 years of practical work experience or secondary school degree in traditional Chinese medicine, and more than 5 years of practical work experience.
*0502	Whether the person in charge of production management and quality management department concurrently in charge of each other.
0601	Whether the personnel engaged in the processing of Chinese medicine decoction pieces are trained in the professional knowledge of Chinese medicine processing, and have the professional knowledge and practical operation skills of Chinese medicine processing.
0604	Whether the personnel engaged in quality inspection have knowledge of inspection theory, master relevant quality standards and practical inspection operation skills, and have the ability to experience identification ability.
0605	Whether the production and operation personnel engaged in toxic raw Chinese medicine (including raw Chinese medicine managed according to narcotic drugs) and other special requirements have relevant professional knowledge and practical operation skills, and are familiar with relevant labor protection requirements.
0606	Whether the personnel engaged in warehouse storage and conservation have the knowledge and skills to master the storage and conservation of raw Chinese medicine and Chinese medicine decoction pieces.
0701	Whether personnel at all levels engaged in the production of Chinese medicine decoction pieces are trained and evaluated in accordance with the requirements of this specification.
0801	Whether the production environment of Chinese medicine decoction pieces is tidy, whether the factory floor, roads, and transportation have caused pollution to the production, and whether the overall layout of the production, administration, living, and auxiliary areas is reasonable and and interferes with each other.
0901	Whether the factory equipment are reasonably arranged in accordance with the technological process, and whether the operation rooms such as cleaning, cutting, stir-baking are suitable for their production scale.
0902	Whether production operations in the same plant and adjacent plants interfere with each other.
1001	Whether the plant has facilities to prevent insects and other animals from entering (the rodenticide shall not be used in the production operation room).
1104	Whether the inner surface of the factory floor, walls, ceiling is flat, easy to clean, not easy to produce falling objects, and not easy to breed mold.
1105	Whether the sorting workbench is set up for the cleaning and selection, and whether the surface of the workbench is flat and not easy to produce falling objects objects.
1201	Whether the production area has an area and space suitable for the production scale.
1202	Whether the workshops for steaming, stir-baking, stir-baking with liquid excipient and calcining of raw Chinese medicine and Chinese medicine decoction pieces are suitable for their production scale.
1204	Whether the storage area has an area and space suitable for the production scale.
1205	Whether there are any measures to prevent errors and cross-pollution in the storage area of materials, semifinished products and products to be tested.
1604	Production plants for crushing, sieving, and inner packaging of directly taken Chinese medicine decoction pieces shall be in accordance with requirements of clean areas.

continued

clause	Inspection contents
2302	Whether there are appropriate ventilation, dust removal, smoke removal, moisture removal, and cooling facilities in the cleaning, cutting, and stir-baking operations.
2304	Whether dust collection and other facilities are installed in the operation room easy to produce dust, such as screening, cutting, crushing, etc.
2305	Whether the waste gas, waste water, dust generated during the production process is discharged after treatment and in accordance with the national environmental protection requirements. And the local unit with environmental inspection and monitoring qualification shall issue relevant certificates in accordance with the requirements.
2601	Whether the storage area is kept clean and dry, and whether lighting and ventilation facilities are installed. Whether the temperature and humidity control in the storage area are in accordance with the storage requirements and regularly monitored as required.
2801	Whether laboratories, specimen rooms, and sample retained observation rooms are separated from the production area.
2901	Whether the instruments and meters with special requirements are placed in a special instrument room, and there are facilities to prevent static electricity, vibration, humidity or other external factors.
3104	Whether to select the equipment that can be in accordance with the requirements of processing parameters according to the different characteristics of raw Chinese medicine and Chinese medicine decoction pieces and the needs of processing technology.
3201	Whether the surface of equipment, tools and containers in direct contact with raw Chinese medicine and Chinese medicine decoction pieces is easy to clean and sterilize, and is not easy to produce falling objects, does not cause chemical reactions with raw Chinese medicine, Chinese medicine decoction pieces, and does not adsorb raw Chinese medicine, Chinese medicine decoction pieces.
3206	Whether the lubricants and coolants are used in the equipment contaminating the Chinese medicine decoction pieces or containers.
*3207	Whether the production of Chinese medicine decoction pieces with special requirements such as toxic raw Chinese medicine (including raw Chinese medicine managed according to narcotic drugs) is in accordance with relevant national regulations. There shall be special equipment and production lines for the production of toxic raw Chinese medicine.
3301	Whether the main fixed pipeline connected to the equipment is marked with the material name and flow direction in the pipeline.
3501	Whether the application scope and precision of production and inspection instruments, meters, measuring tools and weighing instruments are in accordance with the production and inspection requirements, whether there are obvious conformity marks, and whether they are regularly verified.
3601	Whether the production equipment has obvious status mark.
3602	Whether production equipment is regularly repaired and maintained. Whether the operation of equipment installation, repair, maintenance affects the quality of the product.
3701	Whether the production and inspection equipment has use, repair and maintenance records, and is managed by a specially assigned person.
3801	Whether there is a management system for the purchase, storage, distribution and use of materials.
3802	Whether raw materials and auxiliary materials are stored separately according to variety, specification and batch number.
*3901	Whether the materials shall be in accordance with the drug standards, packaging material standards and other relevant standards, and must not have an adverse effect on the quality of Chinese medicine decoction pieces.

continued

clause	Inspection contents
*3903	Whether the imported medicinal materials have the certification documents approved by the State Food and Drug Administration.
4001	Whether the raw Chinese medicine used in production were purchased according to quality standards and whether their origins remained relatively stable.
4002	Whether the purchased raw Chinese medicine have detailed records, whether there are obvious labels on the packaging, and indicate the product name, specifications, quantity, origin, source, and date of collection (initial processing). Whether the raw Chinese medicine implementing the approval number indicate the approval number of the drug.
4101	Whether the materials are purchased from the qualified units and put into storage as required.
4201	Whether the materials to be inspected, qualified and unqualified are strictly managed.
*4202	Whether the unqualified materials are stored in a dedicated area, and whether there are obvious signs that can be easily identified, and timely handle according to the relevant regulations.
4301	Whether materials, semifinished products and finished products with special requirements are stored according to specified conditions. Whether the temperature of shady and cool storage is not higher than 25℃.
4302	Whether volatile materials avoid contaminating other materials, whether clean containers or packaging are used after processing and finishing, and whether the clean raw Chinese medicine are strictly separated from the unprocessed and processed raw Chinese medicine.
4303	Whether raw Chinese medicine and Chinese medicine decoction pieces are separately stored, and Whether they are stored and conserved as required.
*4401	Whether toxic raw Chinese medicine (including raw Chinese medicine managed according to narcotic drugs) and other special requirements medicinal materials are accepted, stored, and conserved in accordance with regulations, and whether there is a special warehouses or counters set up.
*4411	Whether toxic raw Chinese medicine (including raw Chinese medicine managed according to narcotic drugs) and other medicines with special requirements are marked with obvious signs.
4501	Whether the material is stored within the specified period of use, and whether it is re-inspected after the expiration. If there are special circumstances during the storage period, whether it is re-inspected in a timely manner.
4601	Whether the Chinese medicine decoction pieces use packaging materials and containers that can ensure the quality during storage and transportation.
4602	Whether the is label printed, issued and used after proofreading by the quality management department.
4603	Whether the package is printed or pasted with a label, indicating the product name, specification, origin, manufacturer, product batch number and production date. Whether the Chinese medicine decoction pieces that implement the approval number management indicate the drug approval number.
4701	Whether the label is kept and used by a special person.
4702	Whether the labels are stored in the special counter according to the varieties and specifications, and whether they are collected according to the actual demand.
4703	Whether the label is counted and issued shall be checked and signed by the recipient. Whether the sum of the number of label used, the number of damages and the remaining number matches the number of claims.
4704	Whether the damaged or residual labels printed with batch number are destroyed by special personnel, whether there are records of counting, distribution, use and destruction.
4801	Whether there are sanitation measures to prevent pollution and various sanitation management systems, and special personnel shall be responsible for them.

continued

clause	Inspection contents
4904	Whether there are cleaning procedures for plant, equipment, and containers, including cleaning methods, procedures, intervals, cleaning agents or disinfectants used, cleaning methods and storage locations for cleaning tools.
5001	Whether non-produced items and personal sundries are stored in the production area, and whether the waste in production is disposed of in a timely manner.
5201	Whether the personnel engaged in toxic and harmful operations to the human body wear protective clothing according to the regulations, whether their special work clothes and other workers' work clothes are washed and sorted separately, and cross-pollution is avoided.
5402	Whether the personnel entering the production area change clothes and wash hands as required.
5601	Whether the production personnel have health records, and whether the production personnel who have direct contact with Chinese herbal pieces have physical examination at least once a year. Whether the patients with infectious diseases, skin diseases and body surface wounds are engaged in the production of Chinese herbal pieces in direct contact.
5701	Whether to carry out production verification of Chinese medicine decoction pieces, whether to establish a verification team according to the verification object, propose a verification project, develop a verification plan, and organize the implementation.
*5704	Whether equipment verification and process verification are performed for key processes in the production process.
5801	Whether to re-verify after a certain period of production.
5901	Whether the verification report is written after the completion of the verification work shall be reviewed and approved by the person in charge of the verification work.
6001	Whether the data and analysis content in the verification process are archived and stored in a file, and whether the verification file includes a verification plan, a verification report, evaluations and recommendations, approver, etc.
6401	Whether to establish a management system for the drafting, revision, review, approval, revocation, printing and storage of documents.
6402	Whether the documents distributed and used are the approved current documents, and whether the cancelled and obsolete documents appear on the work site except for archived file.
6501	Whether the formulation of documents is in accordance with the regulations.
*6601	Whether there are production process regulations, post operation methods or standard operating procedures, whether they are arbitrarily changed, and whether they are implemented according to the specified procedures if they need to be changed.
6602	Whether the production process specification includes the name, specifications, operating requirements and technical parameters of the processing technology, quality standards and storage considerations for materials, semifinished products, finished products, calculation methods for material balance, packaging specifications.
*6603	Whether the Chinese medicine decoction pieces are processed in accordance with national drug standards. If there is no national drug standard, whether they are processed in accordance with the processing standards formulated by Food and Drug Administration departments of provinces, autonomous regions and municipalities.
6701	Whether the product undergoes a material balance check. The material balance exceeds the prescribed limit, the cause shall be found out, and the normal product can be treated only after reasonable explanation is obtained and no potential quality accident is confirmed.

continued

clause	Inspection contents
6801	Whether the standard operation procedures and batch production records are prepared according to the process procedures. Whether batch production records are filled in time, with clear handwriting, authentic content and complete data, and signed by the operator and reviewer.
6802	Whether batch production records are kept tidy, must not be torn up and arbitrarily altered. If the batch production record is incorrectly filled, whether to change it as required. Whether batch production records are archived by batch number and kept for three years.
*6901	Whether the batch number of Chinese medicine decoction pieces is a batch of relatively homogeneous Chinese medicine decoction pieces produced by the same batch of raw Chinese medicine in the same continuous production cycle.
7001	Whether there is no remnant of the last production before production.
7003	Whether there are isolation measures or other facilities to effectively prevent pollution and confusion when production operations of different product varieties and specifications are carried out in the same operation room at the same time.
7009	Whether there is a product or material name, batch number, quantity and other status signs in each production operation room or production equipment and container.
7015	Whether raw Chinese medicine directly touch the ground after cleaning and selection.
7016	Whether there are special measures to prevent cross-pollution in the production of toxic raw Chinese medicine (including raw Chinese medicine managed according to narcotic drugs) and other special requirements.
7017	Whether mobile water is used for washing the selected raw Chinese medicine, and whether the used water is used for washing other raw Chinese medicine.
7018	Different raw Chinese medicine must not be washed together, and Chinese medicine decoction pieces processed cannot be dried in the open air.
7021	Whether the auxiliary materials are absorbed completely in the infiltration of raw Chinese medicine.
*7101	Whether the quality standard of production water is lower than that of drinking water.
7202	Whether the Chinese medicine decoction piece package is limited to two batches in one box, Whether all batch numbers are marked on the outside of the box and establish a combined box.
7301	Whether the production operator clears the field after completing each stage of production of Chinese medicine decoction pieces, and fills in the field clearance records. Whether the clearance records are complete and whether they are included in the batch production records.
7401	Whether the quality management department is directly led by the person in charge of the enterprise.
7402	Whether the number of quality management and inspection personnel is suitable for the scale of production of Chinese medicine decoction pieces.
7403	Whether the quality management department has set up equipment suitable for the scale, type and quality inspection requirements of Chinese medicine decoction pieces.
7406	Whether the quality department effectively monitor the entire process of raw Chinese medicine processing with special requirements such as toxic raw Chinese medicine (including raw Chinese medicine managed according to narcotic drugs).
*7501	Whether there are quality standards for raw Chinese medicine, auxiliary materials, packaging materials, semifinished products, and Chinese medicine decoction pieces in the quality documents and their inspection and operating procedures.
7502	Whether the quality management department fulfills the responsibility of formulating the sampling and retention system.

continued

clause	Inspection contents
7503	Whether the quality management department has fulfilled the responsibility of formulating management measures for inspection equipment, instruments, reagents, test solutions, standards (or reference materials), titration solutions, etc.
*7504	Whether the quality management department fulfills the responsibility of determining the use of materials and intermediate products.
*7505	Whether the relevant records are reviewed by the quality management department before the Chinese medicine decoction pieces are released and signed by the reviewers. Whether the audit content includes the review of the counterweight and weighing process, inspection records of each production process, clearance records, semifinished product quality inspection results, deviation treatment, finished product inspection results, etc.
*7506	Whether the quality management department fulfills the responsibility of reviewing the procedures for handling non-conforming products.
*7507	Whether the quality management department fulfills the responsibility of sampling, testing, retaining samples of materials, semifinished products and finished products, and issuing inspection reports.
7511	Whether the quality management department fulfills the responsibility of formulating the duties of quality management and inspection personnel.
7601	Whether the quality management department evaluates the major material suppliers together with relevant departments.
7701	Whether there are sales records for each batch of Chinese medicine decoction pieces. According to the sales records, the sales of each batch of Chinese medicine decoction pieces can be tracked, and if necessary, can all be recovered in time. Does the sales record include product name, batch number, specifications, quantity, receiving unit and address, and delivery date, etc.
7801	Whether sales records are kept for three years.
7901	Whether written procedures for drug returns and withdrawals are established and documented. Whether the contents of the drug return and withdrawal records include the product name, batch number, specifications, quantity, unit and address of the return and withdrawal, the reason and date of the return and withdrawal, and treatment opinions.
7902	Whether the Chinese medicine decoction pieces returned and recovered due to quality reasons are destroyed under the supervision of the quality management department, and whether other batches are involved, are they also treated at the same time.
8101	Whether there are detailed records, investigation and handling of complaints about the quality of Chinese herbal pieces from users.
8201	If there are major quality problems occur in the production of Chinese medicine decoction pieces, whether to report to the local Food and Drug Administration departments in a timely manner.
8301	Whether the company regularly organizes self-inspection and whether the self-inspection comprehensively inspects the enterprise in accordance with predetermined procedures.
8401	Whether there is a record of self-inspection. Whether the self-inspection report are in accordance with the requirements.